The Founders of Operative Surgery

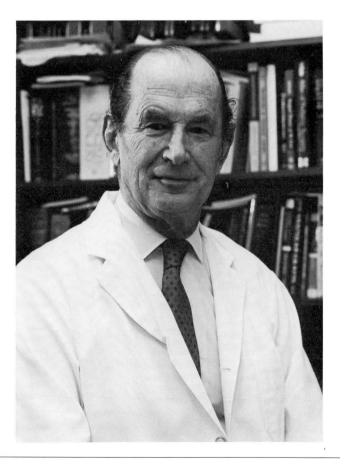

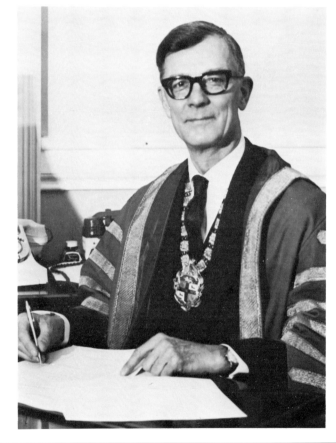

Charles Granville Rob MC, MChir, FRCS, FACS
Professor of Surgery, East Carolina University
Quondam: Professor of Surgery, St Mary's Hospital Medical
School, London 1950–1960;
Professor and Chairman, Department of Surgery, University of
Rochester, New York, 1960–1978

Lord Smith of Marlow KBE, MS, FRCS, Hon DSc (Exeter
and Leeds), Hon MD (Zurich), Hon FRACS, Hon FRCS(Ed.),
Hon FACS, Hon FRCS(Can.), Hon FRCS(I.); Hon FRCS(SA),
Hon FDS.
Honorary Consulting Surgeon, St George's Hospital, London
Quondam: Surgeon, St George's Hospital, London,
1946–1978;
President of the Royal College of Surgeons of England,
1973–1977

Rob & Smith's

Operative Surgery

General Principles, Breast and Extracranial Endocrines

Fourth Edition

Rob & Smith's
Operative Surgery

General Editors

Hugh Dudley ChM, FRCS(Ed.), FRACS, FRCS
Professor of Surgery, St Mary's Hospital, London

Walter J. Pories MD, FACS
Professor and Chairman, Department of Surgery, School of Medicine,
East Carolina University, Greenville, North Carolina

Rob & Smith's

Operative Surgery

General Principles, Breast and Extracranial Endocrines

Fourth Edition

Edited by

Hugh Dudley ChM, FRCS(Ed.), FRACS, FRCS
Professor of Surgery, St Mary's Hospital, London

Walter J. Pories MD, FACS
Professor and Chairman, Department of Surgery, School of Medicine,
East Carolina University, Greenville, North Carolina

Butterworth Scientific
London Boston Sydney Wellington Durban Toronto

© Butterworth Scientific 1982

First edition published in eight volumes 1956–1958
Second edition published in fourteen volumes 1968–1971
Third edition published in nineteen volumes 1976–1981
Fourth edition published 1982

British Library Cataloguing in Publication Data

Rob, Charles
    Rob & Smith's operative surgery. — 4th ed.
    General principles, breast and extracranial endocrines
    1. Surgery, Operative
    I. Title   II. Smith, Rodney, *Baron*
    III. Dudley, Hugh   IV. Pories, Walter J.
    617'.91   RD32

    ISBN 0-407-00650-8

Photoset by Butterworths Litho Preparation Department
Printed and bound in England by Butler and Tanner Limited, London and Frome

Volumes and Editors

Accident Surgery

Not yet appointed

Cardiac Surgery

Stuart W. Jamieson MB, BS, FRCS
Assistant Professor of Cardiovascular Surgery,
Stanford University School of Medicine, California

Norman E. Shumway MD, PhD, FRCS
Professor and Chairman, Department of Cardiovascular Surgery,
Stanford University School of Medicine, California

Colon, Rectum and Anus

Ian P.Todd MS, MD(Tor), FRCS, DCH
Consulting Surgeon, St Bartholomew's Hospital, London;
Consultant Surgeon, St Mark's Hospital and
King Edward VII Hospital for Officers, London

L. P. Fielding MB, FRCS
Chief of Surgery, St Mary's Hospital, Waterbury, Connecticut;
Associate Professor of Surgery, Yale University, Connecticut

The Ear

John C. Ballantyne FRCS, HonFRCS(I.), DLO
Consultant Ear, Nose and Throat Surgeon,
Royal Free and King Edward VII Hospital for Officers, London;
Honorary Consultant in Otolaryngology to the Army

Andrew Morrison FRCS, DLO
Senior Consultant Otolaryngologist, The London Hospital

General Principles, Breast and Extracranial Endocrines

Hugh Dudley ChM, FRCS(Ed.), FRACS, FRCS
Professor of Surgery, St Mary's Hospital, London

Walter J. Pories MD, FACS
Professor and Chairman, Department of Surgery, School of Medicine,
East Carolina University, Greenville, North Carolina

Gynaecology and Obstetrics

D. W. T. Roberts MA, MChir, FRCS, FRCOG
Consultant Gynaecologist, The Samaritan Hospital for Women
and the Soho Hospital for Women, London

The Hand

Rolfe Birch FRCS
Consultant Orthopaedic Surgeon, PNI Unit and Hand Clinic,
Royal National Orthopaedic Hospital, London;
Consultant Orthopaedic Surgeon, St Mary's Hospital, London

Donal Brooks MA, MB, FRCS, FRCS(I.)

Neurosurgery

Lindsay Symon TD, FRCS, FRCS(Ed.)
Professor of Neurological Surgery, Institute of Neurology,
The National Hospital, Queen Square, London

Nose and Throat

John C. Ballantyne FRCS, HonFRCS(I.), DLO
Consultant Ear, Nose and Throat Surgeon,
Royal Free and King Edward VII Hospital for Officers, London;
Honorary Consultant in Otolaryngology to the Army

D. F. N. Harrison MD, MS, FRCS, FRACS
Professor of Laryngology and Otology,
Royal National Throat, Nose and Ear Hospital, London

Ophthalmic Surgery

Ronald G. Michels MD
Assistant Professor, The Wilmer Ophthalmological Institute,
The Johns Hopkins University and Hospital, Baltimore, Maryland

Thomas A. Rice MD
Associate Professor, The Wilmer Ophthalmological Institute,
The Johns Hopkins University and Hospital, Baltimore, Maryland

Walter W. J. Stark MD
Associate Professor of Ophthalmology and Director of Corneal
Services, The Wilmer Ophthalmological Institute,
The Johns Hopkins University and Hospital, Baltimore, Maryland

Orthopaedics (in 2 volumes)

George Bentley ChM, FRCS
Professor of Orthopaedic Surgery, Institute of Orthopaedics,
Royal National Orthopaedic Hospital, London

Paediatric Surgery

L. Spitz PhD, FRCS
Nuffield Professor of Paediatric Surgery and Honorary Consultant
Paediatric Surgeon, The Hospital for Sick Children,
Great Ormond Street, London

H. Homewood Nixon MA, MB, BChir, FRCS, Hon FAAP
Consultant Paediatric Surgeon, The Hospital for Sick Children,
Great Ormond Street, London and Paddington Green Children's
Hospital, St Mary's Hospital Group, London

Plastic Surgery

T. L. Barclay ChM, FRCS
Consultant Plastic Surgeon, St Luke's Hospital,
Bradford, West Yorkshire

Desmond A. Kernahan MD
Chief, Division of Plastic Surgery,
The Children's Memorial Hospital, Chicago, Illinois

Thoracic Surgery

J. W. Jackson MCh, FRCS
Formerly Consultant Thoracic Surgeon, Harefield Hospital, Middlesex

D. K. C. Cooper MD, PhD, FRCS
Department of Cardiac Surgery, University of Cape Town
Medical School, Cape Town, South Africa

Upper Gastrointestinal Surgery

Hugh Dudley ChM, FRCS(Ed.), FRACS, FRCS
Professor of Surgery, St Mary's Hospital, London

Urology

W. Scott McDougal MD
Associate Professor of Surgery (Urology),
Dartmouth-Hitchcock Clinic, Hanover, New Hampshire

Vascular Surgery

James A. DeWeese MD
Chairman, Division of Cardiothoracic Surgery,
University of Rochester Medical Center, Rochester, New York

Contributors

J. Wesley Alexander MD, ScD
Director, Transplantation Division,
University of Cincinnati Medical Center, Cincinnati, Ohio;
Director of Research, Shriners' Burn Institute, Cincinnati Unit

J. Alexander-Williams MD, ChM, FRCS
Consultant Surgeon, The General Hospital, Birmingham

W. K. Blenkinsopp MD, MB, BChir, FRCPath
Consultant Histopathologist, Watford General Hospital, Hertfordshire

Allen F. Bowyer MD
Professor of Medicine and Chief, Division of Cardiology,
Department of Medicine, School of Medicine,
East Carolina University, Greenville, North Carolina

Dulcie V. Coleman MBBS, MD, MRCPath
Senior Lecturer in Cytology, Department of Pathology,
St Mary's Hospital, London

Ernest D. Cronin MD, FACS
Plastic Surgery Section, St Joseph Hospital, Houston, Texas

Thomas D. Cronin MD, FACS
Clinical Professor of Plastic Surgery,
Baylor College of Medicine, Houston, Texas

Hugh Dudley ChM, FRCS(Ed.), FRACS, FRCS
Professor of Surgery, St Mary's Hospital, London

Brian W. Ellis MB, FRCS
Senior Registrar in Surgery, St Mary's Hospital, London

Caldwell B. Esselstyn, Jr MD
Department of General Surgery,
The Cleveland Clinic Foundation, Cleveland, Ohio

L. P. Fielding MB, FRCS
Chief of Surgery, St Mary's Hospital, Waterbury, Connecticut;
Associate Professor of Surgery, Yale University, Connecticut

Edward G. Flickinger MD
Associate Professor of General Surgery, School of Medicine,
East Carolina University, Greenville, North Carolina

A. P. M. Forrest MD, ChM, DSc, FRCS, HonFACS
Regius Professor of Clinical Surgery, University of Edinburgh

Eugene D. Furth MD
Chairman, Department of Medicine, School of Medicine,
East Carolina University, Greenville, North Carolina

Carl E. Haisch MD
Department of Surgery, School of Medicine,
East Carolina University, Greenville, North Carolina

M. M. Hares FRCS
Research Fellow, The General Hospital, Birmingham

Robert E. Hermann MD
Department of General Surgery,
The Cleveland Clinic Foundation, Cleveland, Ohio

L. E. Hughes DS, FRCS, FRACS
Professor of Surgery, Welsh National School of Medicine, Cardiff

C. W. Jamieson MS, FRCS
Consultant Vascular Surgeon, Hammersmith Hospital, London;
Surgeon, St Thomas's Hospital, London

Edward Janosko MD
Section of Urology, School of Medicine,
East Carolina University, Greenville, North Carolina

C. R. Kapadia MB, FRCS
Lecturer in Surgery, Academic Surgical Unit,
St Mary's Hospital Medical School, London

L. P. Le Quesne DM, MCh, FRCS, HonFRACS
Professor of Surgery and Director of Surgical Studies,
The Middlesex Hospital, London

R. G. Lightwood FRCS
Senior Surgical Registrar, St Mary's Hospital, London

J. F. Mainland FFARACS, BSc
Associate Professor (Anaesthesia), Monash University,
Alfred Hospital, Melbourne

James A. Majeski PhD, MD
Assistant Professor of Surgery,
Medical University of South Carolina, Charleston, South Carolina

John Masterton FRCS, FRACS
Associate Professor of Surgery, Monash University,
Alfred Hospital, Melbourne

Diane Meelheim RN, FNP
Department of Surgery, School of Medicine,
East Carolina University, Greenville, North Carolina

Bryan C. Mendelson FRCS(Ed.), FRACS
Lecturer in Surgery, Monash University Department of Surgery;
Alfred Hospital, Melbourne

Douglas Millar FRCS, FRCS(Ed.)
Surgeon and Surgical Tutor, Essex County Hospital, Colchester

Euan Milroy MB BS, FRCS
Consultant Urologist, The Middlesex Hospital, London

W. P. Morgan BSc, FRCS
Senior Registrar in Surgery, University Hospital of Wales, Cardiff

J. Nayman ChM, FRCS, FRCS(Ed.), FRACS
Chief of Surgery, Royal Southern Memorial Hospital; Associate
Professor, Department of Surgery, Monash University, Melbourne

G. B. Ong MB BS, DSc, FRCS(Ed.), FRCS, FRACS, FRSE
Professor of Surgery, University of Hong Kong; Head of the
Department of Surgery, Queen Mary Hospital, Hong Kong

A. G. Poole FRACS, FACS
Visiting Surgeon, Royal North Shore Hospital,
St Leonards, New South Wales;
Clinical Tutor, Department of Surgery, The University of Sydney

Walter J. Pories MD, FACS
Professor and Chairman, Department of Surgery, School of Medicine,
East Carolina University, Greenville, North Carolina

Mary Raab MD
Division of Hematology/Oncology, Department of Internal Medicine,
East Carolina University, Greenville, North Carolina

Spencer Raab MD
Division of Hematology/Oncology, Department of Internal Medicine,
East Carolina University, Greenville, North Carolina

T. S. Reeve CBE, FACS, FRACS
Professor and Chairman, Department of Surgery, The University of
Sydney, Royal North Shore Hospital, St Leonards, New South Wales

Charles G. Rob MD
Professor of Surgery, Department of Surgery, School of Medicine,
East Carolina University, Greenville, North Carolina

Russell C. Romero DDS, MD
Resident, Plastic Surgery Section, St Joseph Hospital, Houston, Texas

R. C. G. Russell MS, FRCS
Consultant Surgeon, St John's Hospital for Diseases of the Skin
and The Middlesex Hospital, London

P. C. Rutter MB, FRCS
Registrar, Academic Surgical Unit, St Mary's Hospital, London

Hilliard F. Seigler MD
Professor of Surgery and Associate Professor of Immunology,
Duke University Medical Center, Durham, North Carolina

Sydney Selwyn MD, BSc, FRCPath, FIBiol
Professor of Medical Microbiology,
University of London (at Westminster Medical School);
Consultant Microbiologist, Westminster Hospital, London

Anne B. Sutherland MD, MB ChB, FRCS(Ed.)
Consultant Plastic Surgeon, Regional Plastic and Maxillofacial Surgery
Unit, Bangour General Hospital, Broxburn, West Lothian, Scotland

Francis T. Thomas MD, FACS
Professor of Surgery, Department of Surgery, School of Medicine,
East Carolina University, Greenville, North Carolina

A. M. van Rij FRACS
Senior Lecturer in Surgery, University of Otago, New Zealand

Major General W. J. Watson MBE, QHP, FACMA, RAAMC
Director General, Army Health Services, Canberra

George T. Watts ChM, FRCS
Consultant Surgeon, United Birmingham Hospitals

R. B. Welbourn MA, MD(Cantab.), HonMD(Karolinska), FRCS,
FCS(West Africa), HonMRCS(Denmark)
Professor of Surgical Endocrinology, Royal Postgraduate
Medical School and Hammersmith Hospital, London

D. J. Williams FRCS
Consultant Orthopaedic and Trauma Surgeon,
Queen Elizabeth II Hospital, Welwyn Garden City,
Hertfordshire and Hertford County Hospitals

Contributing Medical Artists

Anne Barrett
Medical Illustrator, 43 Vineyard Hill Road, London SW19

Cynthia Clarke AIMBI
Medical Illustrator, Wallets, Great Worley, Brentwood, Essex

Michael Courtney
Medical Illustrator, 78 Alfred Road, Hastings

Kate Crowle NDD, AIMBI
127 Viewmount Road, Glenwaverley 3150, Victoria, Australia

Paul Darton NDD, MAA
Medical Artist, The Middlesex Hospital Medical School, London

Patrick Elliott
Senior Medical Artist, Department of Medical Illustration;
Royal Hallamshire Hospital, Glossop Road, Sheffield

Ray Elmore MFA
Assistant Professor of Art, School of Art,
East Carolina University, Greenville, North Carolina

Shian Hartshorn
Medical Illustrator, 67 Park Lane, Congleton, Cheshire

Barbara Hyams MA, AMI
Medical Illustrator, 82 Kingsland Road,
Boxmoor, Hemel Hempstead, Herts

Russell Jones
Jones-Pointer-Winn Inc., Design and Illustration, Dallas, Texas

Sheila Jones
Academic Surgical Unit, St Mary's Hospital, London

Robert Lane
Medical Illustrator, Studio 19A, Edith Grove, Chelsea, London SW10

Gillian Lee AIMBI, MMAA
Medical Illustrator, Burnham, 15 Little Plucketts Way,
Buckhurst Hill, Essex

Geoff Lyth
Medical Illustrator, 15 Gunthorpe Road, Lowdham, Notts

Ann McNeill
Medical Artist, The Royal Infirmary, Glasgow

A. Malpass IMMBIA
Medical Illustrator, Royal Southern Memorial Hospital, Melbourne

Kevin Marks
Illustrator, 29 Vancouver Road, Forest Hill, London

Oxford Illustrators Ltd
Aristotle Lane, Oxford

Carol J. Pienta BS
Medical Illustrator, Audio-Visual Services Center, School of Medicine,
East Carolina University, Greenville, North Carolina

Donald G. Powell
Medical Illustrator, VA Medical Center, Durham, North Carolina

Frank B. Price
Medical Illustrator, 5 Tudor Cottage, Lovers Walk, Finchley, London

Robert M. Reed
Manager of Biomedical Communications,
The Cleveland Clinic Foundation, Cleveland, Ohio

D. D. Simmonds
Chief Medical Artist, Royal Postgraduate Medical School, London

Contents

Preface

The general principles of surgery are both undefined and large in their scope. No single text could hope to encompass them and there would be disagreement from individual to individual about the necessary principles that should be encompassed by any surgeon in training or in practice. In assembling the fourth edition of this work we have sought principally to consider matters which are in direct relationship to the conduct of an operation and have but rarely strayed into other therapeutic fields. The one major exception is adjuvant treatment of malignant disease which now marches in step with surgery in many fields.

This volume also contains operations from the field of so-called 'general' surgery which are ill accommodated in other special areas and thus would not have fitted in well in different volumes of this series. The surgery of the breast and the extracranial endocrines, the management of the burn wound and some simple aspects of reconstruction are examples. Thus, though at first glance the contents of this volume may appear somewhat disparate, we feel there is a unity about them which supports the title.

Hugh Dudley
Walter Pories

Illustrations by Gillian Lee

Bacteriology and preparation of the skin

Sydney Selwyn   MD, BSc, FRCPath, FIBiol
Professor of Medical Microbiology,
University of London (at Westminster Medical School);
Consultant Microbiologist, Westminster Hospital, London

Historical background

Simple cleansing of the operation site and of the surgeon's hands was advocated in a number of ancient medical texts. The most notable of these are from India and the Middle East where ritual purity was a religious duty. Unfortunately, hygienic standards in surgery declined to a very low ebb in medieval Europe when the body was neglected in favour of the soul. Indeed no improvement can be discerned until the last quarter of the nineteenth century, with occasional exceptions – notably the obscure German surgeon, Caspar Stromayr, who over 300 years earlier subjected his patients to a preoperative bath and shaving of the operation site[1].

1a, b & c

The first deliberate disinfection of the operator's skin is usually ascribed to Ignaz Semmelweis (a), who in the 1840s achieved a considerable reduction in the incidence of puerperal fever among his patients in Vienna by hand-washing with chlorinated solutions. His aim was, however, the mere removal of malodorous organic debris – bacteria played no part in his concept of infection. Even when, some 20 years later, Joseph Lister (b) for the first time deliberately directed a chemical agent – 5 per cent phenol – against bacteria on the skin of the patient as well as the surgeon, the microbial target was a nebulous and indefinite one. Lister's pioneer bacteriological studies, first in Glasgow then in Edinburgh, were not clinically orientated, but instead were intended to settle general scientific controversies such as the possibility of spontaneous generation. It was not until 1880 that the major causes of wound sepsis – the pathogenic staphylococci and streptococci – came clearly into focus as a result of the work of another surgeon, Alexander Ogston (c), in the more northerly Scottish city of Aberdeen.

Curiously, the rapid growth in bacteriological knowledge during the next few decades did not extend to that most accessible and largest of organs, the human skin. The first quantitative studies of the skin microflora and of the efficiency of the conventional surgical 'scrub' were delayed until 1938. In that year the American surgeon P. B. Price reported his pioneer observations and differentiated between the 'resident' and the 'transient' bacteria of the skin. However, many basic facts relating to skin microbiology remained in doubt until the early 1970s[2]. Those of surgical importance may be usefully summarized before the practical aspects of skin preparation are considered.

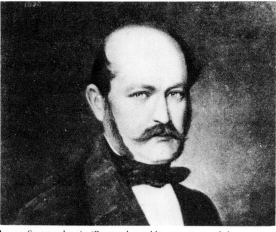

1a

Ignaz Semmelweis *(Reproduced by courtesy of the Wellcome Trustees)*

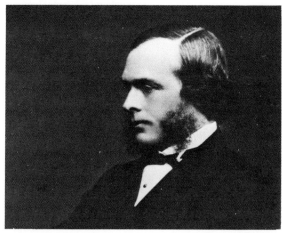

1b

Joseph Lister *(Reproduced by courtesy of the Audio Visual Department, St Mary's Hospital Medical School and Professor H. Dudley)*

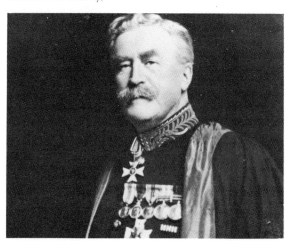

1c

Alexander Ogston *(Reproduced by courtesy of the Wellcome Trustees)*

Skin microbiology

There are several surgically relevant aspects of the skin's bacterial population. These are the total bacterial numbers at different sites on the body surface, the exact location of bacteria on or in the skin, the range of different micro-organisms which may be regarded as normal skin commensals, the significance of *Staphylococcus aureus* and Gram-negative bacilli on the epidermis, and the natural control mechanisms which limit microbial survival and colonization on the skin.

Population densities

2

The remarkable divergencies in the published estimates of bacterial numbers – ranging from 14 to over half a million bacteria per cm^2 – are due to the motley collection of sampling methods used. Most of these have been both inadequately standardized and incapable of yielding more than 0.5 per cent of the accessible microflora. However, optimal and highly reproducible results have been obtained using a radical procedure which involves agitation of fresh biopsy specimens in a suitable detergent (0.1 per cent Triton X-400) followed by quantitative culture of the suspended bacteria[2]. Average bacterial counts have ranged from approximately a million 'colony-forming bacterial units' per cm^2 in the axilla or on the scalp, around 40000 on the abdomen, thigh or interscapular region, reducing to about 10000 on the breast or forearm. These counts are higher than most previous estimates, but are nevertheless considerably lower than the bacterial densities observed on the mucosa of the oropharynx, female lower genital tract or, most spectacularly, the large intestine.

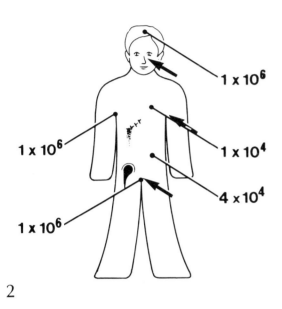

2

Histological location

As with the bacterial counts, the precise location of the skin microflora has been the subject of much controversy. Qualitative studies have often led to a firm conclusion in the literature that virtually all of the bacteria are superficially situated and can be readily removed by disinfection[3]. This view has been evenly balanced by confident statements such as that of Lovell, for whom the majority of bacteria were 'situated so deep in hair follicles and sebaceous glands that they cannot be removed without injuring the skin'[4]. Detailed microscopic studies more recently seem to have provided partial support for Lovell's conclusions[5].

3

Personal studies using quantitative methods have shown that on glabrous skin more than 20 per cent of the total flora is inaccessible to disinfection. In the axilla or on the scalp the proportion rises to over 50 per cent. The organisms not only lurk in pilosebaceous units (C) but find protection also in skin lipids or within microscopic crevices (B) and beneath keratinized debris (A). Normal sweat glands (D) are essentially sterile.

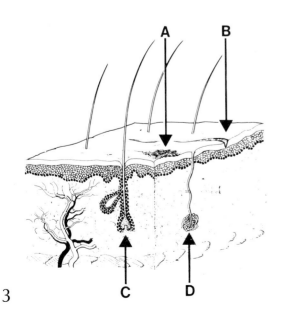

3

Skin commensals and intruders

Healthy skin under normal conditions is colonized by a remarkably limited range of micro-organisms. The 'resident' bacteria usually consist only of Gram-positive bacilli of the diphtheroid (or 'coryneform') group and Gram-positive cocci of the *Staphylococcus/Micrococcus* group. The predominant species is usually *Staphylococcus epidermidis* (formerly *'albus'*). This can cause low grade infections of wounds, assisted by sutures or other foreign bodies, and it is an opportunistic pathogen around surgical implants, such as hip joint prostheses and Spitz-Holter valves. Insidious bacteraemia may follow such infections. A less prominent commensal, *Staphylococcus saprophyticus*, is now recognized to be an important potential pathogen of the urinary tract.

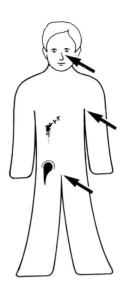

4

4

The coagulase-positive primary pathogen, *Staphylococcus aureus*, is normally unable to grow on healthy intact skin, except in three specialized areas – the nostrils, axillae and perineum – from where it may infect wounds and prostheses. Even so, less than 30 per cent of the general population are persistent 'carriers' of this organism.

Diphtheroid bacilli have minimal pathogenic potential. A notable exception is the anaerobe, *Propionibacterium* (formerly *Corynebacterium*) *acnes*, which plays an important part in the pathogenesis of acne vulgaris and related skin disorders, probably due to the production of lipases, and both leukotactic and complement-activating factors.

Apart from the two groups of Gram-positive bacteria only two other kinds of micro-organism – one a fungus and one an animal – can be regarded as true residents of the skin. Yeasts of the genus *Pityrosporum* live in large numbers on the scalp but occasionally produce the widespread skin disease pityriasis (tinea) versicolor. The causative species is often labelled *Malassezia furfur* but this is merely a form of *Pityrosporum orbiculare*. The curious worm-like mite *Demodex folliculorum* flourishes harmlessly in the pilosebaceous units of the face. This sole member of the normal skin fauna probably produces irritation when it proliferates under the particularly luxuriant conditions of rosacea and related disorders.

In contrast to the very restricted range of true residents, the transient microflora of the skin can include virtually any pathogenic micro-organism. Those of major surgical importance are the Gram-positive species *Staph. aureus*, *Streptococcus pyogenes*, *Streptococcus faecalis*, anaerobic streptococci and clostridia – notably *Clostridium perfringens* (previously *welchii*) in the form of spores. The main Gram-negative 'transients' are *Escherichia coli* and other 'coliforms', *Klebsiella* and *Proteus* species, *Pseudomonas aeruginosa* (formerly *pyocyanea*) and the anaerobic *Bacteroides* group. *Actinobacter* species are unusual among the Gram-negative bacilli since they sometimes colonize normal skin, notably on the feet.

Most of the transient bacteria are of endogenous origin, chiefly from the large bowel. Members of the hospital staff are, however, readily contaminated with these bacteria which can then survive, notably on the hands, for several hours in the case of *Staph. aureus*, and for about 3 h with *Klebsiella*[6]. The continued importance of hand-borne infection more than 130 years after Semmelweis's observations underlines the need for efficient and well tolerated skin disinfection procedures.

While the transient flora can survive only passively and for relatively short periods on healthy skin, active multiplication of any of these organisms can occur if the epidermis is damaged or diseased. Colonization or subclinical infection by pathogenic bacteria can then lead to dangerous dispersal[7] and alarming outbreaks of postoperative sepsis have been produced by such inapparent sources of infection on surgeons' skin[8].

Control factors

In comparison to the mucous membranes of the oropharynx, female lower genital tract and large bowel, the relatively small microbial population on healthy skin – despite frequent contamination from inside and outside the body – together with the very limited variety of commensal organisms emphasizes the efficiency of the skin's natural antimicrobial mechanisms. These include the relative dryness, low pH (around 5.5), high sodium chloride concentration, low nutrient content and continuous microscopic desquamation of the epidermis, as well as the production of inhibitory substances – notably fatty acids and even true antibiotics – by the normal flora[9]. The very considerable protective effect of the commensal bacteria points to a potential dilemma in the preoperative preparation of the skin. Suppressing the normal flora can be shown to encourage colonization and infection by pathogens; moreover, most antiseptics even in very low concentrations have been found to delay wound healing[10]. Nevertheless, under the special conditions of a surgical operation small inocula of pathogens – and even commensals in high risk procedures – can produce sepsis. Consequently, the benefits of efficient skin disinfection greatly outweigh any possible drawbacks.

Skin disinfection

The microbial population requires reduction to a minimum both at the operation site and on the hands and forearms of the surgical team. The use of ordinary soap and water is considerably less efficacious than the application of detergent-based or alcoholic solutions of iodine (or iodophors), chlorhexidine or alcohols alone[11]. Hexachlorophane preparations are less satisfactory. The traditional, colourful organic mercurials and acridine dyes are no longer recommended, nor are the quaternary ammonium cationic compounds or chloroxylenol.

Preoperative patient care

Admission to hospital several days before the operation for preparation of the skin (and possibly the bowel) is undesirable because of the risk that the patient will acquire antibiotic-resistant 'hospital' pathogens. This is apart from direct economic objections. There is, however, evidence that bathing combined with the application of chlorhexidine-detergent solution over the entire body surface 24h before the operation leads to a reduced wound infection rate, particularly in vascular or orthopaedic surgery[12]. The bathing procedure is, logically, repeated on the morning of the operation, and indeed this seems a reasonable routine when the patient is only admitted the evening before surgery. The chlorhexidine will greatly decrease the transient microflora and will have a smaller but useful effect on resident organisms, including any pathogens that have colonized areas of abnormal skin. A moderate residual action may contribute to the beneficial effect.

Shaving of the operation site allows more efficient cleansing and disinfection of the skin, and it facilitates accurate incision and closure. However, the production of minor epidermal damage by razors or depilatory creams encourages colonization of the skin by hospital pathogens in proportion to the time elapsing before the operation[13]. Therefore patients should be shaved only immediately before surgery. In addition, shaving brushes have occasionally been vehicles for cross infection with *Ps. aeruginosa* and other organisms.

Disinfecting the operation site

5 & 6

Highly efficient disinfection of non-sporing bacteria is achieved if alcoholic solutions of 1.5 per cent iodine, 10 per cent povidone-iodine or 0.5 per cent chlorhexidine are applied to the operation site for 30s, using either sponges or preferably the gloved hand. An acceptable colouring agent such as carmoisine is helpful in indicating the area of chlorhexidine treatment. Comparable disinfection has been obtained with alcohols alone (70–95 per cent ethanol, or 60 per cent *n*- or *iso*-propanol)[11].

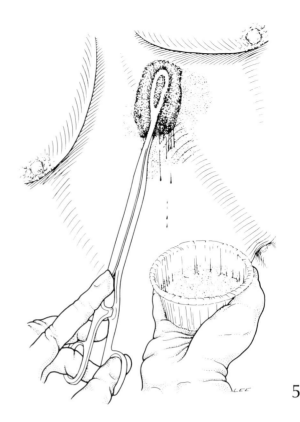

5

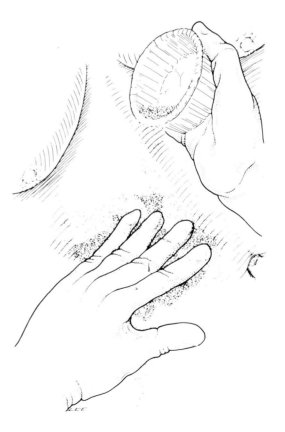

6

7

Alternatively, and traditionally in North America, the operation site is washed with soap or detergent for 5 or more minutes.

Although few comparative studies have been reported, bacteria seem to be more readily killed on ordinary abdominal skin compared to the umbilicus – or hand. Surface complexity is probably the main factor, and for this reason disinfection should continue for at least twice as long on the scrotum, vulva and perianal region as on less convoluted surfaces.

The destruction of clostridial spores is particularly desirable at sites on the lower limb in patients with vascular disease, but is also advisable at and around the anus. Iodine requires at least 15 min – in the moist state – to exert an adequate sporicidal action; and povidone-iodine needs at least 2 h, necessitating the repeated application of compresses. To avoid possible skin irritation, elemental iodine when dried should be removed with alcohol.

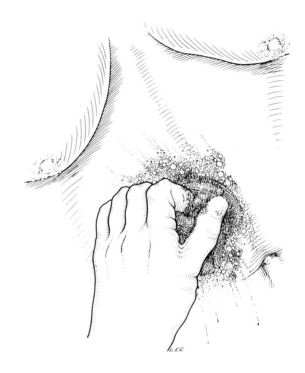

7

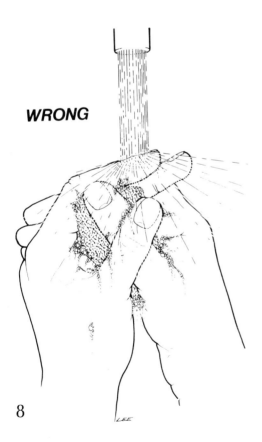

WRONG

8

The surgeon's skin

Paradoxically, a shower or bath taken by the surgeon or his assistants shortly before the operation may lead to a temporary rise in dispersal of skin bacteria. This is probably due to increased desquamation and perhaps increased bacterial multiplication following the temporary reduction in skin lipids. The effect is minimized by showering at least 2 h earlier and by using antibacterial soaps.

8

The traditional 'surgical scrub' involves prolonged washing under a running tap of the hands and arms with soap and water aided by the use of a scrubbing brush. This procedure is not only time-consuming but is likely to produce minor skin damage which then facilitates colonization by pathogenic organisms. The use of a brush should be restricted to cleaning the nails, but a pointed plastic spatula is gentler and to be preferred.

9

Before the beginning of an operating list a combination of thorough skin cleansing and disinfection is required. This is readily achieved by washing with two consecutive applications of 4 per cent chlorhexidine-detergent solution and water over a period of 2 min. A moderately firm sponge may be useful at the start of the procedure. Finally, a rinse with 95 per cent ethanol (containing emollients such as glycerol) allows rapid drying and also enhances the initial disinfection[14]. Povidone-iodine in surfactant, hexachlorophane-detergent or Irgasan-detergent solutions have been found by one group to be significantly less efficient than the chlorhexidine preparation[15, 16], but povidone-iodine has been shown to be equally efficacious in my own studies[17].

After initial disinfection, the antimicrobial effect of chlorhexidine, povidone-iodine and alcohols continues under gloves for 3 h or more. Consequently, between subsequent cases on the operating list, a brief rinse in ethanol or propanol is adequate if there have been no obvious glove punctures. Where gloves have been damaged a repeat of the original cleansing and disinfection procedure is advisable.

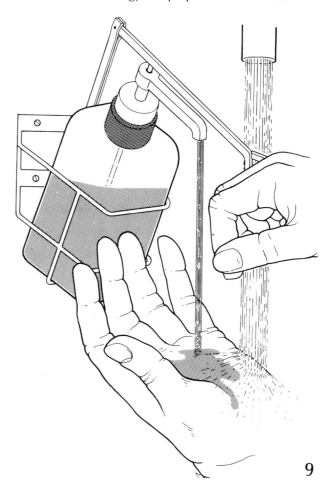

9

References

1. Stromayr, C. Die Handschrift des Schmitt-und Augenarztes Caspar Stromayr, [Practica copiosa] 1559. Reprinted in 1925, von Brunn, W., ed. Berlin: Idra-Verlagsanstalt

2. Selwyn, S., Ellis, H. Skin bacteria and skin disinfection reconsidered. British Medical Journal 1972; 1: 136–140

3. Pecora, D. V., Landis, R. E., Martin, E. Location of cutaneous microorganisms. Surgery 1968; 64: 1114–1118

4. Lovell, D. L. Skin bacteria: their location with reference to skin sterilization. Surgery, Gynecology and Obstetrics 1945; 80: 174–177

5. Montes, L. F., Wilborn, W. H. Anatomical location of normal skin flora. Archives of Dermatology 1970; 101: 145–159

6. Casewell, M., Phillips, I. Hands as route of transmission for Klebsiella species. British Medical Journal 1977; 2: 1315–1317

7. Selwyn, S., Chalmers, D. Dispersal of bacteria from skin lesions: a hospital hazard. British Journal of Dermatology 1965; 77: 349–356

8. Shanson, D. C., McSwiggan, D. A. Operating theatre acquired infection with a gentamicin-resistant strain of Staphylococcus aureus: outbreaks in two hospitals attributable to one surgeon. Journal of Hospital Infection 1980; 1: 171–172

9. Selwyn, S. Microbiology and ecology of human skin. Practitioner 1980; 224: 1059–1062

10. Brånemark, P.-I., Ekholm, R. Tissue injury caused by wound disinfectants. Journal of Bone and Joint Surgery 1967; 49: 48–62

11. Ayliffe, G. A. J. The effect of antibacterial agents on the flora of the skin. Journal of Hospital Infection 1980; 1: 111–124

12. Brandberg, A., Holm, J., Hammarsten, J., Schersten, T. Post-operative wound infections in vascular surgery: effect of pre-operative whole body disinfection by shower bath with chlorhexidine soap. In: Newsom, S. W. B., Caldwell, A. D., eds. Problems in the control of hospital infection. Royal Society of Medicine International Congress and Symposium Series, Vol. 23, p. 71. London and New York: Academic Press and Royal Society of Medicine, 1980

13. Seropian, R., Reynolds, B. M. Wound infections after preoperative depilatory versus razor preparation. American Journal of Surgery 1971; 121: 251–254

14. Lilly, H. A., Lowbury, E. J. L., Wilkins, M. D. Limits to progressive reduction of resident skin bacteria by disinfection. Journal of Clinical Pathology 1979; 32: 382–385

15. Lowbury, E. J. L., Lilly, H. A. Use of 4% chlorhexidine detergent solution (Hibiscrub) and other methods of skin disinfection. British Medical Journal 1973; 1: 510–515

16. Lilly, H. A., Lowbury, E. J. L. Disinfection of the skin with detergent preparations of Irgasan DP300 and other antiseptics. British Medical Journal 1974; 4: 372–374

17. Selwyn, S., Anderson, I. S., Rogers, T. R. Quantitative studies on the decontamination of skin and mucous membranes in relation to immunological patients. In: Clinical and experimental gnotobiotics, pp. 281–284. Stuttgart, New York: Gustav Fischer Verlag, 1979

Bowel preparation

M. M. Hares FRCS
Research Fellow, The General Hospital, Birmingham

J. Alexander-Williams MD, ChM, FRCS
Consultant Surgeon, The General Hospital, Birmingham

Editor's note

Adequate bowel preparation is a *sine qua non* of colonic surgery. In addition and increasingly it is required in other fields – e.g. biliary tract surgery, oesophageal replacement by colon and in any anastomoses where it is desirable for the bowel not to move. Accordingly we include in the general principles section the preparation of the colon with particular, but not exclusive, emphasis on colonic surgery.

Introduction

Septic complications are the commonest that occur after large bowel operations. The normal and, particularly, the obstructed colon contain large amounts of residue from the diet, desquamated cells and bacteria. The presence of faeces poses two problems in colonic surgery: obstructive and infective.

The faecal bulk, mainly composed of cellular residue, is dirty and aesthetically undesirable. However, obstruction is the principal problem posed by any formed hard faeces remaining in the colon at operation. Their presence proximal to an anastomosis constitutes a danger, for when bowel function returns a bolus of faeces may become impacted at the anastomosis, resulting in tension at the suture line which may increase the risk of anastomotic leakage or breakdown.

Faeces containing large numbers of bacteria are potentially infective. The large bowel contains aerobic and anaerobic bacteria, the latter being 10000 times more numerous. So great is the risk that, in the absence of antibiotic prophylaxis after large bowel operations, a greater than 50 per cent incidence of sepsis has been reported[1]. After gastrointestinal operations wound infections are nearly always caused by intestinal organisms that have contaminated the wound during operation[2]. The greater the bacterial contamination, the higher is the incidence of wound sepsis[3].

The dangers posed by the presence of faeces in the colon at the time of operation are such that bowel preparation is required in all patients undergoing elective colorectal surgery, except perhaps for those with acute inflammatory bowel disease, when purgation or enemas may be dangerous. An absolute contraindication to bowel preparation via the oral route is the presence of obstruction of the colon, though colonic lavage distal to the obstruction may be used.

The objectives of bowel preparation before operation are to reduce the amount of faeces and, if possible, the concentration of micro-organisms within the colon. From an empty bowel the risk of faecal spillage at operation is minimized and, should such spillage occur, the low concentration of micro-organisms reduces the risk of sepsis. Preparation of the colon involves some form of mechanical bowel preparation to remove solid faecal matter, with or without the administration of oral antibiotics. Mechanical preparation of the colon does not by itself alter significantly the concentration of colonic micro-organisms but, without the removal of faeces, the concentration of colonic micro-organisms is unlikely to be reduced by oral antibiotics.

Mechanical bowel preparation

The following techniques are used for preoperative mechanical bowel preparation.

Conventional bowel preparation

This method of bowel preparation requires the admission of the patient some 3–5 days before operation. A low residue diet is started and progresses to a 'fluid only' diet 1–2 days before surgery. Purgation with one of a variety of laxatives (senna, magnesium sulphate, castor oil, etc.) is given for 2 days followed by enemas and rectal lavage on the last day. This method provides an excellent clearance of the bowel but it is exhausting for the patient, results in electrolyte loss[4], is time-consuming for nurses and is therefore expensive.

Elemental diets

Elemental diets are designed to be totally absorbed, providing nitrogen and energy but leaving no residue. They do not empty the colon of faeces and neither do they reduce the concentration of colonic micro-organisms within the colon[5]. Their value, however, is to maintain adequate preoperative nutrition in the debilitated patient[6].

To reduce the time required to prepare the colon and the length of time of preoperative admission, within the last few years two methods of orthograde colonic lavage have been introduced: whole bowel irrigation (WBI) and oral mannitol bowel preparation (MBP).

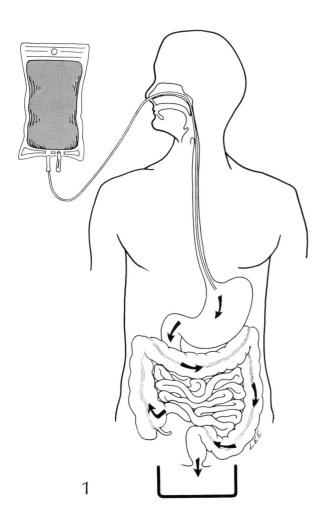

1

1

Whole bowel irrigation

The day before operation an isotonic electrolyte solution is perfused through a nasogastric tube into the stomach at a rate of 4 litres/h and is continued until the material passed per rectum is entirely free of faecal matter[7, 8]. The irrigation takes approximately 4 h and, if the bowel is not obstructed, results in an impeccably clean bowel[8, 9]. The technique is usually preferred by patients who have had previous conventional bowel preparation[10]. Antimicrobial agents can be added to the perfusate to reduce the concentration of colonic micro-organisms[7].

Oral mannitol bowel preparation

2

Mannitol bowel preparation depends upon the fact that mannitol is poorly absorbed. If it is given as a hypertonic solution (10–20 per cent) it draws fluid into the lumen of the bowel by its osmotic action. If given as an isotonic solution (5 per cent) the fluid is retained within the bowel[11] and the catharsis is produced by irrigation of the colon. Mannitol is less unpalatable than other osmotic cathartics, such as magnesium sulphate. On the day before operation 200 g of mannitol, diluted in 1 litre of water (20 per cent), 2 litres of water (10 per cent) or 4 litres of water (5 per cent) is drunk over 4 h. A hypertonic solution results in less abdominal distension than an isotonic solution, but the patient becomes dehydrated. This dehydration can be countered by an intravenous infusion. Provided there is no intestinal obstruction, an excellent colonic clearance results[12, 13]. Patients prefer the oral mannitol method of bowel preparation to whole bowel irrigation principally because it avoids nasogastric intubation[12].

Despite the fact that MBP is easier to use than WBI, we think that it is unacceptable in its present form because it predisposes to infection. We observed that following the introduction of MBP into our unit there has been a significant increase in the incidence of postoperative sepsis. In a recent trial in which both MBP and WBI were used, the incidence of sepsis following MBP was 41 per cent compared with 16 per cent after WBI despite postoperative antibiotic prophylaxis. The excess postoperative sepsis in the MBP group was due almost entirely to aerobic micro-organisms. We also found that in those patients who received MBP there was a significant rise in the colonic concentration of *Escherichia coli* to $\geq 10^8$ organisms/ml compared with a colonic concentration of the same organism of $\geq 10^5$/ml in those patients who received WBI[13]. We believe that mannitol, some of which remains in the colon[14], acts as a bacterial nutrient facilitating growth of *E. coli* within the colon. It is possible that the addition of oral neomycin or kanamycin to the mannitol may reduce this growth of *E. coli* or that other non-absorbed polysaccharides will be found which do not act as culture media and which prepare the colon as well as mannitol. We are investigating these hypotheses.

Antimicrobial prophylaxis

Sepsis after colorectal operations is due to both aerobic and anaerobic organisms[15]. Therefore, it is desirable, if possible, to reduce the concentration of these organisms within the colon. Thus the second aim of bowel preparation is 'bacterial cleanliness of the colon. Oral antibiotics, active against both aerobic and anaerobic bacteria, are given for 48 h before operation. Oral antibiotics suitable for the suppression of most aerobic colonic micro-

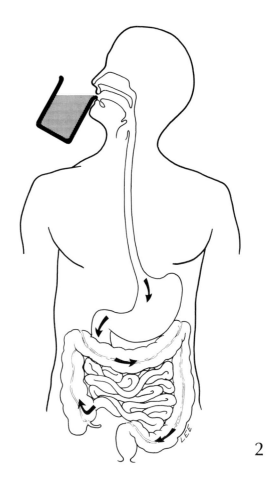

2

organisms are neomycin and kanamycin (1 g three times a day for 2 days preoperatively), and oral metronidazole (400 mg three times a day for 2 days preoperatively) is best for the suppression of the colonic anaerobic micro-organisms. Such a regimen has been shown to reduce postoperative sepsis to approximately 16 per cent compared with 42 per cent in a control group[15].

Recently the wisdom of attempting suppression of the colonic micro-organisms has been questioned. Keighley et al.[16] found that the incidence of postoperative sepsis in patients who received oral kanamycin and metronidazole (suppressed colonic micro-organisms) was 36 per cent compared with 7 per cent in those patients who received a short course of preoperative systemic kanamycin and metronidazole (unsuppressed colonic micro-organisms). Furthermore, it was found that bacterial resistance to kanamycin developed following oral administration. The evidence of a higher incidence of postoperative sepsis when oral antibiotic prophylaxis is used, together with the knowledge that the colon cannot be 'sterilized', suggests that it is more important to achieve high serum and tissue levels of antibiotic at the time of operation than to inhibit the colonic micro-organisms preoperatively.

Our present recommended policy for bowel preparation is to use whole bowel irrigation on the day before operation and antibiotic prophylaxis by a 3-dose course of intravenous gentamicin (120 mg) and metronidazole (500 mg). The first dose of antibiotic is given at the time of the induction of the anaesthetic.

References

1. Burton, R. C. Post-operative wound infection in colonic and rectal surgery. British Journal of Surgery 1973: 60: 363–365

2. Jackson, D. W., Pollock, A. V., Tindal, D. S. The value of a plastic adhesive drape in the prevention of wound infection. British Journal of Surgery 1971; 58: 340–342

3. Cruse, P. J. E., Foord, R. A five year prospective study of 23 649 surgical wounds. Archives of Surgery 1973; 107: 206–210

4. Mikal, S. Metabolic effects of preoperative intestinal preparation. American Journal of Proctology 1965; 16: 437–442

5. Arabi, Y., Dimock, F., Burdon, D. W., Alexander-Williams, J., Keighley, M. R. B. Influence of bowel preparation and antimicrobials on colonic microflora. British Journal of Surgery 1978; 65: 555–559

6. Glotzer, D. J., Boyle, P. J., Silen, W. Preoperative preparation of the colon with an elemental diet. Surgery 1973; 74: 703–707

7. Hewitt, J., Reeve, J., Rigby, J., Cox, A. G. Whole gut irrigation in preparation for large bowel surgery. Lancet 1973; 2: 337–340

8. Grace, R. H. Whole gut irrigation. Colo-Proctology 1980; 2: 297–299

9. Crapp, A. R., Tillotson, P., Powis, S. J. A., Cooke, W. T., Alexander-Williams, J. Preparation of the bowel by whole gut irrigation. Lancet 1975; 2: 1239–1240

10. Levy, A. G., Benson, J. W., Hewlett, E. L., Herdt, J. R., Doppman, J. L., Gordon, R. S. Saline lavage: a rapid, effective, and acceptable method for cleansing the gastrointestinal tract. Gastroenterology 1976; 70: 157

11. Hindle, W., Code, C. F. Some differences between duodenal and ileal sorption. American Journal of Physiology 1962; 203: 215–220

12. Minervini, S., Alexander-Williams, J., Donovan, I.A., Bentley, S., Keighley, M. R. B. Comparison of three methods of whole bowel irrigation. American Journal of Surgery 1980; 140: 400–402

13. Hares, M. M., Greca, F., Youngs, D., Bentley, S., Burdon, D. W., Keighley, M. R. B. Failure of antimicrobial prophylaxis with cefoxitin, or metronidazole and gentamicin in colo-rectal surgery. Is mannitol to blame? Journal of Hospital Infection 1981; 2: 127–133

14. Getman, P. M., Gagnon, O., Iber, F. L. Controlled diarrhea in the treatment of cirrhosis. Journal of the American Medical Association 1966; 197: 257–260

15. Matheson, D. M., Arabi, Y., Baxter-Smith, D., Alexander-Williams, J., Keighley, M.R.B. Randomized multicentre trial of oral bowel preparation and antimicrobials for elective colorectal surgery. British Journal of Surgery 1978; 65: 597–600

16. Keighley, M. R. B., Arabi, Y., Alexander-Williams, J., Youngs, D., Burdon, D. W. Comparison between systemic and oral antimicrobial prophylaxis in colorectal surgery. Lancet 1979; 894–897

Illustrations by Carol J. Pienta

Respiratory management of the surgical patient

Carl E. Haisch MD
Department of Surgery, School of Medicine, East Carolina University, Greenville, North Carolina

The importance of respiratory management in surgical patients is indicated by the finding that 5–7 per cent of all postoperative patients have respiratory complications causing either morbidity or mortality. About 25 per cent of all postoperative deaths are caused by pulmonary complications, and the figure increases with the age of the patient and with a history of smoking, emphysema, obesity or malnutrition.

The severity and frequency of respiratory complications vary in relation to the surgical site, being most frequent in patients who have undergone thoracic procedures and least often seen in those who have had extremity surgery. Upper abdominal and lower abdominal operations incur an intermediate number of complications.

Preoperative assessment

The major objective of respiratory management is the identification of high-risk patients and development of a plan to prevent pulmonary complications. Numerous studies show that postoperative pulmonary complications can be decreased by prophylactic measures in poor-risk patients. An accurate history, the physical examination and a routine chest roentgenogram will generally signal the problem patient. In taking the history one should look especially for a significant smoking history (20 cigarettes a day for 20 years), shortness of breath, old chest injuries, exposure to occupational dust, obesity or advanced age. In carrying out the physical examination, the physician should pay particular attention to dyspnoea, cyanosis, lack of diaphragmatic excursion (noted by percussion), or prolonged exporation or wheezing. On the chest film, one is looking for evidence of bullous disease, previous scarring or fibrosis. If any of the above are present and especially if thoracic or upper abdominal surgery is contemplated, pulmonary function tests should be performed.

Table 1 Patients requiring preoperative pulmonary evaluation[1]

Previous or anticipated thoracic surgery
Significant smoking history (20 cigarettes a day for 20 years)
History consistent with pulmonary disease
Significant obesity
Elderly patients

The basic *pulmonary function tests* are *forced vital capacity* (FVC) and *forced expiratory volume* in 1s (FEV$_1$). The FVC is the total volume of air which the patient can forcibly exhale. Normal values are 30–50 cm^3/kg body weight. The FEV$_1$ is the air a patient can exhale forcibly in 1s. Normal values for the FEV$_1$ are $\simeq$ 85 per cent of FVC. The *maximum voluntary ventilation* (MVV), formerly called the maximum breathing capacity (MBC), is also useful. The MVV is the amount of air which can be moved by a patient during a 15 or 20s interval, expressed as litres per minute. Normal values are 150–500 l/min. In addition, *arterial blood gases* should be done for an assessment of oxygenation and carbon dioxide retention. Normal values for patients breathing room air are as follows: pH 7.35–7.45, PaO_2 75–100 mmHg, $PaCO_2$ 35–45 mmHg.

Table 2 Findings which indicate a high risk[1]

Spirometric measurements
MVV less than 50 per cent predicted
FEV$_1$ less than 2 litres

Arterial blood gases
$PaCO_2$ greater than 45 mmHg

Preoperative therapy should include cessation of smoking, preferably for 3 weeks, a full course of ampicillin or tetracycline for purulent bronchitis, intensive chest physiotherapy and preoperative teaching of respiratory therapy.

Chest physiotherapy includes percussion of the chest and postural drainage of the segmental bronchi by having the patient assume the dependent position. Preoperative teaching includes acquainting the patient with postoperative respiratory exercises such as deep breathing and use of a deep breathing device. The patient is usually instructed to take as deep a breath as possible and hold it for 2 or 3s. The physician should delay surgery until the patient is judged to be in the best possible condition[1, 2].

Intraoperative care

Intraoperative care is as important as pre- and postoperative care. Proper intubation prevents collapse of a portion of the lung, and blood gases may need to be monitored periodically. Adequate ventilation, suction and appropriate position are essential to prevent atelectasis during surgery. Intraoperative fluid management is crucial. Too much fluid will cause pulmonary oedema, and too little will result in dryness of the mucous membranes, with alveolar plugging and subsequent atelectasis.

Postoperative care

Postoperative pulmonary therapy should aim to prevent or correct alveolar collapse and eventually restore normal pulmonary function. As Bartlett[1] has stated, this means that the ideal respiratory manoeuvre would be one which would maintain high alveolar inflating pressure for a sustained period of time (2–4s).

Various postoperative manoeuvres have been suggested, including intermittent positive pressure breathing (IPPB), coughing, CO_2 breathing, and deep breathing with incentive spirometry. IPPB appears to be a relatively ineffective form of postoperative therapy and in fact can cause alveolar rupture and decreased venous return to the heart, thereby decreasing cardiac output. The other disadvantage of IPPB is that it is pressure-limited rather than volume-limited. Thus a patient with increased airway resistance caused by splinting (because of pain, dressings or atelactasis) will not get the full volume of gas desired.

Rebreathing carbon dioxide with a 1000 ml tube can increase respiratory rate and tidal volume. To ensure maximum benefit, the patient's lips must seal around the mouthpiece and the nares must be pinched closed by the patient or an attendant. The major difficulty with CO_2 rebreathing is that it does not allow for sustained expansion of alveoli; thus there can still be microatelectasis.

Expiratory manoeuvres such as the use of blow bottles and the various products which require lifting one or several balls by air pressure are helpful in removing secretions, as is coughing; however, sustained opening of alveoli is prevented by such efforts. Blow bottles, like coughing, bring about a positive pleural pressure so that the alveoli do not inflate. Their major recommendation may be that the patient is forced to inspire deeply before beginning the blow-up exercise, so as to inhale enough air to compensate for the deficit caused by expiration. The benefit from these manoeuvres is mobilization of secretions, with improvement of pulmonary toilet.

Maximal inhalation is considered by many to be the most useful and effective means of preventing or minimizing postoperative respiratory complications. Patients can be instructed in the technique of maximal inspiration without any special equipment. Used postoperatively, this measure has been successful in reducing pulmonary complications, and when it is undertaken preoperatively as well as postoperatively the incidence of postoperative atelectasis is even lower. Use of the incentive spirometer has also been found to decrease postoperative complications[3].

Correct postoperative respiratory management calls for maintenance of proper fluid balance and optimal nutrition, early ambulation, and prevention of sepsis. Proper induction of analgesia is crucial and must be individualized to the particular patient as well as to the specific procedure. Dressings must not bind so tightly as to prevent pulmonary expansion. Coughing and chest physiotherapy to mobilize secretions both play major roles in direct pulmonary care.

Optimal respiratory management of the surgical patient thus begins in the preoperative period, with identification of high-risk patients and proper preparation, continues into and through the operation, and finishes in the postoperative period, with attention to general as well as to specific pulmonary measures.

The adult respiratory distress syndrome

The adult respiratory distress syndrome (ARDS), identified by the findings of hypoxia, decreased compliance, decreased lung volume, and a chest roentgenogram showing diffuse bilateral infiltrates, is most common in patients with chest trauma, sepsis, soft-tissue injuries, or disseminated intravascular coagulation. These patients are usually critically ill with more than one major problem, but many of them are young and with aggressive care they can often be saved[4, 5].

ENDOTRACHEAL INTUBATION

The common indications for intubation of patients with ARDS are listed in *Table 3*. In essence, intubation is required for deficiencies in oxygenation, as in ARDS, or for problems with ventilation which occur with elevations in $PaCO_2$. A patient who does not have chronic CO_2 retention (defined as $PaCO_2$ of 50 mmHg or greater) should be considered for intubation and ventilation.

Endoscopy requires careful preparation. The endotracheal tube should be as large as possible and should be equipped with a large low-pressure cuff. Suction must be available and working; the laryngoscope light should be checked and be operational; the endotracheal tube should be the proper size; and the cuff should be inflated with air and checked for leaks[6].

Table 3 Indications for ventilatory support in ARDS

	Normal	*Acceptable*	*Begin therapy*
Oxygenation			
PaO_2	100 mmHg on room air	>90 mmHg on 40% FIO_2*	<90 mmHg or decreasing on 40% FIO_2
$(A–a)\,DO_2$†	30 mmHg on room air	<200 mmHg on 40% FIO_2	>200 mmHg or increasing on 40% FIO_2
Ventilation			
$PaCO_2$	40 mmHg	30–40 mmHg	30 mmHg or decreasing
Minute volume	6 l/min	<12 l/min	>12 l/min and increasing
V_D/V_T‡		0.25–0.40	>0.6
Mechanics			
Rate		12–15/min	>25/min or increasing
Compliance	100 cm³/cmH₂O	50–100 cm³/cmH₂O	<50 cm³/cmH₂O or decreasing

*FIO_2 = fraction of inspired oxygen
†$(A–a)\,DO_2$ = difference in alveolar–arterial oxygen tension
‡V_D/V_T = volume of dead air space/tidal volume

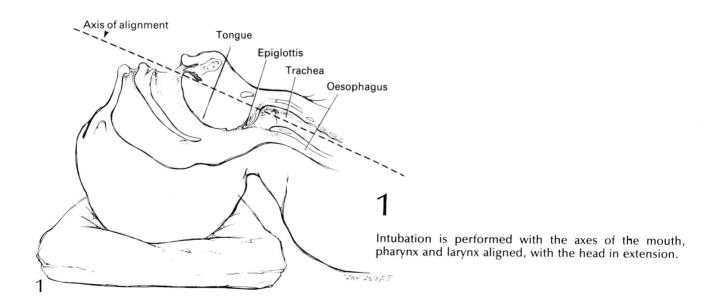

Intubation is performed with the axes of the mouth, pharynx and larynx aligned, with the head in extension.

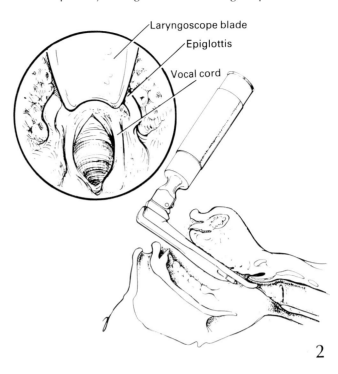

2

The laryngoscope is inserted through the right side of the mouth with the tip aimed in the midline. The tip of the laryngoscope is then placed posterior to the epiglottis with a straight blade.

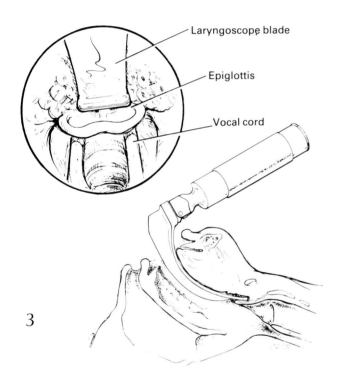

3

Alternatively, with a curved blade, the tip is placed between the epiglottis and the tongue.

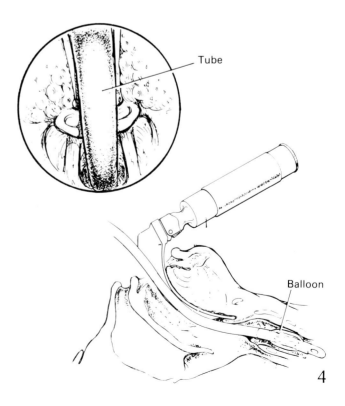

4

After the vocal cords are seen, the tube is inserted and the balloon inflated.

Welch (personal communication) has recently introduced an important advance in intubation, a technique that dispenses with the laryngoscope, which can cause trauma to the teeth and laceration of the oropharyngeal and laryngeal tissues. Welch's 'chin lift method' overcomes mechanical failure of the laryngoscope, is quick, avoids mucosal and dental damage, and is particularly helpful in patients whose head cannot be extended. The method is contraindicated in patients with hoarseness, dysphonia or tumours; in these patients, the cords and areas in the pathway of the tube should be inspected.

5

The endotracheal tube is prepared with lubrication and stiffened with a curved stylet which does not protrude beyond the tip.

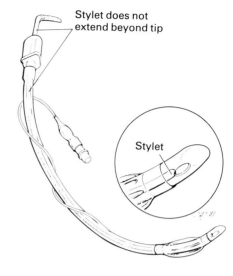

Stylet does not extend beyond tip

Stylet

5

6

The chin is lifted by grasping the anterior mandible between thumb and index finger.

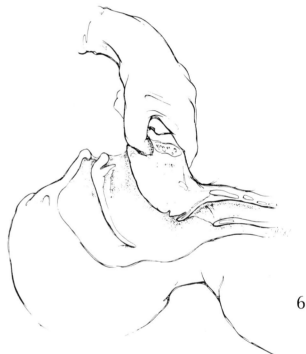

6

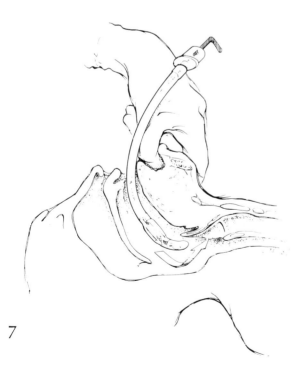

7

7

The tube is inserted precisely in the midline with the delicacy of a safe-cracker. Resistance to movement will be encountered if the tip of the tube lies in the pyriform fossa or if it is halted by the epiglottis.

8

The thyroid cartilage is the critical landmark. It will deviate if the tube is misdirected but will remain in the midline as long as intubation proceeds properly.

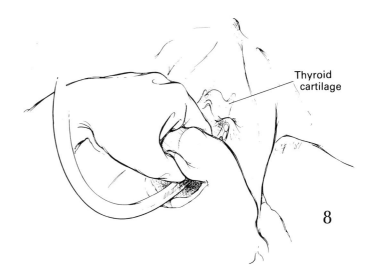

8

9

In addition, the neck will show a bulge if the tube is off centre. In this event, the tube should be withdrawn and redirected either to the right, to the left, or posteriorly; it can then be made to enter either the trachea or the oesophagus.

The tactile sensations differ according to whether the tube is in the trachea or in the oesophagus: in the oesophagus, the tube moves with a sticky sensation; in the trachea it 'gives' and then drops in effortlessly with a loss of resistance. With an experience of more than 9000 cases, Welch maintains his method is a safe and satisfactory means of intubation.

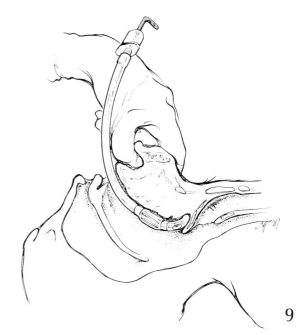

9

Complications of endotracheal intubation

A potential complication associated with intubation, gastric distension, is likely to occur when prolonged attempts at intubation have been made. Should gastric distension develop, the stomach must be quickly decompressed by means of a nasogastric tube. Another complication, occlusion of the left lung, is caused by advancing the tube into the right main-stem bronchus. This situation will have serious results if it is not corrected. A roentgenogram of the chest should be made immediately after intubation to determine the location of the the endotracheal tube.

Other problems associated with the use of the endotracheal tube may include leakage from the cuff as well as such complications as nasal necrosis, epistaxis, hoarse-

ness after extubation and airway obstruction secondary to inspissated secretions or herniation of the cuff over the end of the tube[7].

Tracheal erosion and stenosis, once common, have been much decreased. The small high-pressure balloon formerly used on the endotracheal tube has been replaced by a large-volume, low-pressure cuff which completely occludes the trachea without distension. Some authors now report the use of an endotracheal tube for as long as 3 weeks before tracheostomy is considered. Skilled nursing care, careful stabilization of the tube, sterile technique and adequate humidification are the main factors necessary for success in prolonged intubation[4].

Ventilators

Ventilators are of three basic types: (1) patient-sensitive pressure-limited; (2) patient-insensitive volume-limited; and (3) patient-sensitive volume-limited. In the pressure-limited ventilator, the lungs are inflated to a predetermined pressure, regardless of the volume delivered to the patient. Accordingly, pressure-limited ventilators are unsatisfactory when the patient's lungs are of low compliance. Volume-limited ventilators deliver a set volume into a patient regardless of the pressure required and are therefore unsatisfactory for patients with emphysema or bullous lung disease. Patient-sensitive volume-limited ventilators deliver a preset volume within a preset pressure limit, permitting control of both the tidal volume and the pressure limit; thus their use can be tailored to each patient's needs. The patient-sensitive volume-limited ventilator is the type of ventilator most commonly used at present.

The usual tidal volume used is 10–15 ml/kg of body weight. Smaller volumes may be necessary for the patient with emphysema, decreased usable lung, or a single lung. A large tidal volume decreases atelectasis and mitigates the necessity for the sigh mode on the ventilator. A respiratory rate of 12–16 is usually selected initially; when the patient seems ready, he can be carefully advanced to an assist mode. Measurements of blood gases serve as a guide to adjustment of the ventilator rate and the percentage of oxygen. The ventilator rate is adjusted in accordance with the Pa_{CO_2}. Inspired oxygen can usually be started at 40 per cent and then adjusted, according to the Pa_{O_2} value. Patients should generally be maintained at a Pa_{O_2} level of 75–125 mmHg. Prolonged elevation of oxygen levels above 60 per cent is probably detrimental and should be avoided if possible. When an inspired oxygen level greater than 60 per cent is required for longer than 24h, positive and expiratory pressure (PEEP) should be considered.

PEEP

The primary indication for PEEP is hypoxia (defined as Pa_{O_2} < 60 mmHg with F_{IO_2} > 50 per cent), a change generally associated with ARDS, hydrostatic pulmonary oedema or pneumonia. Contraindications to PEEP are relative, depending upon the clinical situation. PEEP increases risk for patients with emphysema, bronchitis and asthma and may cause rupture of bullous portions of the lung, leading to tension pneumothorax. Patients with head trauma may be made worse by PEEP because of increased cerebrospinal fluid pressure, the PEEP pressure being transmitted to the central nervous system via the internal jugular veins. A third contraindication is shock, which may be deepened by PEEP through a decrease in venous return and subsequent decreased cardiac output.

MONITORING PEEP EFFECTIVENESS

Before a patient is started on PEEP, an arterial line and Swan-Ganz catheter with cardiac output capabilities should be placed. The cardiac output measurements reflect the influence of the PEEP on the cardiac status. When the level of PEEP exceeds left atrial pressure, the wedge pressure will be influenced more by PEEP than by the left atrial pressure; an artificially high wedge pressure will result. The arterial line is placed for accurate blood pressure monitoring and for ease in obtaining blood gas determinations.

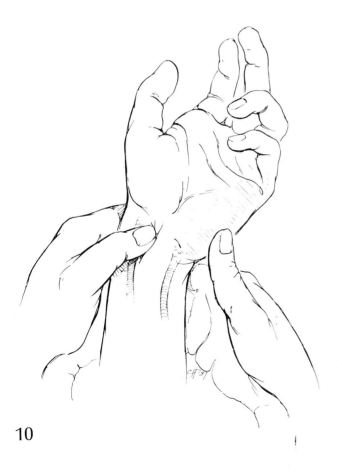

Arterial lines

10

Arterial lines may be placed in the radial, brachial or femoral artery. If the radial artery is to be used, the collateral circulation must first be tested by the Allen test. The patient is asked to clench his fist in order to evacuate the blood from the hand, and both the radial and ulnar arteries are occluded by the examiner.

11

The hand should regain its colour quickly when the ulnar artery alone is released.

The radial artery can then be cannulated percutaneously or via a cutdown.

Percutaneous cannulation

12

The skin is prepared with organic iodine solution (Betadine), a sterile field is established and approximately 1 cm³ of 1 per cent lignocaine is injected over the site for needle insertion.

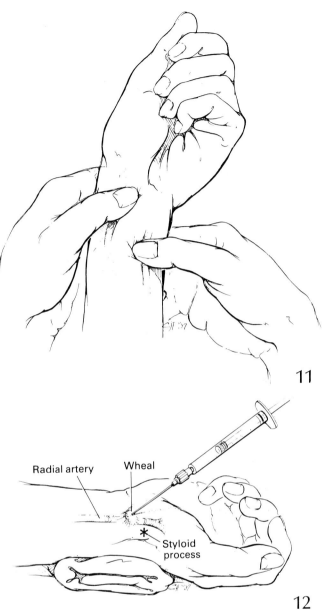

11

Radial artery   Wheal

*

Styloid process

12

13

A 20 gauge plastic sheath needle (Abbocath) is used. The artery is located between the index and middle fingers of the left hand, and the catheter needle is placed through the local anaesthetic wheal.

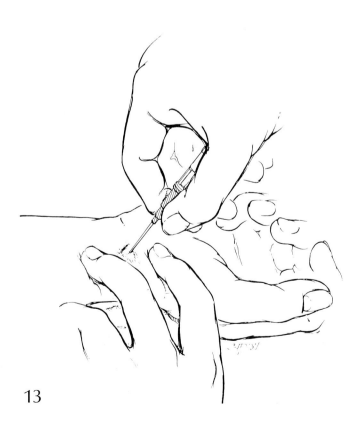

13

14

The needle impales the artery and is slowly withdrawn.

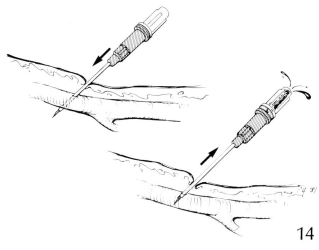

14

15

When blood is seen in the needle, the plastic sheath is slipped off the needle and is advanced into the artery. When the catheter is properly positioned, a suture is placed through the skin, securing the catheter.

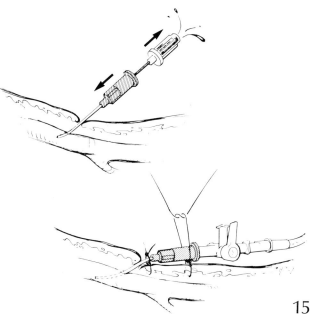

15

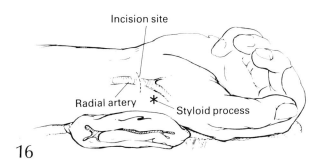

Incision site

Radial artery   *   Styloid process

16

Cannulation via a cutdown

16

A transverse incision is made at the proximal end of the styloid process and the artery located.

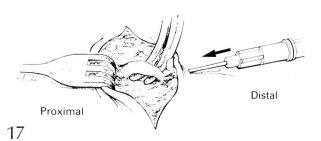

Proximal   Distal

17

17

The catheter needle is pushed through the skin distal to the incision.

18

The artery is cannulated under direct vision and the needle withdrawn.

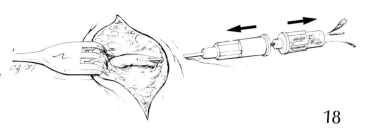

18

19

The wound is then closed and the catheter securely anchored with two sutures, one about the hub of the needle.

19

Complications

Complications associated with arterial line catheters can be disastrous. The most common complication, infection, can be prevented by strict aseptic technique during insertion and good nursing care after insertion. Thrombi can form on the end of the catheter, causing small infarcts in the hand; this complication can be prevented by careful choice of material of low thrombogenic potential, such as Teflon in the artery, and a small-sized cannula. Catheters with non-tapered shafts are preferable because they are less likely to cause thrombosis. The most dangerous complication, inadvertent haemorrhage from disconnected lines, can be prevented by proper securing of the catheter and the lines, accompanied by careful observation. An alarm system is essential if the catheter is to be used for blood pressure monitoring.

The Swan-Ganz catheter

20

The Swan-Ganz catheter is preferably of the thermodilution type with a distal port (a) for measuring pulmonary artery and wedge pressures. The inflatable balloon will hold 1–1.5 cm³ of air. Proximal to the balloon is the thermistor (b) for measuring pulmonary artery temperatures, and 30 cm from the distal tip is the proximal port (c) for central venous pressure measurements and for the injection of cold saline or 5 per cent dextrose in water.

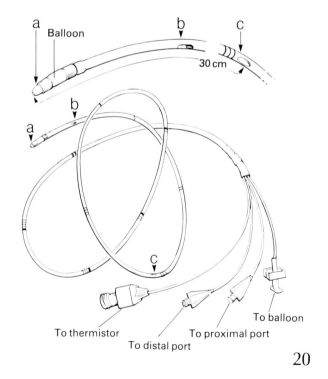

20

Testing of the Swan-Ganz catheter

The catheter is thoroughly checked before insertion; once it is in place, if a malfunction is discovered, replacement will be necessary. The first step is to connect the catheter to the cardiac output machine to make sure that the catheter is intact electrically. Next a TB syringe is used to add 1 cm³ of air to the balloon. The inflated balloon is placed in a sterile container filled with sterile saline. If no air bubbles are seen one may assume that the balloon is intact and the catheter may then be inserted.

The Swan-Ganz catheter is placed through the subclavian, brachial or femoral vein.

21

The subclavian vein is preferred because this location is out of the patient's way and also because the catheter in this position is rather difficult to dislodge. The Sorensen introducer is used for a 7 French catheter (the size of the Edwards Swan-Ganz catheter with cardiac output capabilities).

Insertion of the Swan-Ganz catheter

A sterile field on the chest is prepared after the subclavian area has been shaved.

22

The needle is inserted at the junction of the inner and middle thirds of the clavicle and directed toward the sternal notch. A syringe must always be attached to prevent entry of an air embolus. When the needle is in the vein, the steel wire is placed through the needle with the floppy lead end foremost.

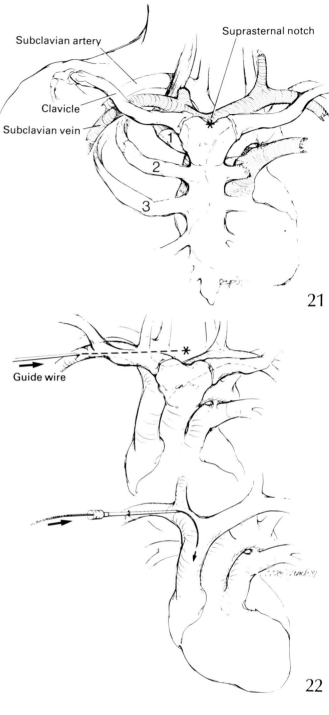

21

22

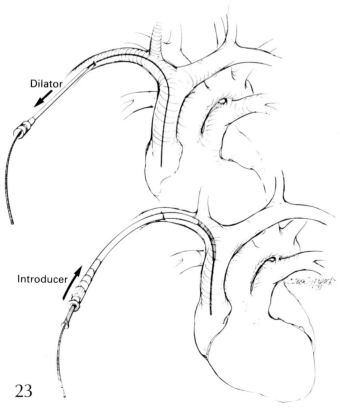

23

23

The needle is then withdrawn from the guide wire. The dilator and introducer are then threaded over the guide wire as a single unit.

24

Care must be taken not to lose hold of the guide wire. The dilator and introducer are pushed over the guide wire until the introducer is at the hub on the skin. When the dilator and guide wire are removed, a free backflow of blood should then follow through the introducer.

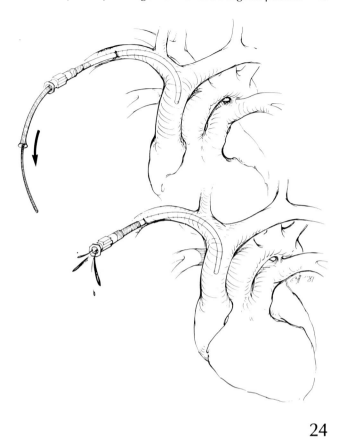

24

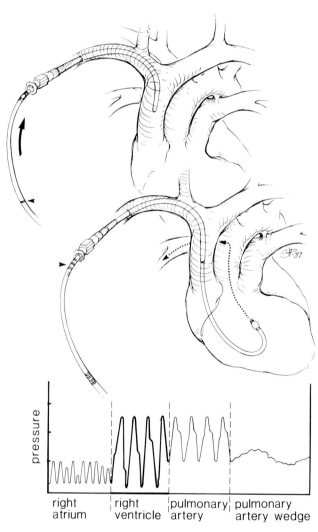

25

The Swan-Ganz catheter is placed through the introducer and, when the catheter is at the 20 cm mark, 1 cm^3 of air is introduced into the balloon. The distal tip of the catheter is connected to a pressure transducer and pressure monitor. The proximal port is filled with saline from a syringe which is left in place to prevent blood clotting in the lumen. The typical tracing of the right ventricular pressures is shown.

25

26

The change in tracing from the right ventricle to that of the pulmonary artery is demonstrated by the accented line. Note that there is a change in the diastolic pressure as well as in the shape of the curve.

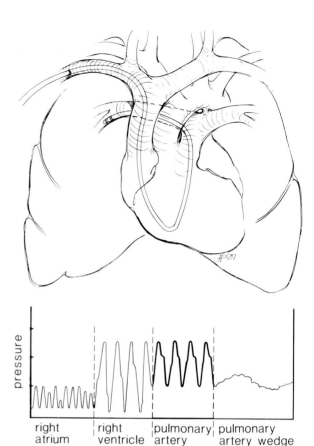

26

27

The advance of the catheter is continued until a wedge tracing is seen on the pressure monitor.

The balloon is then collapsed by removing the syringe. If the pulmonary artery tracing is seen and the wedge tracing is easily obtainable with less than 1.5 cm³ of air, the introducer is moved back over the catheter and the catheter is sutured into place. An occlusive dressing is then placed at the Swan-Ganz insertion site.

After the catheter is secured, a chest roentgenogram should be obtained to exclude a pneumothorax and check that the Swan-Ganz tip is correctly placed in the mid-third of the hemithorax.

Swan-Ganz catheterization can bring about a number of complications, most frequently arrhythmias during insertion, thromboemboli and infection. Other reported complications include perforation of the pulmonary artery, massive haemorrhage and intracardiac knotting. These complications decrease with experience and can be avoided in some measure by monitoring of the ECG during insertion.

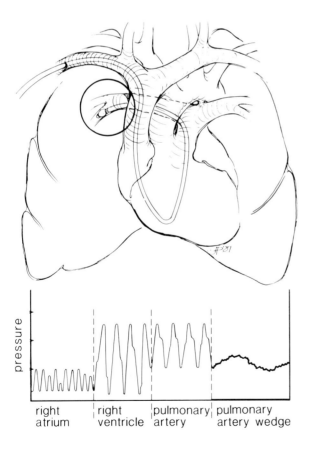

27

PEEP trial

With the Swan-Ganz catheter in place, a trial of PEEP can be begun. A number of parameters must be followed and reviewed (*Table 4*), including arterial and mixed venous

Table 4 Parameters to follow while patient is on PEEP

Blood pressure	Pulmonary artery wedge
Pulse	pressure
PEEP level	Pa_{O_2}
Respiratory rate	Pa_{CO_2}
Tidal volume	Arterial pH
Static pressure	% Arterial saturation
Compliance	$P\bar{v}_{O_2}$
Fi_{O_2}	% Venous saturation
Pulmonary artery pressure	Cardiac output

blood gases, which should be processed as quickly as possible for optimum accuracy. An Fi_{O_2} is chosen which is adequate for the individual patient at a PEEP level of zero. The level of PEEP may then be increased by increments of $5\,cmH_2O$, the listed parameters being checked at each new level of PEEP. PEEP is then increased until there is adequate oxygenation, until compliance either decreases or stops improving, or until cardiac output falls significantly (usually a 20 per cent decrease from baseline). If adequate oxygenation ($Pa_{O_2}>80$) has not been achieved by increasing the PEEP before the cardiac output decreases, a fluid challenge may be necessary to increase intravascular volume and thus increase cardiac output. By this means, a higher level of PEEP can be used and oxygenation may then be improved.

PEEP COMPLICATIONS

The most common complication of the use of PEEP is a decrease in cardiac output. Pressure on the great vessels and increased vascular resistance in the pulmonary vessels decreases venous return to the heart. Administration of increased quantities of intravenous fluids will generally correct the decreased venous return to the heart. Barotrauma, pneumothorax and pneumomediastinum are also complications of PEEP. The likelihood of their occurrence can be decreased by following the static compliance,

$$\frac{\text{tidal volume}}{\text{change in static pressure minus PEEP level}}$$

If compliance is found to be improving as PEEP is increased, the incidence of barotrauma will be small. If compliance begins to plateau or decrease, however, the danger of barotrauma increases markedly. A large-bore needle on a syringe should be kept at the bedside for relief of tension pneumothorax, should it occur. Blood pressure is a valuable indicator: sudden decrease frequently means a tension pneumothorax has occurred. When the patient is stable, with the appropriate level of PEEP, a chest roentgenogram should be made, to rule out barotrauma.

A patient maintained on PEEP should be monitored with daily chest roentgenograms. Arterial blood gases, blood pressure and urinary output should be monitored closely. Once the patient is brought to a stable level of PEEP, with subsequent decrease in the Fi_{O_2} to 40 per cent, weaning from PEEP can begin.

WEANING FROM PEEP

Before weaning from PEEP, the patient should be clinically stable, with no recent increase in white blood cells, no decrease in Pa_{O_2}, no increase in temperature and no new cardiac difficulties. An Fi_{O_2} of 40 per cent is ideal and the

Table 5 Preconditions for weaning the patient from PEEP[8]

Clinically stable patient
Stable temperature, cardiac status, fluid, electrolyte and
  complete blood count values for 24 h
$Fi_{O_2} = 40\%$
$Pa_{O_2} \geqslant 80\,mmHg$
Compliance $\geqslant 25\,cm^3/cmH_2O$

Pa_{O_2} should be $80\,mmHg$ or greater. The static compliance should be $25\,cm^3/cmH_2O$ or greater. The first step is to decrease the PEEP by $5\,cmH_2O$, check the arterial blood gases in 3 min, and then re-establish the same PEEP level. If the Pa_{O_2} falls less than 20 per cent from baseline and the change is tolerated well, the PEEP may be safely moved down by $5\,cmH_2O$. This manoeuvre may be repeated every 12 h until the patient is at zero PEEP[8].

Patients who are taken off PEEP too quickly or who do not do well when the level is decreased have a high incidence of complications when PEEP is reinstituted.

Intermittent mandatory ventilation

Once the patient is off PEEP, he can be advanced to intermittent mandatory ventilation (IMV). IMV requires the patient to take some breaths on his own, but if he is unable to maintain his own rate of respiration at, say, 15 respirations per minute, the ventilator will maintain a preset minute ventilation as a safeguard. Thus the patient is gradually weaned from the ventilator and forced to breathe on his own, which is particularly advantageous for the patient with ARDS, because the lungs are stiff and assistance in ventilation is usually required at first. Both Pa_{CO_2} and Pa_{O_2} must be watched, because the patient required to take over increasing amounts of ventilation may tire easily and be unable to maintain adequate ventilation. The fatigue will be reflected by an increase in Pa_{CO_2}. The Fi_{O_2} is then adjusted to maintain an acceptable Pa_{O_2}[9].

Extubation

The criteria for extubation have been well outlined and are noted in *Table 6*. After extubation a patient must still be closely observed because he may not be able to maintain his ventilations and may require reintubation as late as 18 h after the initial extubation[10, 11].

Table 6 Criteria for extubation

$(A–a)\,D_{O_2}$ (on 100%) $< 300\,mmHg$
Vital capacity $10–15\,cm^3/kg$
Maximum inspiratory force $< -20\,cmH_2O$
$V_D/V_T < 0.6$
Cardiovascular stability
Minute ventilation < 10 litres

Flail chest

Flail chest, or loss of the mechanical structure of the rib cage due to multiple rib or sternal fractures, frequently occurs in patients with other underlying disease processes who have also sustained a pulmonary contusion. Flail chest is best managed by 'internal splinting', that is ventilator settings that allow no patient-initiated respirations, with rate and tidal volume set to deprive the patient of respiratory drive. This will usually require a $PaCO_2$ in the low 30s. The patient is maintained in this manner until there is no paradoxical motion of the chest when he is disconnected from the ventilator. Patients with underlying pulmonary contusion may require PEEP. Recent studies suggest that patients do not require 2 weeks of continuous ventilation; rather, treatment of the underlying pulmonary injury with IMV is adequate.

References

1. Tisi, G. M. Preoperative evaluation of pulmonary function: validity, indications, and benefits. American Review of Respiratory Disease 1979; 119: 293–310

2. Stein, M., Cassara, E. L. Preoperative pulmonary evaluation and therapy for surgery patients. Journal of the American Medical Association 1970; 211: 787–790

3. Bartlett, R. H., Gazzaniga, A. B., Geraghty, T. R. Respiratory manoeuvers to prevent postoperative pulmonary complications: a critical review. Journal of the American Medical Association 1973; 224: 1017–1021

4. Blaisdell, F. W., Lewis, F. R. Respiratory distress syndrome of shock and trauma: post-traumatic respiratory failure. Philadelphia: W. B. Saunders, 1977

5. Pontoppidan, H., Geffin, B., Lowenstein, E. Acute respiratory failure in the adult. New England Journal of Medicine 1972; 287: 690–698, 743–752, 799–806

6. Salem, M. R., Mathrubhatham, M., Bennett, E. J. Difficult intubation. New England Journal of Medicine 1976; 295: 879–881

7. Zwillich, C. W., Pierson, D. J., Creagh, C. E., Sutton, F. D., Schatz, E., Petty, T. L. Complications of assisted ventilation. A prospective study of 354 consecutive episodes. American Journal of Medicine 1974; 57: 161–170

8. Weaver, L. J., Hudson, L. D., Carrico, C. J. Prospective analysis of PEEP reduction. Chest 1980; 78: 544

9. Downs, J. B., Klein, E. F., Desautels, D., Modell, J. H., Kirby, R. R. Intermittent mandatory ventilation: a new approach to weaning patients from mechanical ventilators. Chest 1973; 64: 331–335

10. Feeley, T. W., Hedley-Whyte, J. Weaning from controlled ventilation and supplemental oxygen. New England Journal of Medicine 1975; 292: 903–906

11. Hedley-Whyte, J., Burgess, G. E., Feeley, T. W., Miller, M. G. Applied physiology of respiratory care. Boston: Little, Brown & Co, 1976

Cardiac evaluation of the surgical patient

Allen F. Bowyer MD
Professor of Medicine and Chief, Division of Cardiology, Department of Medicine,
School of Medicine, East Carolina University, Greenville, North Carolina

Introduction

The cardiac evaluation of the surgical patient is best undertaken with the following three patient groups in mind.

1. No history or current findings of cardiac disease.
2. History of cardiac disease but no current findings of heart disease.
3. Signs and symptoms of current cardiac problems.

Subjects for elective or emergency surgery without previous history of heart disease or signs or symptoms of current heart disease should have limited cardiac evaluation. For a man aged under 40 years or a woman aged under 50 years, a routine resting 12-lead electrocardiogram (ECG) should be sufficient for detection of a previous 'silent' myocardial infarct. Of all patients with myocardial infarctions, approximately 20 per cent have no classical precordial pain, but their lesions may be signalled by changes in a standard resting ECG.

Symptoms of previous infarction or ischaemic heart disease indicate the need for a cardiac examination, resting 12-lead ECG, and exercise stress test to determine the ischaemic state. A patient with a history of previous congenital or acquired valvular heart disease or history of cardiac surgery should undergo echocardiography. If echocardiography demonstrates a significant heart valve or myocardial problem, invasive cardiac catheterization is indicated.

The patient with current signs and symptoms of heart disease should have a more complete cardiovascular examination prior to surgery. Before emergency surgery, such evaluation may necessarily be limited to auscultation and a brief echocardiographic examination. Before elective surgery, a careful physical examination, resting 12-lead ECG, stress test, and echocardiography are basic, followed by cardiac catheterization and coronary arteriography if the patient demonstrates evidence of coronary artery, valve or myocardial disease. Such studies establish priorities and risks.

The patient with signs and symptoms of ischaemic heart disease should undergo a progressive exercise stress test, to determine the following points.

1. Relative risk of developing myocardial infarction during or following an elective procedure.
2. Probability that he has significant underlying heart disease.
3. Whether coronary angiography should precede the elective surgery.

If non-critical, low-risk coronary lesions are seen on arteriography, the elective surgery may proceed. If critical, high-risk coronary stenoses are present, myocardial revascularization surgery should be considered before elective non-cardiac surgery.

In general, a stable cardiac condition (defined as one in which the signs and symptoms have not altered for a period of 3 months) without evidence for arterial desaturation (normal range for arterial haemoglobin saturation is 92–98 per cent) adds but a small risk for elective surgery.

History of ischaemic heart disease

All surgical patients should be questioned carefully about previous myocardial infarction, abnormal ECG, episodes of chest pain, or hospitalization in intensive or coronary care units. Angina pectoris must be suspected when a patient describes precordial pain reproducibly provoked by activities which increase heart rate, systolic pressure or both. Pain brought on by exercise, anger, anxiety, excitement, sexual arousal or sudden exposure to cold air and which subsides within 5 min after the activity or exposure is terminated must be assumed to be angina pectoris. A history of predictable precordial pain indicates 90–95 per cent probability that the patient has coronary artery stenosis. If precordial pain has been increasing over a 3 month period the patient has unstable progressive angina, and elective surgery should be postponed until coronary arteriographic assessment of the extent of his coronary stenosis is made. If left main stenosis, left main equivalent stenosis or three-vessel disease is found, then myocardial revascularization is advised prior to elective non-cardiac surgery. Conversely, if distal, single-vessel or no coronary stenosis is found, then elective surgery can proceed.

If the precordial pain has not progressed in intensity, severity or frequency over the previous 3 months, stable angina pectoris may be diagnosed, and a progressive exercise stress test will determine the degree of effort limitation. If the stress test is markedly positive at low levels of exercise, less than 5 Mets (1 Met = resting metabolic rate of $3.5 \, ml \, O_2 \, kg^{-1} \, min^{-1}$), the patient should be considered for coronary arteriography before elective surgery. If the stress test shows ischaemic change at high levels of exercise or at or near the patient's fatigue limit, surgery can usually be undertaken without great risk.

A subject who provides a history of precordial pain that is atypical in type, location and predictability has an approximately 50 per cent likelihood of having underlying coronary artery disease and should have progressive exercise stress testing. If the stress test is positive at low levels of exercise, coronary arteriography should be done; if the stress test is negative, elective surgery can be undertaken.

History of congenital or valvular heart disease

Subjects with a history of previous congenital or valvular heart disease should have the diagnosis confirmed or denied with echocardiography or nuclear cardiography. Echocardiography provides an excellent non-invasive tool for examining the form and function of the aortic and mitral valves; it indicates, less consistently, pulmonic and tricuspid valve disease. If echocardiography indicates significant cardiac structural abnormality, cardiac catheterization should precede elective surgery. Typically, cardiac catheterization should usually precede elective surgery in patients with suspected right-to-left shunts, severe ventricular hypertrophy, significant aortic or mitral valve disease, or significant loss of ventricular function (i.e. ejection fraction less than 40 per cent). If cardiac catheterization demonstrates right-to-left shunt, loss of ventricular function, or significant valvular disease, elective surgery should be postponed until the cardiac problem has been corrected. If catheterization reveals no clinically significant problem, then the elective surgery should proceed.

Resting electrocardiogram

The standard resting 12-lead ECG does not assist in the diagnosis of angina pectoris, but it is extremely useful in documenting arrhythmias, the presence of a previous myocardial infarction or suspected acute ischaemia. The ECG rhythm strip is the single most important aid to diagnosis of cardiac arrhythmia. If findings of acute myocardial infarction or ischaemia are present, surgery should be postponed until the stability of the condition has been established by enzymatic study and serial ECG. If new Q waves with a width of 0.04 s are seen, myocardial infarction may have occurred, and efforts should be made to determine its age. If the patient provides no history of myocardial infarction, electrocardiographic patterns are helpful in establishing the severity and stability of the lesion. If there are no changes in ST segments or T waves for 3 days and if creatinine kinase and lactic dehydrogenase values are normal, one may assume the infarction is stable. Changing ST-T wave pattern or elevation of serum enzymes is an indicator of unstable, evolving infarction, and elective surgery should be postponed. Stable ST-T wave changes, hypertrophies or bundle branch blocks need not delay surgery.

Complicated ventricular premature beats, however, indicate a need to delay surgery until the rhythm is under control. Complicated ventricular beats consist of the following.

Multiple ventricular beats (2 premature beats in sequence).
Multifocal premature ventricular beats (PVCs from 2 or more localities).
R-on-T phenomenon (R wave of the premature beat firing on or in close proximity to the T wave of the previous beat).
Ventricular tachycardia.

The patient with complicated ventricular beats is at high risk for the development of severe ventricular tachycardia, flutter or fibrillation, and his elective surgery should be delayed until the rhythm has been corrected and any underlying cardiac cause has been treated. In conditions of emergency surgery which are life-threatening, therapy with cardiac anti-arrhythmic drugs can proceed simultaneously with surgery, but a greater surgical risk must be accepted.

Exercise stress test

The two types of progressive exercise stress test currently performed are bicycle ergometry and treadmill stress testing. Although the mode of exercise is different in each, there are advantages and disadvantages to either method for detection of underlying cardiovascular disease not evident at rest. Both stress tests define functional status according to age, sex and peer group. Symptoms developing from exercise stress can be related to external work load, ECG change and arterial pressure. Stress testing is best applied to those patients with suspected ischaemic heart disease or myocardial disease or to those who have had myocardial infarction or cardiac surgery. Of several testing methods available, the Bruce treadmill protocol has been widely used in a variety of subjects; normal values for this protocol are well defined.

Bruce protocol

Following a resting control 12-lead ECG and 30 s hyperventilation cardiogram, the patient exercises on a treadmill at 6 per cent elevation at a belt speed of 0.93 km/h. Exercise continues for 3 min, at which point the treadmill is elevated to 10 per cent and speed is increased to 1.24 km/h. At each 3 min interval, elevation, speed or both are further increased. Elapsed time, estimated oxygen uptake, heart rate, arterial pressure, rate-pressure index, ST segment change and symptoms are usually recorded throughout exercise and during 6–10 min of post-exercise rest. Throughout exercise, a continuous dialogue is conducted with the patient; exercise is terminated when the patient reaches an effort-limiting fatigue state or develops symptoms that would normally terminate exercise at home or at work. The normal ranges for maximum exercise for normal men are shown in *Table 1*.

Table 1 Treadmill exercise stress test; variation of maximal exercise with age for normal men (adapted from Bruce, Kusumi and Hosmer[1])

Stage	Elapsed time (min)	Speed (km/h)	Elevation (%)	Computed oxygen uptake* (ml O_2 kg^{-1} min^{-1})	Age range	Maximal oxygen uptake† (ml O_2 kg^{-1} min^{-1})	n
0	0	0	0	3.5			
1/2	3	0.93	6	9.6			
1	6	1.24	10	16.7			
					81–90	22.0	4
2	9	1.55	12	23.3			
					71–80	28.0	12
					61–70	33.0	43
3	12	2.17	14	35.0			
					51–60	36.0	142
					41–50	39.0	127
					31–40	42.0	64
4	15	2.49	16	47.2			
					21–30	48.0	222
					11–20	49.0	60
					9–10	53.0	26
5	18	3.11	18	61.1			
6	21	3.42	20	72.5			
7	24	3.73	20	84.9			

* Computed from: $V_{O_2} = (48.28)(S)(0.073 + E/100)$
   where
   V_{O_2} = oxygen uptake in ml O_2 kg^{-1} min^{-1}
   S = treadmill speed in mph
   E = treadmill elevation in %
   (From Balke and Ware[2])
† Data from 700 normal men (From Dehn and Bruce[3])

Bicycle ergometer stress test

This form of exercise stress testing provides cardiovascular stress different in several aspects from that produced by treadmill exercise. Heart rate and rate-pressure product (systolic pressure × heart rate ÷ 100) tend to be greater than values achieved with treadmill testing. When the subject stops exercising on the bicycle, the power load is off immediately. Power requirements are identical for all subjects and are not a function of height or weight, as they are with treadmill testing. Bicycle ergometer testing results, like those from treadmill testing, indicate the status of the total cardiovascular system and the patient's capability for performing exercise. The indications for ergometry testing are similar to those for treadmill, but because the work loads and work load increment are less with the bicycle, the patient with more severe disease states may better be exercised on the bicycle. Bicycle testing is the preferred method if significant weight alteration is contemplated.

The patient is studied during a progressive exercise programme, usually on a computer-controlled ergometer system. Power requirements begin with 50 W (3 Mets) and increase by steps of 25 W every 3 min until clinical fatigue or exercise-limiting symptoms appear. Heart rate, arterial pressure, ECG change and symptoms are continuously monitored during control rest, exercise stress and 6 min of post-exercise recovery. The exercise protocol shows that the oxygen requirement increases every 3 min by approximately 1 Met, as shown in *Table 2*.

Table 2 Bicycle ergometer stress test

Stage	Elapsed time (min)	Power (W)	Computed oxygen uptake (ml O_2 kg^{-1} min^{-1})
0	0	0	3.5
1	3	50	9
2	6	75	12
3	9	100	15
4	12	125	18
5	15	150	21
6	18	175	24
7	21	200	28
8	24	250	35
9	27	300	42
10	30	350	50

Stress testing can suggest the probability of coronary artery disease, as *Table 3* demonstrates. The likelihood that the subject has underlying coronary disease varies according to age, sex and symptoms developed during the test. For example, a man aged 45 years who develops chest pain during stress testing has greater than 60 per cent probability of having significant coronary disease (defined as 75 per cent or greater stenosis of one, two or three vessels). A woman aged 45 years who develops chest pain alone, however, has approximately 24 per cent probability

Table 3 Probability of coronary artery disease indicated by specific results during stress testing

Pop.	ST segment elevation (> 1.0 mm)	ST segment depression (> 1.0 mm)	Chest pain	No signs or symptoms
Men				
20	96.9	26.6	16.6	3.2
30	99.0	54.0	39.2	7.9
40	99.6	74.5	61.6	15.6
50	99.7	81.9	71.3	22.1
60	99.7	80.3	69.2	20.5
70	99.9	92.7	87.4	45.3
Women				
20	73.7	3.1	1.7	0.2
30	92.6	12.5	7.3	0.9
40	98.0	36.3	23.9	3.5
50	99.2	58.8	43.9	8.2
60	99.2	59.5	47.7	8.5
70	99.6	75.9	63.4	16.6

of having significant coronary disease. If an elective surgical patient has 75 per cent or greater probability for underlying significant coronary disease, coronary arteriography should precede the elective surgery.

Echocardiography

Time motion (TM) or two-dimensional echocardiography provides a completely non-invasive method of visualizing the normal or pathological anatomy of the heart. The structures most easily visualized include the aortic root and valve, mitral valve structure, left atrium, right ventricle, interventricular septum, left ventricle and pericardium. Occasionally the tricuspid and pulmonary valves may be seen.

Patients with severe mitral or aortic valve disease or heart muscle disease should be evaluated by cardiac catheterization before elective non-cardiac surgery. Patients with prolapse deformity or mild aortic or mitral valve disease and normal ventricular function need not undergo cardiac catheterization but can proceed directly to elective surgery.

Invasive cardiac testing

Invasive cardiac testing should be limited to those patients who before elective cardiac surgery are found to have significant or unstable coronary or cardiac structural disease. A patient with mild cardiac disease who has no arrhythmia and no unstable angina pectoris may proceed to elective non-cardiac surgery. Under conditions of emergency surgery, a judgement will have to be made in each case regarding the advisability of delay for cardiac evaluation or proceeding with surgery and accepting the increased surgical risk. Three broad categories of invasive testing are available today: right heart catheterization, left heart catheterization, and coronary angiography.

Right heart catheterization using balloon-tip, flow-directed catheters and thermistor cardiac output devices can be done at the bedside. A portable fluoroscopic device, if one is available, is an aid to catheter positioning. The right antecubital or brachial vein can be cut down in either the right or the left arm, or percutaneous entrance may be made at the groin (see chapter on 'Respiratory management of the surgical patient', pp. 12–26).

Left heart catheterization is usually performed by cutdown in the right or left brachial artery or by percutaneous entrance using a Seldinger needle in the right or left femoral artery. Contrast medium can be injected under pressure during cineangiographic filming, to determine the volume, shape and contractile sequence of the left ventricle.

Coronary arteriography today is done by selective introduction of catheters into the left and right coronary ostia and injection of 8–10 ml of contrast medium during 35 mm cineangiography or 105 mm serial angiography. The morbidity and mortality of this procedure is usually less than 0.1 per cent and vessels down to 0.2 mm in diameter can be seen with it. The stenosis of coronary arteries is usually expressed in percentage of lumen lost: for example, 75 per cent stenosis indicates the diameter of the lumen is only 25 per cent of the diameter of the immediate upstream or downstream normal vessel. An unobstructed vessel would have 0 per cent stenosis, and a completely blocked vessel would demonstrate 100 per cent stenosis. Patients with 75 per cent or greater stenosis of one or more coronary arteries often develop angina pectoris;

patients demonstrating 90 per cent or greater stenosis of a coronary artery may have abnormal left ventricular function. If the coronary stenotic lesions involve the left main coronary, all branches of the left main coronary or three coronary vessels, myocardial revascularization surgery is indicated prior to an elective non-cardiac procedure. Conversely, the patient with single-vessel distal coronary disease or stenosis of 75 per cent or less in one or two arteries may undergo elective surgery with relatively little risk.

Conclusion

Cardiac evaluation of the surgical patient should proceed systematically from history and physical examination through those tests likely to indicate the relative risk for surgery. Patients with suspected myocardial ischaemia should undergo exercise stress testing. Patients with suspected left ventricular function abnormality should undergo echocardiography and, possibly, left ventricular function study. Patients with significantly positive stress tests should undergo coronary arteriography, and patients with congenital or valvular disease should have echocardiography. If echocardiography shows significant abnormality, right and left heart catheterization is the next procedure. Invasive cardiac studies will indicate whether patients should first undergo corrective cardiac surgery prior to elective non-cardiac surgery, or whether they may proceed to the elective non-cardiac surgery. Patients requiring emergency non-cardiac surgery will obviously undergo an abbreviated evaluation to assess the risks and dangers and as a guide to therapy for any cardiac problem.

The underlying principle of any cardiac evaluation should be the progressive, logical uncovering and assessment of cardiac risk, accomplished with the minimum amount of testing required for complete diagnosis.

Table 4 Left ventricular volume and function

Measurements	Units	Normal range
Heart rate	beats/min	60–100
LV ejection time	s	0.250–0.352
Septal wall thickness	cm	0.7–1.1
Septal wall excursion	cm	0.5–1.0
End-diastolic diameter	cm	3.8–5.6
End-systolic diameter	cm	2.2–4.0
Change in diameter	%	24–46
Velocity of circumferential fibre shortening	circ/s	0.88–1.55
Posterior wall thickness	cm	0.7–1.1
Posterior wall excursion	cm	0.5–1.2
End-diastolic volume	ml	62–155
End-systolic volume	ml	16–70
Stroke volume	ml	30–70
Ejection fraction	%	53–78
Mean ejection rate	vol/s	1.7–3.1

References

1. Bruce, R. A., Kusumi, F., Hosmer, D. Maximal oxygen intake and nomographic assessment of functional aerobic impairment in cardiovascular disease. American Heart Journal 1973; 85: 546–562

2. Balke, B., Ware, R. W. An experimental study of physical fitness of Air Force personnel. US Armed Forces Medical Journal 1959; 10: 675

3. Dehn, M. M., Bruce, R. A. Longitudinal variations in maximal oxygen intake with age and activity. Journal of Applied Physiology 1972; 33: 805–807

Illustrations by Carol J. Pienta

Perioperative urological care

Edward Janosko MD
Section of Urology, Department of Surgery, School of Medicine,
East Carolina University, Greenville, North Carolina

Preoperative evaluation

The best way to eliminate perioperative urological complications is by adequate preoperative assessment of the urinary tract. In a healthy patient undergoing routine surgery, the urinalysis may be all that is necessary; in patients undergoing such procedures as abdominoperineal resection, abdominal aneurysmectomy or radical hysterectomy, a more complete evaluation may be needed. This evaluation should include the history, physical examination, laboratory tests, X-ray studies and, in some instances, cystoscopy.

Urological history

The urological history should take note of the following points: urinary frequency, nocturia, stranguria or decreased stream, flank pain (acute and chronic), urgency, haematuria, pneumaturia, potency, incontinence (urgency, overflow, stress, neurogenic). The physician should also inquire about previous history of stone disease, family history of renal disease, urinary tract infections or prior renal disease.

Physical examination

In the male, the physical examination of the urinary tract should include examination of the penis for phimosis, meatal stenosis, warts and carcinomatous lesions. The testes should be examined for masses, hydrocele, hernia and varicocele. The prostate should be examined to estimate the size and consistency and to note any nodular areas suspicious for carcinoma. Finally, the bulbocavernosus reflex should be tested to rule out neurogenic bladder disease.

In the female, the external genitalia should be examined for warty lesions and signs of atrophy. The meatus is inspected, and a pelvic examination is done, the urethral floor being specifically examined for diverticula or carcinomatous lesions. The cervix is inspected to rule out cervical carcinoma. Again, the bulbocavernosus reflex is tested, to rule out neurogenic bladder disease.

Laboratory examination

Basic to the laboratory studies is the urinalysis, including pH, specific gravity, protein, glucose and blood; the sediment should be examined for casts, blood cells and crystals. Pyuria calls for a culture and its cause should be determined before any operative procedure. The blood urea nitrogen and creatinine levels provide an estimate of renal function.

Other studies

When symptoms of urinary tract obstruction are present, a post-voiding residual should be obtained to rule out stricture or urinary retention from prostatism. Further urological instrumentation may be necessary. When the anticipated major surgery may involve the urinary tract, an intravenous urogram (IVU) should be performed to differentiate possible ureteral obstruction from other conditions, for example, to rule out ureteral entrapment from lymphoma, or to detect a horseshoe kidney and renal ectopia before graft surgery or radical pelvic surgery. Finally, cystoscopic examination may be necessary: in cases of carcinoma of the colon and cervix, to rule out extension; in diverticulitis, to rule out fistula; or to evaluate possible prostatic obstruction.

Traumatic haematuria

1

Patients with haematuria who have sustained blunt abdominal trauma need a systematic evaluation. When the patient presents with a history of blunt abdominal trauma, the physician should look for signs of renal trauma (flank discoloration or haematoma), pelvic fracture (haematoma) and displacement of the pelvic fragments, and disruption of the prostate (established by rectal examination). The urinary meatus should be examined for blood. If the patient is unable to void, or if there is blood at the urinary meatus, retrograde urethrography (RUG) should be performed *before* catheterization, because a partial urethral tear can be made complete by faulty catheterization. If the

retrograde urethrogram is abnormal, showing extravasation, the patient should next have an IVU, to rule out upper tract problems. If none is found, the patient should then be taken to the operating room for suprapubic cystostomy drainage. If the retrograde urethrogram is normal, a catheter should be gently passed and cystography carried out. If the cystogram is normal in turn, the IVU should then be done, to rule out upper tract trauma and, if this examination is negative, conservative management should be employed. If the IVU affords poor visualization, however, arteriography and exploration may be warranted. This course of evaluation will serve to identify all significant urological trauma without harm to the patient.

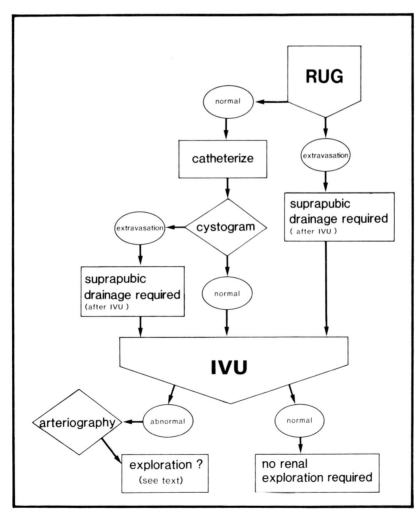

Postoperative care

Catheterization for urinary retention

2

Urinary retention is the most common urological problem for postoperative surgical patients. Acute urinary retention is an obvious emergency and the physician must relieve the urinary retention by drainage of the bladder in the least traumatic and painful manner. This effort should be approached systematically.

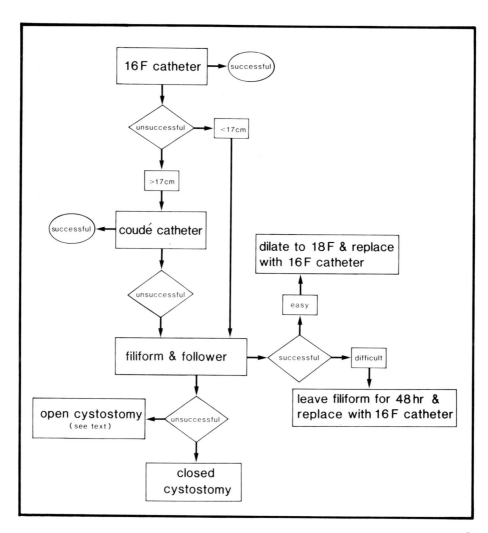

2

3

The illustrated instruments should be available.

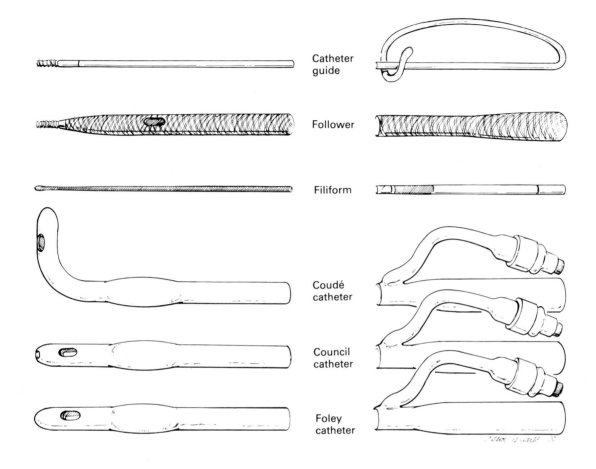

Catheter guide

Follower

Filiform

Coudé catheter

Council catheter

Foley catheter

3

In the female, catheterization is rarely difficult; obstacles might be a retracted or hypospadiac meatus, or significant meatal stenosis. When the patient is placed in the lithotomy position, catheterization with a 16 French catheter, with or without a catheter guide, should be easily accomplished.

In the male, the most common obstacles to easy catheterization are urethral stricture disease, prostatic disease (either benign or carcinomatous) or bladder neck contracture secondary to prostatectomy. If a 16 French catheter cannot be easily introduced into the bladder, all efforts to insert it should be stopped immediately, before significant urethral trauma occurs, and the physician must continue the diagnostic investigation.

The patient must be asked whether his urinary stream has been decreased and whether he has hesitancy or voiding problems which suggest prostatism or urethral stricture. He should be asked about past history of urethral trauma, instrumentation, gonorrhoeal disease or prostatectomy. The patient should then be examined to determine the degree of retention and the size of the bladder. Rectal examination should be performed to evaluate the size and consistency of the prostate gland. Next, the perineum is prepared with an antiseptic solution. A water soluble jelly (Lubafax) or, if available, an anaesthetic jelly (1 per cent lignocaine; Anesticon) is introduced into the urethra gently with a syringe. A 16 Foley catheter is then gently introduced. If the catheter cannot be passed beyond the first 17 cm, the problem is most likely to be a urethral stricture. If the obstruction lies beyond 17 cm, it is most probably secondary to prostatism, carcinoma of the prostate or bladder neck contracture.

4

If prostatism is suspected, one should try to pass a 16 French Coudé catheter, which will usually slip over the median lobe.

If this fails, urethrography should be performed, but if it is not available, one must then proceed with the use of filiforms and followers.

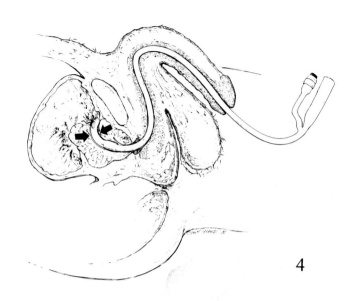

4

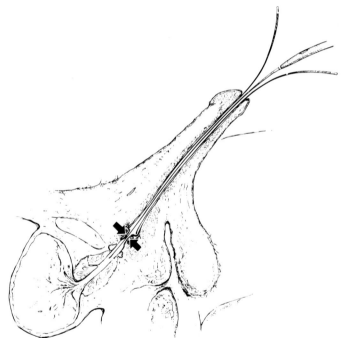

5

5

The filiform, from 3 to 6 French, should be introduced slowly until resistance is met; it is then passed back and forth until it falls through the stricture and enters the bladder. If the filiform will not pass the stricture, it should be advanced as far as it will go and left in place; other filiforms should then be passed sequentially until one finally falls through the stricture into the bladder.

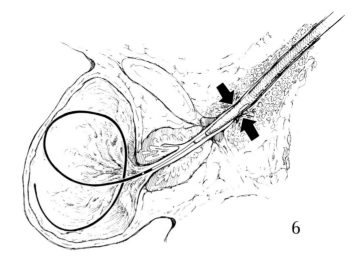

6

6 & 7

Once this filiform is in the bladder, the remaining filiforms are removed and the stricture is dilated gently, starting with an 8 French follower.

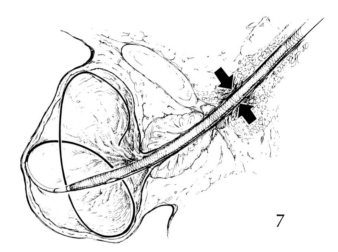

7

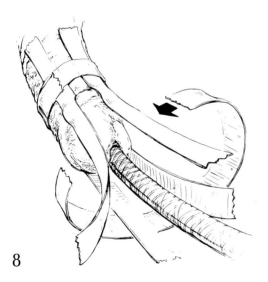

8

8

If the passage of either the filiform or the follower has been especially difficult, the follower should be taped in place to drain for 48h. During this interval, the stricture will soften and the urethra will mould around the follower. Later, after 48h, one should have no difficulty in introducing a catheter into the bladder.

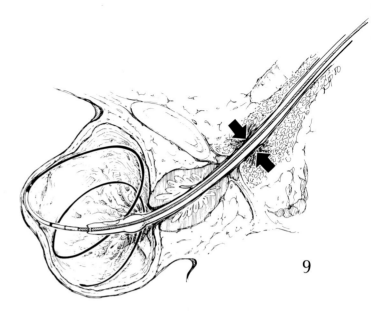

9

9 & 10

Often the stricture is easily dilated from 8 to 18 French by filiform-and-follower technique, with progressively larger followers screwed onto the initial filiform. An ordinary catheter or a Council catheter may then be placed in the bladder. The Council catheter, placed over a catheter guide screwed onto the filiform and adequately lubricated, is gently passed into the bladder. The balloon is then inflated. The filiform and the catheter guide are then removed, leaving the Council catheter in the bladder.

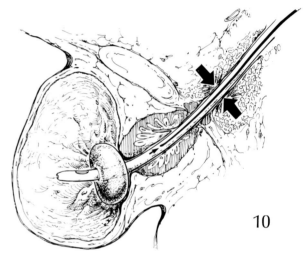

10

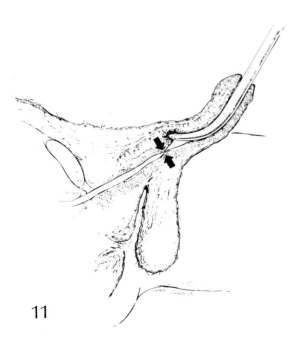

11

11

When neither a catheter nor filiform can be passed and bladder neck contracture seems likely, a 20 French urethral sound should be gently inserted, but never pushed forcibly. This manoeuvre is generally not successful, but with bladder neck contracture the sound will sometimes pass over the lip of the contracture, after which a catheter can be moulded on a catheter guide and passed.

It is imperative that sounds and catheter guides be inserted with great care because they can cause extensive damage. The most common sites of urethral perforation by these instruments are just proximal to a urethral stricture or just below the prostate. For difficult situations, or if the physician is not familiar with sounding, suprapubic cystostomy is strongly recommended.

12

In the rare case of an impassable urethra, suprapubic cystostomy will be called for. For placement of a catheter in this manner, the bladder is palpated just above the pubic ramus. The lower abdomen is prepared with an antiseptic solution, and lignocaine is infiltrated at approximately one-third the distance between the pubic ramus and the umbilicus.

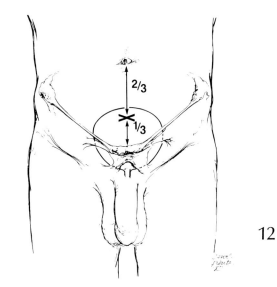

12

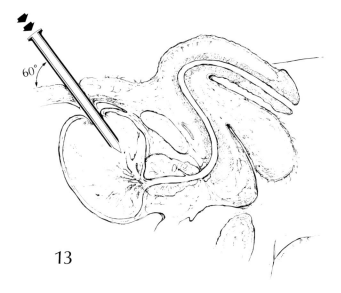

13

13, 14 & 15

A Cystocath catheter is introduced through a trocar at a 60° angle toward the pubic tubercle and passed gently through the skin and rectus sheath into the bladder. This catheter is secured in place and left indwelling, and a voiding cystourethrogram or retrograde urethrogram can later be performed unhurriedly to define the disease. Contraindications to the closed suprapubic technique would be previous pelvic surgery, bladder carcinoma, or an impalpable or small bladder. In these cases, an open cystostomy is generally required.

One may occasionally have to deal with severe phimosis or oedema of the foreskin, from anasarca or localized infection. In such cases, a dorsal slit must be created to expose the glans and the meatus.

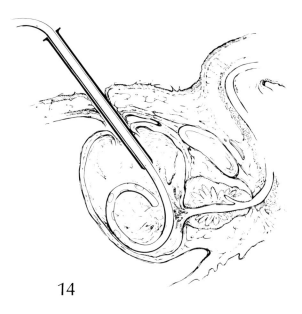

14

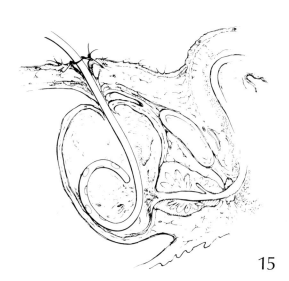

15

Oliguria

If the catheter is successfully passed into the bladder and little or no urine is obtained, the problem is seen to be oliguria, rather than urinary retention, and the aetiology must be determined. The most common cause of oliguria in the perioperative period is dehydration which, if uncompensated, may lead to renal dysfunction. Acute renal failure may occur in conjunction with nephrotoxic drugs, hypotension, incompatible blood transfusion, X-ray contrast material, renal artery occlusions or bilateral ureteral obstruction. Evaluation in such cases must include careful review of the history and physical examination. The urine sediment should be examined for casts, blood and protein. Urine sodium content (U_{Na}), creatinine urine-to-plasma ratio ($U_{Cr}:P_{Cr}$), and urine molality (U_m) should then be measured. A test dose of frusemide (furosemide; Lasix) should be administered. The table illustrates differences between prerenal and renal azotaemia. If the problem is prerenal azotaemia, the patient should be hydrated. If the problem is acute renal failure, the patient will have to be restricted in fluids, potassium and protein; dialysis may be required. Postrenal obstruction from bilateral

ureteral obstruction or renal artery thrombosis is rare. Diagnosis can be made by ultrasonography of the kidneys or retrograde pyelography and renal scanning techniques.

In summary, if one systematically evaluates the urinary tract preoperatively and postoperatively, the common problems can usually be managed successfully, with minimal complications.

Table 1

	Prerenal	*Renal*
Urinalysis	Normal sediment	Casts present
$U_{Cr}:P_{Cr}$	>10 usually >20	5–10
U_{Na}	<20 mmol/l	>40 mmol/l
U_m	>280 mmol/kg	Never hyperosmotic
Frusemide	Diuresis	No response

Illustrations by Gillian Lee

Techniques in intravenous therapy

Brian W. Ellis MB, FRCS
Senior Registrar in Surgery, St Mary's Hospital, London

L. P. Fielding MB, FRCS
Chief of Surgery, St Mary's Hospital, Waterbury, Connecticut;
Associate Professor of Surgery, Yale University, Connecticut

The principles and techniques used for peripheral short cannula intravenous infusion are important in their own right and are the foundation for the management of central venous catheters.

INSERTION OF PERIPHERAL SHORT CANNULA

1

1. Explanation to and preparation of the patient in a comfortable position with adequate light. Preparation and checking of the equipment.
2. *Selection of vein.* Mid-forearm vein away from the elbow or wrist joints.
3. Use of intradermal bleb of local anaesthetic – self experience on one occasion only is enough to convince most people of the necessity for this.
4. *Fixation.* Firm anchorage with tape at the hub of the cannula and separate fixation of the drip tubing. Thereafter a flexible bandage should be all that is required to maintain the position of the cannula and the comfort of the patient.
5. At least daily inspection of the arm and in particular the puncture site. If any tenderness or redness is present the cannula should be removed immediately and re-sited.

The complications of peripheral infusions – local venous thrombosis and thrombophlebitis – have, as their counterpart with central venous catheters, major axial vein thrombosis and systemic sepsis; these iatrogenic complications can be avoided by careful management.

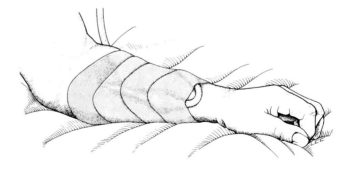

1

Central venous catheterization

Indications

1. Central venous pressure measurement.
2. Intermediate to long-term fluid infusions including parenteral nutrition.

When the need for a central venous catheter can be predicted, for example before major surgery, it should be inserted in sufficient time to allow a chest radiograph to be taken to check the catheter tip position in the mid-superior vena cava.

CHOICE OF APPROACH

This depends on the estimated duration of use and the experience of the operator.

Long catheter placed from cubital fossa

Suitable for relatively short-term use (up to but not exceeding 1 week) by those unfamiliar with subclavian or internal jugular vein puncture. It is accredited with the lowest immediate complication rate, but thrombophlebitis is common.

Internal jugular vein puncture

Favoured by anaesthetists for short-term use, carries a low risk of catheter misplacement, but it is sometimes uncomfortable for the patient because of the strapping required to maintain the position of the tubing and cannula in the neck.

Subclavian vein puncture

This site is the most comfortable for the patient. Catheters may be left *in situ* for 6 weeks or more and are, therefore, suitable for long-term fluids and parenteral nutrition. However, subclavian vein puncture should only be carried out by experienced operators so that the immediate complications of the technique (pneumothorax and hydrothorax) may be avoided.

By separating the puncture sites in skin and vein, the risk of sepsis is reduced. Patients have been fed intravenously for more than 3 years by such tunnelled catheters.

Other methods

The external jugular vein can sometimes be punctured under direct vision, but it is often difficult to 'turn the corner' into the subclavian vein. The femoral or long saphenous veins should not be used because of the high risk of sepsis and venous thrombosis.

CHOICE OF CATHETER MATERIAL

PVC catheters are commonly used; after long periods they become rather rigid, discoloured and encrusted, and are therefore not suitable for long-term use. Although PTFE (Teflon) and nylon catheters are less irritant to the vein wall, they are unacceptably rigid and carry a real risk of vein perforation, which is an especially serious complication if the tip of the catheter lies within the pericardial reflexion of the superior vena cava. Furthermore, Teflon has poor 'kinking' characteristics. A range of silicone elastomer (Silastic) catheters is now available for medium to long-term central venous catheterization. This material combines exceptionally low tissue reactivity with a softness and pliability impossible to achieve with other material.

COMPLICATIONS OF CENTRAL VENOUS CANNULATION

Pneumothorax

The degree of pneumothorax is often quite small and its onset may be delayed. Patients with chronic respiratory disease are most at risk because the subclavian vein may run in a deep pleural groove in the apex of the lung. Patients who are likely to undergo general anaesthesia or mechanical ventilation are also at risk because positive pressure ventilation may convert a small 'mantle' pneumothorax into a large tension pneumothorax. A chest X-ray is always required after catheter insertion.

Hydrothorax

This complication will occasionally occur because of infusion of fluids outside the venous system. No matter how easily the catheter enters the central veins, the presence of blood in the catheter should always be confirmed by withdrawing blood before connecting the infusion.

Sepsis

The incidence of septic complications is reduced by attention to the following details: suturing the apparatus to the skin; keeping both the catheters and tubing clean and tidy; nominating one or two members of the medical and nursing staff to special responsibility for catheter insertion and management; taking twice-weekly cultures of the puncture site to ascertain the presence and sensitivities of any pathogenic organisms.

HOW TO PREVENT COMPLICATIONS OF CENTRAL VENOUS CANNULATION

1. Accept that this is not a trivial procedure.
2. Aseptic and non-touch techniques should be used for the insertion of this apparatus (tunnelling procedures should be carried out in the operating theatre).
3. Blood sampling from, and the addition of drugs to, the central venous catheter must be avoided – a separate peripheral infusion is advocated for these purposes.

The techniques

2

LONG CATHETER FROM FOREARM VEIN

1. Ensure good illumination and prepare all necessary equipment before starting the procedure. Shave the arm if necessary.
2. Apply a tourniquet or sphygmomanometer cuff to the upper arm.
3. Prepare the skin with antiseptic solution (tincture of iodine is best, but confirm that there is no history of allergy).
4. Tighten tourniquet or inflate sphygmomanometer cuff. Ask the patient to open and close the fist. Gentle tapping will often make the veins stand out; a vigorous assault will lead to venous spasm and alarm the patient.
5. Choose a vein just below the cubital fossa on the medial side so that the catheter will ascend in the basilic vein rather than the cephalic vein. Infiltrate the subcutaneous bleb of local anaesthetic about 3 cm below the proposed site of vein puncture.
6. Insert needle through skin and run up subcutaneously to the chosen vein and enter it as a separate manoeuvre. Advance needle a short way into the vein and then advance the catheter through the needle.
7. When the catheter is a few centimetres into the vein, ask the assistant to deflate the cuff and then to continue to advance the catheter. Occasionally it is necessary to abduct the arm further to get the catheter to advance fully. If the catheter fails to advance, *do not* withdraw the catheter whilst the needle is still in the arm; catheter severance and subsequent embolism is a serious complication which is easily avoided.
8. Finally, withdraw and secure the needle.
9. Back-bleeding around the catheter is common because the hole in the vein wall is larger than the catheter. A few minutes' firm pressure is necessary for control.
10. Clean the arm of blood and secure the catheter and drip tubing with tape.
11. Dress the puncture site with dry povidone-iodine aerosol (an effective way of preventing catheter site sepsis).
12. Cover the arm with flexible bandage from the mid-upper arm to the mid-forearm. A splint is unnecessary.
13. Once the catheter is established arrange a chest radiograph to check the position of the catheter tip.

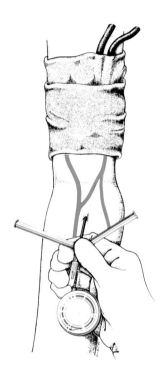

2

Notes

By keeping the skin puncture site well below the skin crease in the cubital fossa the catheter is unlikely to move to and fro with elbow movement and the possibility of catheter contamination is reduced. The risk of basilic vein thrombosis increases with time and therefore the site of the catheter should be changed after not more than 1 week.

The risk of catheter severance using a catheter-through-needle combination is significant. Current opinion favours a catheter-through-cannula device which avoids this serious complication.

INTERNAL JUGULAR VEIN PUNCTURE

(after English *et al.*[1])

Technique 1

3

This is the preferred method in anaesthetized patients who have been given muscle relaxant drugs. A head-down tilt of 30° should be used and for a right internal jugular vein puncture the head is turned to the left. The internal jugular vein can usually be palpated slightly lateral to the line joining the medial edge of the clavicular head of the sternomastoid muscle to the mastoid process and must be distinguished from the carotid artery.

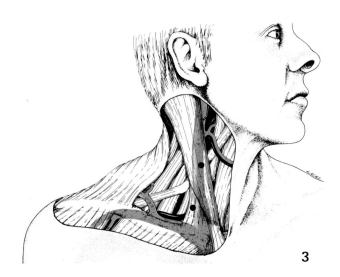

3

4

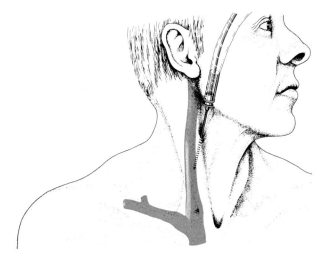

Venepuncture is made at a point where the vein is most easily felt behind the muscle. The needle is inserted through the skin, slightly cephalad and medial to the position where the vein is most easily felt at an angle of 30°–40° to the skin surface and is advanced caudally and laterally. The deep cervical fascia is usually pierced with a definite 'give' followed by the same sensation of 'give' as the vein is entered. It is quite often necessary to insert the needle through the substance of the sternomastoid muscle if the internal jugular vein is felt some way lateral to its medial edge. Whether the muscle is transfixed or not appears to make no difference. Blood reflux into the catheter confirms venepuncture; the catheter is then threaded down the needle into the vein. The needle is withdrawn and placed in its plastic holder. The intravenous infusion is then connected and a folded swab is applied firmly to the puncture site to prevent haematoma formation.

4

5

Technique 2

This was originally developed as an alternative approach to the internal jugular vein in cases where the elective technique failed or the internal jugular vein was not palpated. However, because it does not depend on muscle relaxation it can be used with local analgesia in the conscious patient or in emergency situations (cardiac arrest or severe hypotension). The patient should be positioned as for the first technique. The triangular gap between the sternal and clavicular heads of the sternomastoid, with its base on the medial end of the clavicle, is identified. The terminal part of the internal jugular vein lies behind the medial edge of the clavicular head of the muscle. The catheter needle combination is inserted near the apex of this triangle at an angle of about 30°–40° at the skin surface and advanced caudally and medially towards the inner border of the anterior end of the first rib. The deep cervical fascia is not usually so evident here, though entry into the vein is again often felt. Blood reflux confirms venepuncture and the catheter and the intravenous infusion are secured as previously described.

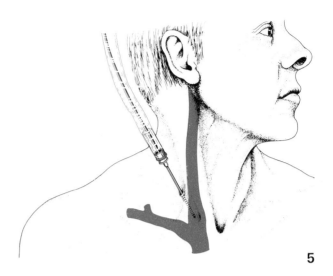

5

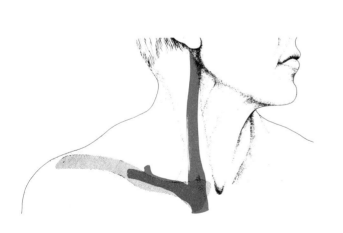

6

SUBCLAVIAN VEIN PUNCTURE – INFRACLAVICULAR ROUTE

6

1. It is worth explaining to the patient that the insertion of such a catheter takes longer than for an ordinary peripheral infusion, but once in place will be much more comfortable. Good illumination and preparation of all equipment is essential before approaching the patient.

2. *Position of patient.* This is perhaps the most vital part of the procedure. It is useful to place a rolled-up hand towel longitudinally behind the patient's spine to allow the shoulders to fall back. The position required of the patient is the 'standing to attention' with the head rotated away from the side of the procedure. Next, the foot of the bed should be considerably elevated, preferably by hydraulic attachment, to at least 25° to the horizontal.

3. The landmark for the skin puncture site is 2 cm below the midpoint of the clavicle. Local anaesthetic is infiltrated subcutaneously and along the proposed track of the introducing cannula (*see below*). The periosteum of the clavicle should also be infiltrated. A small (2 mm) nick is then made in the skin.

7

4. The introducing cannula is then inserted and passed cephalad and medially aiming just above a finger in the suprasternal notch so as to pass under the clavicle at the junction of the middle and medial thirds. At this point the clavicle is quite thick and it is best to strike that bone deliberately, and then, bit by bit, edge the cannula underneath the clavicle, taking care not to tip the cannula too deep. Once under the clavicle, a 'give' is often felt as the cannula passes through the clavipectoral fascia. The vein is usually just behind this structure and therefore the cannula should be advanced slowly with frequent aspirations. If the vein is not entered, withdraw slowly with suction because occasionally both vein walls are punctured at the same time and the lumen is often found during withdrawal.

If the vein is still not found, partially withdraw and try at a slightly different angle. Do not try more than three or four times because the risk of pneumothorax increases considerably.

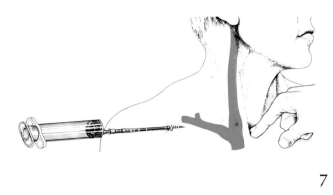

7

8

Once the vein is entered, venous blood is easily aspirated. The cannula and needle should be gently advanced following the curve of the vein so that the entire circumference of the mouth of the cannula is well within the vein lumen. The patient is then requested to stop breathing for a few seconds as the needle is withdrawn and the catheter introduced. The cannula is then withdrawn around the catheter. The syringe attached to the catheter is aspirated to confirm that the tip of the catheter is then still within a vein.

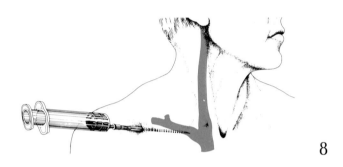

8

9

The drip tubing is next attached via an on/off tap and the catheter flushed. It is then secured by two sutures, one placed about 2 cm from the skin puncture site and the other around the proximal end of the catheter; some devices have eyelets for this purpose. The foot of the bed can be lowered, the chest wall cleaned and dressed. Before applying the dressings it is helpful to spray the chest wall with Tincture Benzoin Co. which, when dry, provides a good surface on which to apply the dressings. Finally, before the puncture site is covered it should be sprayed with dry povidone-iodine aerosol. It is prudent to insert a locking stopcock between the catheter and drip tubing (e.g. Vygon 872). Three-way taps are potentially dangerous due to contamination from the third port.

Before any hypertonic solutions are used, it is essential to confirm with a chest X-ray the correct positioning of the catheter tip. Between 10 and 15 per cent of catheters are likely to go into the internal jugular vein rather than down into the superior vena cava. Hypertonic solutions infused high into the jugular vein have been known to cause thrombosis at this point.

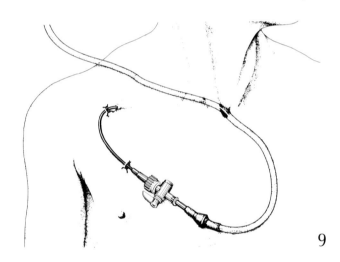

9

Note

As soon as the radiograph is available, it is important to examine: (1) the position of the catheter tip; (2) the presence or absence of pneumothorax; (3) the presence or absence of haemothorax. In experienced hands, the incidence of pneumothorax using this technique is extremely low. However, the danger is always present, particularly if the cannula is angled too deep during insertion. It is worth remembering that the subclavian vein runs over the dome of the pleura and in emphysematous patients, it may run in a groove in the pleura making pneumothorax likely even with apparently uneventful catheter insertion.

Tunnelled catheters

A number of sites exist for the insertion of tunnelled catheters; three will be described. The procedure should be performed in the operating theatre to obtain the best aseptic conditions; an image intensifier is very useful to screen the catheter into the correct position. The patient should be lightly sedated and local anaesthetic used. The catheters of choice for this technique are those made of Silastic and preferably supplied with an introducing cannula.

Only in the 'open' methods described below is the risk of pneumothorax avoided. Thus these are methods of choice for patients being ventilated and those about to undergo general anaesthesia.

TUNNELLED SUBCLAVIAN CATHETER – CLOSED METHOD
(after Titone, Lefton and Sakwa[2])

The techniques of percutaneous infraclavicular subclavian vein puncture and tunnelling are combined in this approach. However, vein puncture is 'blind' and hence the risk of pneumothorax and allied complications is the same as that for standard subclavian puncture. The procedure is best performed in the operating theatre. A special requirement is the use of a catheter with a detachable hub (e.g. Vygon Silastic central venous catheter 2180.20).

After adequate local anaesthesia infiltration and with the patient positioned as for an infraclavicular subclavian puncture, a 5 mm incision is made parallel to and 2 cm below the clavicle at its midpoint.

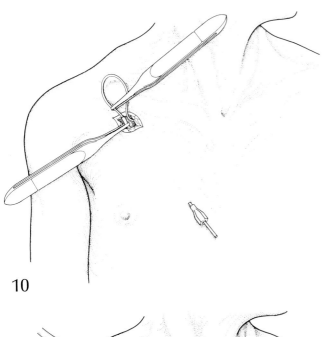

10

10

Subclavian catheterization is then performed (see *Illustrations 7 and 8*). The introducing cannula is then withdrawn and completely removed from the catheter. To prevent air embolism the open end of the catheter is plugged with sterile petroleum jelly or antibiotic ointment. Next, the introducing needle/cannula combination is reassembled and a skin tunnel made so that the tip of the introducing cannula appears in the skin incision. The needle is then withdrawn and the catheter threaded retrograde through the cannula and the latter once again withdrawn completely. The sealed end of the catheter is then cut off and the hub fixed.

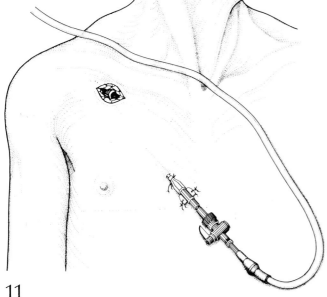

11

11

Finally the wound is closed with a single suture and the catheter hub also secured by suture. Dressings are then applied and a plain radiograph taken. This technique may also be used if a suitable cephalic vein cannot be found (see next technique). Remember that the wound in that case would be placed somewhat more laterally.

TUNNELLED CEPHALIC VEIN

12

After the patient has had the procedure explained he should be positioned supine on the operating table and, if necessary, lightly sedated. The image intensifier, if available, is centred over the medial third of the clavicle. The right upper quadrant of the thorax is prepared with iodine and sterile drapes. Local anaesthetic is then infiltrated along the length of the catheter track.

A 4 cm horizontal incision is made across the delto-pectoral groove 2.5 cm below the clavicle. The dissection is carried down into the groove to the proximal part of the cephalic vein; the vein sometimes lies at a considerable depth between the muscles.

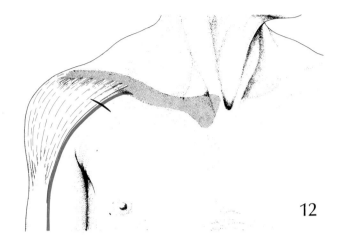

12

13

Once the vein has been adequately exposed, the introducing catheter is passed retrograde from inside the incision, down, and across the chest wall to form the subcutaneous tunnel. When it lies at its full extent, it is pushed outwards through the skin and the needle removed. The catheter is passed carefully backwards through the cannula, which is then removed and discarded.

Two ligatures are now passed under the vein and the distal one tied. A small incision is made between the ligatures with dissecting scissors and the catheter passed up through into the vein.

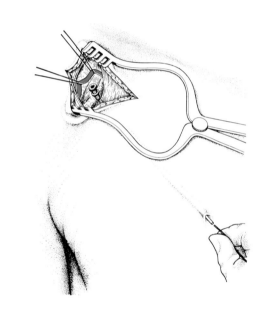

13

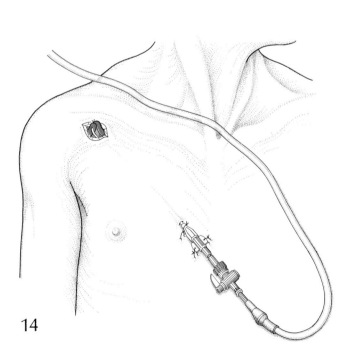

14

14

Under image intensification the catheter is gently advanced through the subclavian and innominate veins and into the superior vena cava. The upper ligature is then tied. The catheter hub assembly is secured by suture. The wound is closed and dressings applied.

TUNNELLED SUBCLAVIAN VEIN CATHETER – OPEN METHOD

(after Oosterlee and Dudley[3])

When the risk must be avoided, e.g. in preoperative patients or those receiving mechanical ventilation, this method provides an alternative to the cephalic vein cut-down technique. Indeed, when the latter method fails, the wound may be extended medially and this method used. As in the previous technique, a similar catheter with a removable hub is required.

15

After adequate local anaesthesia and with the patient 15° head-down, an incision 5 cm long is made 2 cm below the midclavicular point down to the pectoralis major muscle. The muscle is split along the line of its fibres and the areolar space medial to the pectoralis minor is opened by incising the clavipectoral fascia. The subclavian vein can now be readily identified and is dissected free just sufficiently to make its course evident.

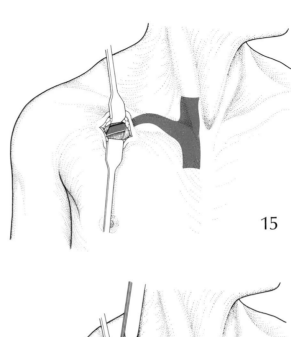

15

16

The subclavian vein is gently steadied and the introducing needle and cannula inserted. When they are well inside the vessel the needle is withdrawn and the catheter passed through for an appropriate distance. The cannula is then withdrawn completely.

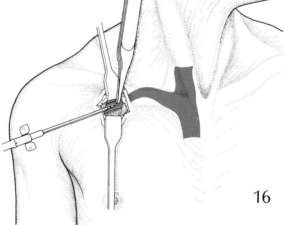

16

17

The catheter is now brought out to a point lower down the chest wall via a subcutaneous tunnel made by passing the reassembled needle and cannula from below upwards and into the incision. The needle is removed and the catheter threaded retrograde through the cannula, which is once again removed completely and the hub attached. It is wise to plug the end of the catheter with sterile petroleum jelly or antibiotic cream to prevent air embolism and then cut this section away before attaching the hub. The wound is closed in layers and the catheter secured by suture. Finally, a radiograph is taken to check the position of the catheter tip.

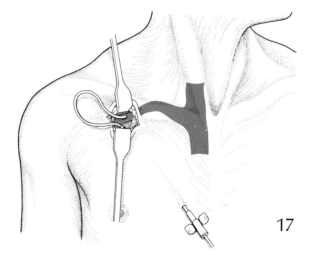

17

Further considerations for patients maintained on parenteral nutrition

The clinician who sets out to nourish patients parenterally must appreciate fully the potential hazards that may arise, not only from non-metabolic problems[4] but also from biochemical, fluid and metabolic disturbances. Strict attention to detail and careful monitoring by medical and nursing staff are mandatory.

Ideally a single clinician should be responsible for the maintenance of balance charts and prescribing. A flexible approach can be adopted by choosing a small range of proprietary solutions and formulating a range of regimens based on different combinations of these solutions[5].

It is to be anticipated that a reduction of septic and metabolic problems will come from the introduction of large-volume delivery systems. All solutions and additives, except for fat emulsion, may be mixed into 3 litre containers. This results in a reduction of bag or bottle changes on the ward and elimination of the need for additions to be made in a contaminated environment. Furthermore, there is a smooth and concurrent delivery of nitrogen and carbohydrate energy, resulting in a decreased requirement for insulin[6].

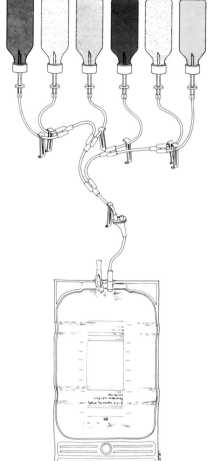

18

18

The 3 litre bag (Travenol Laboratories Ltd) is made of laminated PVC and has a standard outlet port. The inlet port has six leads each with a conventional spike for insertion into commercially available containers of nutrient solutions. An additive port is also available on the inlet side.

The bags are filled in an aseptic pharmacy suite (British Standard Class I Conditions BS5295) under laminar flow conditions. The leads are inserted into the nutrient containers and millipore filters mounted on 21 gauge needles are used as air vents for bottles.

19

The bag is then placed in a vacuum box and allowed to fill. Additions to the 24 h 'mix', such as vitamin solutions, are added through the addition port. When full, the bag is removed, the inlet port sealed and the six leads amputated.

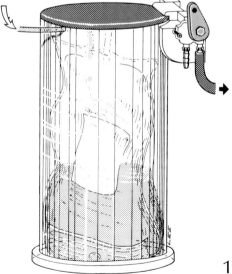

19

20

The bag is labelled with its contents, date of manufacture and expiry date. Bags may be stored for several days at 4 °C and we have chosen an arbitrary 'shelf-life' of one week.

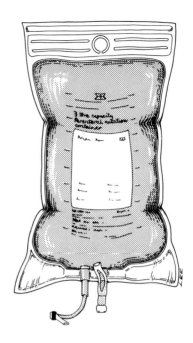

20

References

1. English, I. C. W., Frew, R. M., Pigott, J. F., Zaki, M. Percutaneous catheterisation of the internal jugular vein. Anaesthesia 1969; 24: 521–531

2. Titone, C., Lefton, C., Sakwa, S. A technique for chronic subclavian vein catheterization. Surgery, Gynecology and Obstetrics 1973; 137: 489–490

3. Oosterlee, J., Dudley, H. A. F. Central catheter placement by puncture of exposed subclavian vein. Lancet 1980; 1: 19–20

4. Ellis, B. W., Fielding, L. P. Intravenous technology and non-metabolic complications. In: Hill, G. L., ed. Clinical surgery international, Vol. 2: Nutrition and the surgical patient. London: Churchill Livingstone, 1981

5. Ellis, B. W., Stanbridge, R. de L., Fielding, L. P., Dudley, H. A. F. A rational approach to parenteral nutrition. British Medical Journal 1976; 1: 1388–1391

6. Fielding, L. P., Humfress, A., Mouchizadeh, J., Dudley, H., Gilmour, M. Parenteral nutrition technology: experience with 3 litre bags. The Pharmaceutical Journal 1981; 226: 590–592

Illustrations by Gillian Lee

Gastrointestinal intubation

John Masterton FRCS, FRACS
Associate Professor of Surgery, Monash University, Alfred Hospital, Melbourne

Brian W. Ellis MB, FRCS
Senior Registrar in Surgery, St Mary's Hospital, London

L. P. Fielding MB, FRCS
Chief of Surgery, St Mary's Hospital, Waterbury, Connecticut;
Associate Professor of Surgery, Yale University, Connecticut

Introduction

Upper gastrointestinal decompression or tube feeding is undertaken usually by means of a plastic nasogastric tube passed via the nose or occasionally by mouth. However, there are circumstances where a nasogastric tube may be unsuitable because the patient is uncooperative or unable to accept it or when utilization of the oro-oesophageal route is hazardous or impossible. Then it may be necessary to gain access to the gastrointestinal tract by using a gastrostomy or jejunostomy. Such a procedure can be done safely and simply either as an operation on its own or as an additional procedure at the termination of major intra-abdominal surgery to decompress the stomach and to provide a route by which liquid food supplements or total feeding can be given pending re-establishment of adequate oral feeding. Occasionally it is necessary to establish a jejunostomy beyond a gastric or duodenal fistula in order to reintroduce secretions lost through the fistula and to feed the patient.

There is a special group of patients who are unconscious for prolonged periods for whom nutritional support is often overlooked until they are significantly emaciated. Feeding of these people is mandatory for survival. In many instances tube feeding by nasogastric tube, prefer-ably of 1–2 mm internal diameter, is feasible and sufficient; gastrostomy is an alternative.

There is a small group of patients for whom permanent gastrostomy may be the only practicable way to achieve adequate and continuing nutrition. These are patients who have completely or partly lost the ability to swallow normally because of unrelieved obstruction from oropharyngeal or oesophageal carcinoma, or following major surgery in this region when it may be impossible to restore normal deglutition.

If the patient is still able to lead a meaningful life without, for example, the torture of unremitting pain, a feeding gastrostomy can help, but one should never consider doing this when life expectancy is limited to a few weeks.

Patients can, of course, be fed quite easily by the intravenous route (see chapter on 'Techniques in intravenous therapy', pp. 41–51). However it is important not to overlook the problems of these techniques and the hazard of sepsis and other complications. If the gut is working, one of the following techniques to establish nutrition via the enteric route should be considered.

Non-operative techniques

In its simplest form enteric nutrition, either total or supplemental, may be undertaken with a standard nasogastric tube. The size of the tube depends on the consistency of the feed in use: the larger the tube the greater the patient's discomfort and the likelihood of aspiration. Recently very fine bore tubes (1 mm internal diameter) have become popular. The intubation technique is the same as for a standard nasogastric tube, but because fine bore tubes are very flexible they must be passed with a guide wire. It is imperative to check the correct position of the tube because passage into the bronchial tree is a real danger; by listening over the epigastrium and injecting air down the tube, bubbling will be heard if the tube is in the stomach. If doubt remains a plain radiograph should be taken. Some systems have a reversed male-female Luer system which makes them incompatible with intravenous lines to avoid the danger of intravenous infusion of enteric feeds (Roussel Laboratories).

Another type of tube for enteric feeding is a mercury-weighted (Dobhoff) tube. Some 3 mm in diameter it is relatively comfortable for the patient. They are sometimes easier to pass in an unconscious patient and are said to pass into the duodenum in most patients within 48 h, a further guard against reflux during coma. Polyurethane, from which the tube is made, is also less likely to become rigid in the presence of gastric acid.

At the onset of feeding, particularly in the unconscious patient, it is important to check that the feed is propelled down the gut from its point of delivery. With a standard Ryles tube or the Dobhoff tube simple aspiration usually suffices, but to establish this point for fine bore tubes it is necessary either to inject contrast and take a plain radiograph one hour later, or to have an aspirating tube as well until this point has been verified.

GASTROSCOPIC PLACEMENT OF ENTERIC FEEDING TUBES

On rare occasions it is necessary to place a tube beyond an anatomical problem, e.g. a fistula or stricture. An endoscope allows such placement to be achieved with certainty.

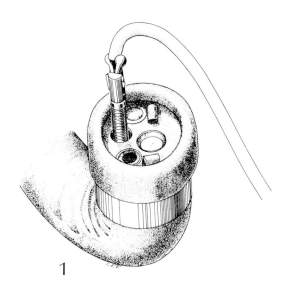

1

1

Technique for fine bore tubes
(after Atkinson, Walford and Allison[1])

The patient is sedated and placed in the left lateral position. The tip of a fine bore tube is passed up a few centimetres retrograde into the biopsy channel of a forward viewing endoscope. The tube is then pulled back to lie alongside the instrument and the guide wire passed so that it lies just proximal to the acute bend at the end of the tube.

The instrument is then steered past the lesion and on into the duodenum. The tube is then freed by pushing the tip clear with the biopsy forceps. Finally, the gastroscope is withdrawn while the tube is held in place with its guide wire.

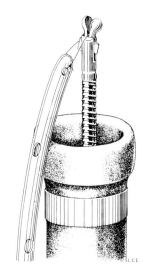

2

2

Technique for small Ryles tubes

If a fine bore tube is not available an alternative method may be used. A fine nylon suture is first passed through the solid tip of a *small* Ryles tube (8 Ch.) and tied as a loose loop. This is then grasped by the biopsy forceps held just protruding from the endoscope. When the endoscope has reached an appropriate position the biopsy forceps is advanced and the tube released. The endoscope is then carefully withdrawn.

Whichever technique is used, the proximal end of the feed tube must then be transferred from the mouth to the nose. It is usually possible, given sufficient sedation, to pass a second nasogastric tube through the nose and retrieve the distal end from the pharynx. The two tubes are tied together and the feeding tube is then pulled back through the mouth, up the nasopharynx and out of the nose.

Operative methods: gastrostomy and jejunostomy

Anaesthesia

When one of these procedures is done as part of a more major operation, it is likely that general anaesthesia will be in use, but when carried out on its own it may be appropriate to use local anaesthesia. If this is so the area of the operative incision is infiltrated down to and includ-

ing parietal peritoneum. The stomach or proximal jejunum can be handled without discomfort to the patient provided there is no stretching or dragging of the mesentery. There are no other special points that need be made about technique of anaesthesia.

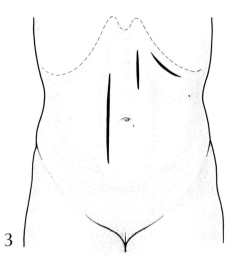

3

3

Choice of incisions

Three types of incision can be used. A right paramedian is one example of an incision used for an unspecified procedure at the conclusion of which a gastrostomy or jejunostomy may be inserted. The short left upper paramedian and left subcostal incisions are both suitable for gastrostomy when this is the only operation. An incision 8–10 cm in length is adequate and both can be done using local anaesthesia. A small paramedian incision sited in the umbilical region is suitable for access to the jejunum. In every instance the gastrostomy and jejunostomy tube must be brought out through a separate stab wound so that it lies comfortably in relation to the viscus it drains.

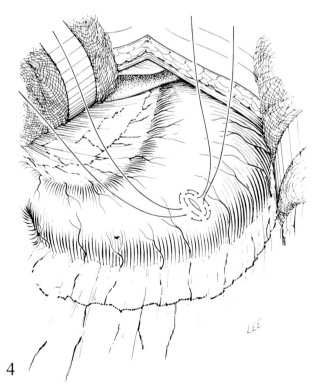

4

GASTROSTOMY

Opening the stomach

4

The anterior surface of the stomach is identified and a point is chosen 10–15 cm from the pylorus. Control is achieved by grasping the stomach wall with Babcock's or similar gentle tissue forceps. Two concentric atraumatic 2/0 or 3/0 chromic catgut purse-string sutures are now inserted leaving a central space of 1.0–1.5 cm in diameter.

5

A short incision is made in the central area through the musculature which reveals the submucosal plexus of vessels – these are then coagulated, the mucosa incised and the lumen opened.

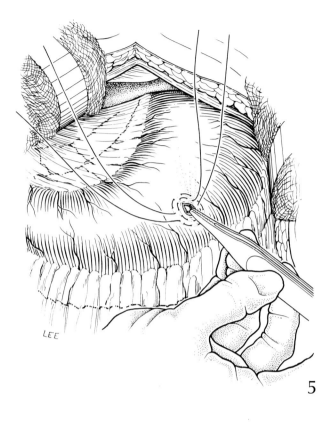

5

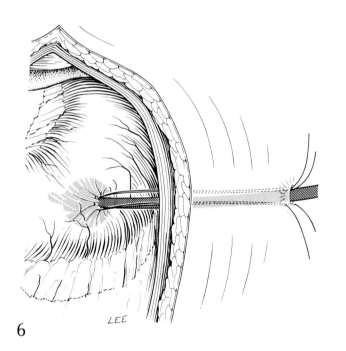

6

Inserting the catheter

6

An 18–22 Ch. Foley balloon catheter, previously checked, is now pulled from the skin surface through a separate stab wound made just big enough to accept the catheter snugly. The catheter is slipped into the stomach several centimetres and the balloon inflated. Five millilitres of water is sufficient for this: too much water in the balloon can cause antral obstruction. The purse-string sutures are pulled tight and tied, the inner one being tied first and then the outer. This achieves an inkwell effect. The ends of the purse-string sutures are left long and threaded back through the stab wound. This is best achieved by passing a straight artery forceps through the stab wound alongside the catheter from the skin inwards.

7

The catheter is now pulled backwards so that the balloon is in contact with the mucosa of the stomach which is then pulled up to the level of the parietal peritoneum by gentle traction on the ends of catgut and the catheter itself. Ideally the stomach should now lie comfortably against the parietal peritoneum without any distortion. The catgut ends are now threaded on to cutting needles each in turn, threaded through the skin, tied to each other and tied around the catheter. This ensures a sound attachment which lasts sufficiently long for the stomach to become adherent to the abdominal wall. In no circumstances should the catheter be changed or removed within 10 days. After this it is safe either to remove it or reinsert a fresh one immediately. Following permanent removal of the catheter there may be a little leakage of gastric contents for several hours but provided there is no obstruction to gastric emptying the gastric fistula will close quite quickly.

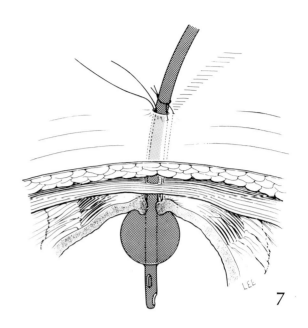

7

8

JEJUNOSTOMY

8

Precisely the same technique is used for this procedure except that it may be necessary to use a smaller volume of water in the Foley balloon to obviate any risk of luminal obstruction of the bowel.

Other intraoperative techniques

NASOGASTRIC ROUTE

The anaesthetist passes through the nose a fine bore tube which can be gently manipulated to an appropriate position well beyond an anastomosis. This is usually easier if the guide wire is left in place until the tube has been finally positioned.

TRANSGASTRIC ROUTE

If the stomach has not been resected a tube may be passed as for or in addition to a gastrostomy. The tube is then manipulated through the pylorus and left with its tip well into the duodenum. It is sometimes possible to position it beyond the duodenojejunal flexure. Such a transgastric feeding tube combined with an aspirating gastrostomy has been well tried for many years by paediatric surgeons.

CATHETER JEJUNOSTOMY
(after Delaney et al.[2])

9

A needle with an internal diameter wide enough for the feeding tube is introduced into the jejunal wall on the antimesenteric border about 10 cm below the ligament of Treitz or an equivalent distance from a jejunal anastomosis. The needle is inserted for its full length into the stretched wall of the jejunum in the seromuscular layer. This relatively avascular plane is easily penetrated by the needle which is then pushed on into the lumen. The catheter, which should be at least 45 cm long, is advanced 10–15 cm into the lumen and the needle withdrawn over it and discarded. A single purse-string or 'Z' stitch secures the catheter. Next a clean needle is passed through the abdominal wall from the outside and the catheter threaded backwards through it and the needle once again withdrawn. Finally the jejunum is sutured to the parietal peritoneum and the catheter or feeding tube sutured on the outside.

Before commencing feeding it is wise to inject 20–30 ml contrast medium to confirm that the catheter tip is still intraluminal and that there is forward propulsion in the jejunum.

When the catheter is finally withdrawn the oblique track through the jejunal wall will close as a flap valve.

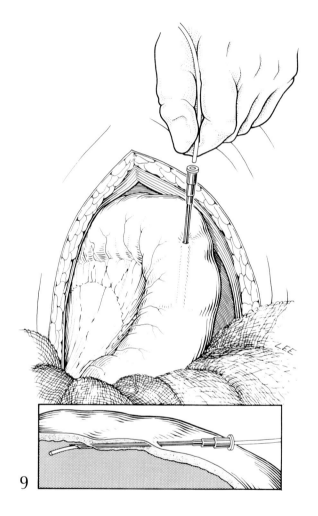

9

Preparation and administration of enteric feeds

Great care must be taken in the preparation and storage of food for enteric use, to prevent contamination by bacteria. Sterile water or cooled boiled water must be used to make up the feeds, which should be stored at 4°C. Alternative commercial preparations are now becoming more widely available.

All feeds should be given by continuous drip rather than bolus injection to minimize the risk of oesophageal reflux and diarrhoea. The best results are achieved by using mechanical peristaltic pumps. If this technique is combined with a cautious phasing in of nutrients (starting with dilute feeds of modest volume) then diarrhoea is less likely.

If diarrhoea persists and the patient is having, or has had, antibiotics the possibility of pseudomembranous enterocolitis should be considered and a sigmoidoscopy plus biopsy and stool culture should be carried out.

Regular biochemical surveillance is as important for a patient being nourished enterally as for those receiving parenteral nutrition.

References

1. Atkinson, M., Walford, S., Allison, S. P. Endoscopic insertion of fine-bore feeding tubes. Lancet 1979; 2: 829

2. Delaney, H. M., Carnevale, N., Garvey, J. W., Moss, C. M. Postoperative nutritional support using needle catheter feeding jejunostomy. Annals of Surgery 1977; 186: 165–170

Illustrations by A. Malpass and Sheila Jones

Pain relief in relation to operations

J. Nayman   ChM, FRCS, FRCS (Ed.), FRACS
Chief of Surgery, Royal Southern Memorial Hospital;
Associate Professor, Department of Surgery, Monash University, Melbourne

P. C. Rutter   MB, FRCS
Registrar, Academic Surgical Unit, St Mary's Hospital, London

Hugh Dudley   ChM, FRCS (Ed.), FRACS, FRCS
Professor of Surgery, St Mary's Hospital, London

Introduction

Surgeons underestimate the pain their incisions cause. This is particularly the case for thoracic and abdominal incisions where respiration necessitates continuous movement and so implies continuous pain. Coughing – a frequent consequence of general anaesthesia and sputum retention – exacerbates the problem. Pain inhibits movement and thus causes difficulty in eliminating sputum; in consequence, unrelieved pain may predispose to respiratory complications after surgery[1] as well as leaving the patient with bad memories of what could have been a relatively atraumatic experience.

Counselling

There is some evidence[2] that the patient who is adequately counselled before operation and to whom the nature and extent of the problems likely to be encountered after operation are explained will be less likely to suffer. It is the duty of the surgical team as a whole and of the surgeon in particular (for he *causes* the pain) to explain not only that there will be pain but also that it can be adequately relieved. In the postoperative period all – the surgeon, anaesthetist and others – must be positive in their attitudes.

There are cultural and individual differences in both the experience and expression of pain. Some patients are stoical; others highly expressive. The surgeon must realize this and not be unduly influenced on the one hand by denial and on the other hand by extravagant behaviour.

The role of anxiolytics in preparing patients for surgery and in providing sound sleep (though the value of this is unknown) has been insufficiently explored scientifically. Most surgeons will have their own 'recipes'; the important principle is to develop a 'feel' for one particular combination and use this to the exclusion of others.

1

Pain pathways

The routes by which a painful stimulus in the periphery reaches expression in consciousness are still incompletely underistood. Those relevant to the control of pain as we understand it today are shown. They may be interrupted in a number of places.

[1–2] Regional block of peripheral nerves

This is effective for short periods. Thus, local analgesia for minor surgery and for (say) hernia repair, permits the patient to walk to his bed or undergo a short journey. Some local anaesthetic agents – e.g. bupivacaine (Marcain) – are said to have a longer action than others, but this is highly variable. Repeated infiltration may be useful – for example, by intercostal local block for severe abdominal pain – but the time and trouble involved makes the method of limited application.

[3] Afferent blockade at dorsal root level

This is achieved by epidural anaesthesia with conventional local anaesthetics – lignocaine, bupivacaine. Pain relief can be virtually complete and, in addition, the blockade of afferent stimuli abolishes some of the metabolic responses to injury[3]. The value of this remains to be determined. The disadvantage of the local anaesthetics is that they may, by paralyzing vasomotor outflow, produce hypotension which, in the presence of compensated hypovolaemia, can be profound. Strict attention to volume replacement and careful avoidance of the head-up position during epidural blockade are essential. The technique is a specialized one. A plastic epidural catheter is inserted at an appropriate space and connected via a filter (Millipore) to a Luer-Lok hub. Analgesia up to T2 can be achieved. 'Top up' doses of the chosen local anaesthetic may be administered as pain occurs. Epidural cannulae can be left in position for up to 3 days.

[4] The alternative to local anaesthesia at dorsal root level is to inject an opiate or opiate-like drug extradurally[4]

Morphine sulphate, bupremorphine (Temgesic) and fentanyl (Sublimaze) have all been used with success. The mechanism of action is not fully known but may be diffusion along nerve roots to occupy receptor sites in the substantia gelatinosa which are modulated by descending pathways (lower arrow in the diagram). The overall physiological impact remains to be explored but the method is effective and said to be devoid of vasomotor problems.

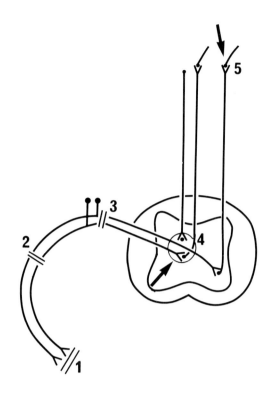

1

As with extradural block, 'top ups' can be used (on average 12-hourly) over a period of 2–3 days.

Intrathecal morphine probably has the some action. The potentially dangerous effects of a catheter in the subarachnoid space make this technique unsuitable for routine use.

Transcutaneous stimulation[5] probably acts at cord level by modulating the signals that pass through the 'gate' of the substantia gelatinosa. The method involves the use either of electrical stimulators in the immediate periphery of the wound or of acupuncture needles. The techniques are of great interest but cannot yet be said to be beyond the experimental stage.

[5] Central relief

The traditional method of relieving pain has been by narcotics (opiates) administered systemically. It is only in recent years that it has become apparent that the mode of action of these agents is to occupy receptor sites which are available to natural substances secreted by the brain (upper arrow in diagram). Origins and sites are still under investigation, but the mental experience of pain can be abolished if receptor sites are fully occupied. This requires that a loading dose of opiate is administered until pain is relieved, followed by continuous administration at a rate sufficient to keep all sites occupied in the face of breakdown of the opiate molecule.

Intravenous administration

The conventional intramuscular administration of morphine, its analogues or pethidine (Demerol) on a 4-hourly basis or *pro re nata* cannot achieve the above aims. Two systems, both based upon intravenous administration, are now in common use.

'On demand' analgesia[6]

The patient senses desaturation by the onset of pain and doses himself with a predetermined amount of agent.

Continuous administration

A 'titration dose' sufficient to relieve pain completely is given and this is then used as a basis for continuous administration[1]. Recent trials have shown this to be effective and its use will be described in detail.

Continuous intravenous infusion of morphine in a dose varied according to the changing needs of the patient is currently the most effective means of controlling postoperative pain and reducing respiratory complications[7]. There is a difference between abdominal pain as a symptom and abdominal pain experienced after an operation: the first is often relieved by movement; the latter is exacerbated by movement. The aim of pain control is a patient who can cooperate with the physiotherapist and move around in bed without discomfort.

Despite improved anaesthetic and surgical techniques, the incidence of postoperative respiratory complications has not decreased and is highest following upper abdominal procedures. The role of pain in the genesis of these complications by reflex splinting of the muscles has been well established, but the traditional approach to the control of this postoperative pain is unchanged. As has been emphasized, conventional administration 4-hourly by intramuscular injection is not adequate. Over this period the serum level rises and falls, and produces corresponding periods of drowsiness and pain. Failure to administer the narcotic on time leads to anxiety and increased perception of pain, and the next routine dose of analgesic will be less effective. There is no provision in these drug schedules for rapid induction of extra analgesia before potentially painful manoeuvres such as turning the patient and physiotherapy are undertaken.

Pharmacokinetic theory predicts that continuous intravenous infusion of drugs will produce a steady concentration in the blood associated with more effective control of pain. Such a concentration can be maintained to keep the patient as alert and pain-free as possible without evidence of respiratory depression.

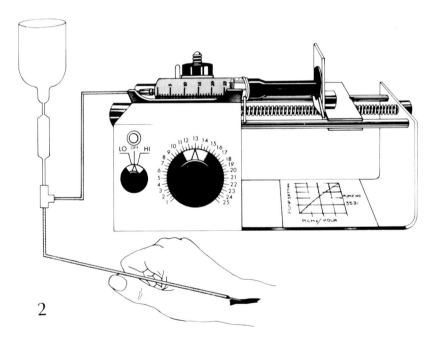

2

2

Using a motor-driven 25 ml syringe containing 3 mg/ml (total 75 mg) of morphine sulphate, an infinitely variable rate of infusion can be adjusted to the degree of pain indicated by the patient and increased to ensure his cooperation. Each pump must be individually calibrated and checked regularly. A graph relating pump setting to rate of infusion in mg/h is attached to the apparatus. An alarm mechanism can be incorporated into the design of each unit so that the motor is turned off when the syringe is almost empty and an audible alarm is activated. Smaller, more portable pumps with a single rate of flow are also available and can be used in conjunction with varying concentrations of morphine.

Guidelines in administration

1. An initial titration or bolus dose is given when the patient returns from the operating room and complains of discomfort. The amount given can then be used to calculate the rate of infusion, which is adjusted to give 2.5 times that dose over the next 24 h[1]. Alternatively, the initial calculations of the infusion setting can be based on patient weight – 0.02 mg morphine/kg bodyweight.
2. Intravenous infusion is then started to allow the establishment of a steady blood concentration of the narcotic.
3. Extra doses can be administered as required.
4. Cessation is usually possible 48–72 h postoperatively. Oral analgesia or intramuscular administration is found to be sufficient for the remainder of the postoperative course.

A prospective study of the amount of morphine administered to surgical patients has led to the following observations.

1. The average amount of morphine administered over 72 h to patients undergoing cholecystectomy differed with age (see graph). Younger patients initially required more morphine than older patients, but after 48 h this relationship is reversed. The older patients required morphine at a relatively constant rate whereas the young required an initially high dose which subsequently quickly dropped off.
2. Requirements varied with different operations and with time elapsed since the procedure: patients undergoing gastric operations required the highest average doses over the longest period; those undergoing cholecystectomy required just over half of their total morphine in the first 24 h after surgery.

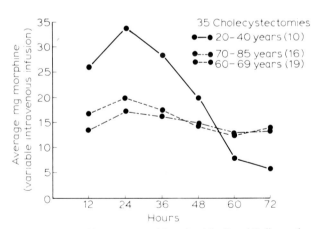

(Reproduced by courtesy of Annals of the Royal College of Surgeons of England[7])

Advantages

The patient is spared the discomfort of repeated intramuscular injections. Before potentially painful procedures the amount given can be turned up or a bolus dose given to raise the serum concentration. This obviates planning of intramuscular administration to coincide with nursing or physiotherapy procedures and gives the nurse more flexibility in managing a patient's pain.

Patients are generally more alert and are able to move themselves in bed. They are told before the operation that they will have less pain with the infusion and that the dosage will be increased according to need and are thus psychologically prepared to be more comfortable and cooperative. Where possible, delegation of authority to the nursing and paramedical staff to increase the infusion rate at their discretion reduces the time spent checking drugs and signing records. Postoperative respiratory complications may also be considerably reduced.

Possible disadvantages

Disadvantages are not encountered as long as normal and careful observation of the patient is maintained and the morphine is decreased if he or she appears drowsy or has depressed respiration. There has been no incidence of addiction and the infusion is usually discontinued by the third postoperative day. Patients receive the same, or in many instances less, overall morphine than those who have conventional medication. Finally, there has been no increased incidence of phlebitis.

Side effects   Nursing staff must monitor patients at all times for side effects just as when using intramuscular morphine; they should be particularly on the alert for depression of respiration, for drowsiness and for nausea.

Minor analgesia

The foregoing relates to major surgical procedures on the abdominal and thoracic cavities. For lesser surgery, lesser analgesia is appropriate. Oral preparations of morphine or pethidine (Demerol) may be used and lesser analgesics such as acetylsalicylic acid are often sufficient. *All should be prescribed on a regular basis designed to keep pain at bay rather than to let it occur and then require relief.* When a patient goes home after a minor procedure it must be with a sufficient supply of pain relief to last for the expected duration of the wound pain.

Conclusions

The relief of pain after surgery can now be regarded as a problem which has found a solution. The pain-free patient is, however, faced with difficulties in sleep which are incompletely explored and understood. Parenteral (preferably intravenous) non-barbiturate sedation (diazepam, chlorpromazine) should be used cautiously but deliberately to ensure a tranquil but cooperative patient. It should be remembered that diazepam's metabolic derivatives have the same activity as the parent compound and build-up of active agents must be avoided. Diazepam is thus less suited to the dynamic circumstances of the postoperative state than is chlorpromazine; the hepatotoxic effects of the latter agent have been exaggerated. Very small carefully adjusted intravenous doses (12.5 mg; 25 mg) are appropriate.

References

1. Rutter, P. C., Murphy, F., Dudley, H. A. F. Morphine: controlled trial of different methods of administration for postoperative pain relief. British Medical Journal 1980; 280: 12–13

2. Egbert, L. D., Lamdin, S. J., Hackett, T. P. Psychologic factors influencing postoperative narcotic administration. Anesthesiology 1967; 28: 246

3. Brandt, M. R., Fernandes, A., Mordhorst, R., Kehlet, H. Epidural analgesia improves postoperative nitrogen balance. British Medical Journal 1978; 1: 1106–1108

4. Behar, M., Magora, F., Olshwang, D., Davidson, J. T. Epidural morphine in treatment of pain. Lancet 1979; 1: 527–529

5. Sternback, R. A., Ignelzi, R. J., Deems, L. M., Timmermans, G. Transcutaneous electrical analgesia: a follow up analysis. Pain 1976; 2: 35–41

6. Anonymous. Patient-controlled analgesia. Lancet 1980; 1: 289–290

7. Nayman, J. Measurement and control of postoperative pain. Annals of the Royal College of Surgeons of England 1979; 61: 419–426

Skin protection in the presence of fistulae

Diane Meelheim RN, FNP
Department of Surgery, School of Medicine,
East Carolina University, Greenville, North Carolina

The location and types of fistula will dictate the care and protection used. In essence, protection of the skin in the presence of fistulae involves collecting the drainage and providing skin barriers if the drainage is irritating in nature. The drainage collection system may consist of dry sterile dressings, ostomy appliances or both.

Commonly encountered types of fistula with the kind of attendant drainage are listed in the table.

Table

Type of fistula	Attendant drainage
Oesophagocutaneous	Saliva
Bronchocutaneous	Pus, usually
Gastrocutaneous	Acidic/digestive
Small bowel cutaneous	Alkaline/digestive
Large bowel cutaneous	
Ascending and transverse	Liquid and irritating
Descending (enterocutaneous)	More solid, less irritating
Rectocutaneous	Chiefly solid, with pus or blood

Oesophagacutaneous

Dressings used to collect non-irritating drainage, such as that from an oesophagocutaneous fistula, may be of dry sterile gauze held in place by tape. No special skin barrier is required though Stomahesive may help. A stomal appliance may be called for if the dressing requires too frequent changing. To affix an ostomy appliance the skin should first be cleansed with soap and water, rinsed well and dried. Temporary packing of the fistula with gauze or tampon while positioning the appliance may maintain the dry skin surface necessary for good adherence. The appliance should fit the fistula snugly. The appliance is then positioned over the fistula and the backing applied directly to the skin. The bag may be worn until it leaks (usually 4–5 days), at which time it is removed. The skin is cleansed again, the appliance replaced and fitted with a new bag. A secure, complete skin seal is vital.

With a tracheo-oesophagocutaneous fistula, an appliance with an antireflux system such as that found in urostomy appliances is helpful. There should be an opening at the bottom for drainage which can be closed between drainages by a rubber band or standard ostomy appliance clip.

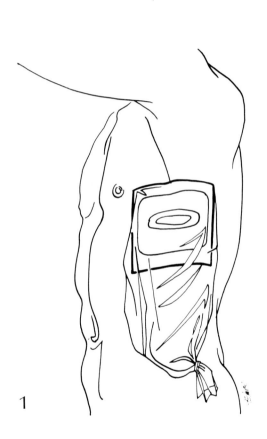

1

1

Bronchocutaneous

The bronchocutaneous fistula, as found in Eloesser flaps, usually drains in such quantities that use of an ostomy appliance is obligatory. The drainage is not usually irritating to the skin and therefore an appliance with a tape seal is the only skin protection required. The location on the chest wall and stress on the tape from pulling and bending call for use of wider margins (about 7.5–10 cm) than are otherwise left. The appliance can usually be left in place for 4–5 days and should be drainable. If it is worn under clothing it should not interfere with the activities of daily living.

Gastrocutaneous

The drainage from gastrocutaneous fistulae can be irritating to exposed skin which must be protected with a skin seal. Skin seals vary in flexibility and can be chosen to suit the tension and movement of the skin around the fistula. Seals need to be changed as soon as they are ineffective. The ostomy appliance is placed on top of the seals and additional support may be given to the appliance using either a tape frame or a belt. Transparent film may be used as the skin barrier, applying the equipment directly over it, but this thin semipermeable membrane must be changed frequently as secretions may find their way under it if the skin is weeping.

2

Small bowel

Drainage from small bowel fistulae and ileostomies is irritating to the skin and skin barriers must be provided. Skin exposed to such drainage may become excoriated, weeping and painful. In such cases ostomy appliances, preferably drainable ones, are worn over the barrier.

Large bowel

Fistulae of the *ascending* and *transverse large bowel* must be treated in the same manner as small bowel fistulae.

Enterocutaneous fistulae of the large bowel or colostomies need not be so treated. With these, the irritating enzymes have been neutralized and no skin barrier is necessary. Drainage from such fistulae is more solid. Appliances with tape backing may be used. Such stomas or fistulae can sometimes be trained to evacuate daily at a certain time by irrigation; in such cases a small patch or small closed-ended bag will suffice for coverage.

With *rectocutaneous* fistulae an appliance is not worn but sanitary napkins may prove useful. The surrounding skin may need the protection of a barrier cream or a skin seal.

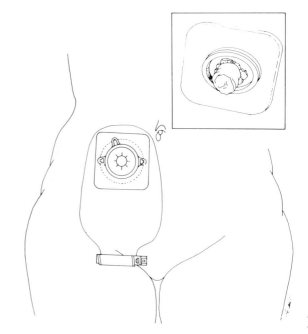

2

Conclusion

There is an extensive range of products available: expertise should be developed with two or three, turning to others only when these few are unsatisfactory. However, none of these products will be effective without constant vigilance to ensure that bags are emptied promptly and seals are intact. Proper use of appliances, together with support for the patient, ensures that most patients with fistulae are kept comfortable and can adjust to a fairly normal round of daily activites.

For a more detailed account of surgical management *see* volumes on *Colon, Rectum and Anus* and *Upper Gastrointestinal Surgery*.

Illustrations by Anne Barrett

Prevention and treatment of decubitus ulcers (pressure sores)

Diane Meelheim   RN, FNP
Department of Surgery, School of Medicine,
East Carolina University, Greenville, North Carolina

Neither pressure sore nor decubitus ulcer is the most appropriate term, though both are hallowed by long usage, because the earlist lesion is a surface abrasion or devascularization of the most superficial layers of the skin. The initial break is red, angry and often painful, but may progress with considerable rapidity to a full-thickness ulcer with necrosis. Pain persists. Though pressure is the predominant cause, other factors exacerbate the deterioration of the skin. These are lack of mobility caused by either physical restriction, e.g. a plaster cast, or the patient's psychological state, e.g. depression. Poor hygiene and nutritional status are often additional factors. In malnourished or paralysed patients who cannot move, such lesions can begin to develop within 30 min to 1 h. Their surgical importance in general is that they may be initiated on the operating table, particularly in the seriously ill.

Prevention

Prevention is far easier than cure. Measures for prevention include the following.

Frequent changes of position
Adequate padding
Cleanliness
Avoidance of local skin irritation
Adequate nutrition
Extreme care on the operating table to avoid points of high pressure, particularly in prolonged operations

Positioning of the patient – particularly on the operating table – should always be done with good body mechanics in mind. Patients should be supported by as many pillows or rolls as required. Off the operating table, change of position should be carried out at least once an hour, preferably every 30 min for immobile patients. Areas to be protected most carefully are the sacrum, shoulders, ankles and hips and any other bony prominence that may be subjected to pressure (see below). In pre- and postoperative care of high-risk patients, foam mattresses, alternating pressure mattresses, water beds and sheepskins all perform the same function – to reduce focal pressure at any one point. The particular virtue of a sheepskin or its synthetic substitute, is that it also provides air circulation and thus evaporation, so preventing skin maceration from moisture.

More elaborate support systems (levitation on an air support or the use of the Clinitron System* using silicone beads activated by air) may be available for very high-risk patients such as those with burns or extensive injuries. However, nursing is difficult and prolonged use of this equipment thus very difficult.

* Support Systems International

Treatment of the established sore/ulcer

1

Decubitus ulcers occur over bony prominences. Locations vary with the patient's disability, but the most common sites overlie the shoulders, sacrum, femoral trochanters, ischiae, knees and ankles.

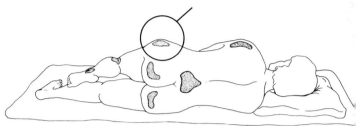

1

Superficial ulcers

All the approaches pertaining to prevention are relevant to therapy of superficial ulcers plus:

avoidance of pressure;
gentle cleansing with soap and water;
keeping the skin dry and free of stool and urine;
application of Op-site or Stomahesive for very superficial lesions;
application of antibiotic ointments and absorptive dressings for full-thickness ulcers;
desloughing with enzymes or surgical debridement (rarely required for superficial ulcers).

Deep ulcers

Deep ulcers require excision when they drain pus, when they connect to deep tracts and when they are suspected to be the cause of sepsis. Excision should be carried out under broad antibiotic coverage. Transfusion is frequently required because patients with decubitus ulcers are usually anaemic.

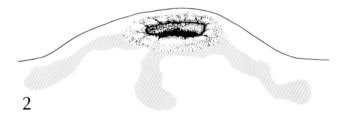

2

2

Even though the opening of the decubitus ulcer may be small, considerable tissue destruction may be hidden underneath the surface with extensive infected sinuses.

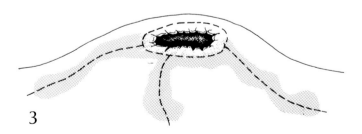

3

3

Incisions are designed to excise a minimum of skin (less than 1 cm) and to uncover each sinus fully.

4

It is essential that all necrotic tissue and exposed tendon is excised so that the entire wound surface is lined by viable muscle or fat. Often full debridement requires entry into the underlying joint. If this is the case, the exposed joint capsule must also be removed.

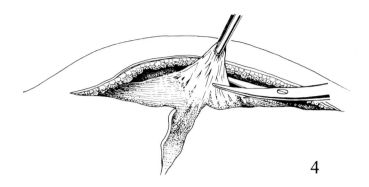

4

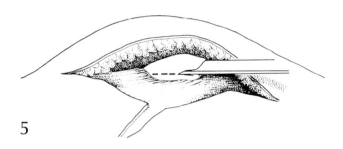

5

5

The bony prominence is chiselled off until a smooth flat plane is created. The chiselling must be done gently as the bone is usually weak and can break easily. Bleeding is controlled with bone wax and the cautery.

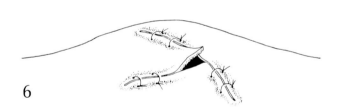

6

6

The wound is closed in two layers. The soft tissues are approximated first with absorbable suture to cover and cushion the bone. The wound edges are then closed loosely with polyethylene sutures to allow drainage. No drain is used.

A bulky absorbent dressing is applied and changed as frequently as needed to keep the wound dry. Allowing the patient to rest on the wound does not interfere with healing. The sutures are left in place for 4 weeks.

Managing the surgical operative specimen

W. K. Blenkinsopp MD, MB, BChir, FRCPath
Consultant Histopathologist, Watford General Hospital, Hertfordshire

Introduction

All too often the procurement of a critical biopsy specimen by surgical means is left to the inexperienced. There are simple procedural, surgical and organizational rules which, though vital, may not have been learnt. Here they are set down. Individual hospital practices may differ slightly but the principles are the same.

Fixatives

The handling of most surgical specimens falls into two familiar categories: the majority are placed in fixative, usually a formalin solution, and a minority are placed in a clean dry container for urgent frozen section. Urgent frozen sections can be cut on tissue which has been in formalin, but the results are less satisfactory and the sections tend to float off the slide.

This basic dichotomy can usefully be extended by consideration of requirements for which formalin-fixed tissue is:

1. *inappropriate*
   (*a*) Tissue for bacteriology, virology or mycology.
   (*b*) Rapid-frozen tissue for immunofluorescence or immunoperoxidase, such as skin or kidney. These specimens must be orientated and frozen rapidly in liquid nitrogen, and this usually requires the presence of a trained technician at the biopsy.
2. *often inappropriate*
   (*a*) Electron microscopy can be done on paraffin-embedded, formalin-fixed, or specially-fixed (usually glutaraldehyde) material, in increasing order of efficiency. Glutaraldehyde fixation requires the presence of a trained technician at the biopsy.
   (*b*) Enzyme histochemistry, such as disaccharidase estimations on small gut mucosa, requires frozen unfixed tissue, and the details must be arranged before biopsy.
   (*c*) Muscle biopsy may require histochemistry (fresh, unfixed, unfrozen tissue), electron microscopy (glutaraldehyde-fixed tissue), and light microscopy of formalin-fixed, paraffin-embedded sections; the details must be arranged before biopsy.
   (*d*) Biopsies for particular purposes may require other fixatives: a testicular biopsy for tumour is satisfactory in formalin, but one for infertility should be put into Bouin's fixative.

Handling of specimens

Large specimens

The handling of large specimens has in the past been a matter for local arrangement – in most hospitals a mixture of fixed and unfixed, opened and unopened, pinned out and packed in. There is still no general agreement on the best method of dealing with them, but safety requirements are now paramount: transport of fresh specimens other than in sealed containers, and transport in containers with a contaminated exterior, can no longer be justified. Transport of fresh specimens in sealed containers such as plastic bags is one solution, but delays in transmission of some hours are common and render some specimens useless.

1

Probably the best method is to put the specimen into a plastic bag (after opening gastrointestinal resections), add at least twice the volume of formalin, seal the bag and place it in a bucket for transportation.

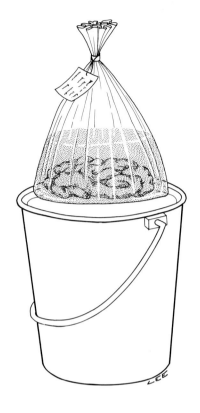

1

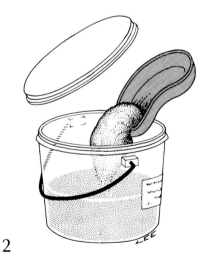

2

Medium-size specimens

2

A kidney, uterus, or specimen of similar size is adequately accommodated in formalin in a plastic container of 0.5 or 1 litre capacity, with a tight-fitting snap closure lid. Larger containers of this type are difficult to handle.

Solid organs such as kidney and uterus should be sliced by the pathologist with a long knife as soon as possible, to improve fixation; this cannot be satisfactorily done by the surgeon with a scalpel blade. Gastrointestinal tubes should be opened cleanly with large scissors and in standard fashion – along the greater curve of the stomach and along the antimesenteric border of the gut.

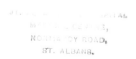

Small biopsies

3 & 4

Most biopsies of epithelial surfaces become very distorted during fixation and processing. This can be virtually eliminated by flattening the biopsy gently, mucosal surface up, on a piece of fine card (coarse fibres such as those in blotting paper can make section cutting impossible) or, better, glass; it should be allowed to adhere for 1–2 min before being placed in fixative. Mucus should not be removed as it may contain giardia, amoebae and inflammatory cells. This orientation takes little time, and except for biopsies of solid tumours it adds considerably to the amount of information obtained.

Degrees of urgency

Reporting time varies from hospital to hospital, but the usual system is overnight processing after the fixed specimen has been cut up, and the sections usually arrive for reporting at around midday; requests marked 'urgent' can often be cut up the same day instead of the following day and can be reported first, so that the report may be available at noon the day after biopsy instead of 17.00 the following day. Heat/vacuum processing machines are available and with these needle biopsies can be processed in 2 h instead of overnight; however, the specimen still requires to be fixed, embedded, cut and stained, and this usually takes a further 3 h. The degrees of urgency, the fixative used and the times involved are summarized in *Table 1*.

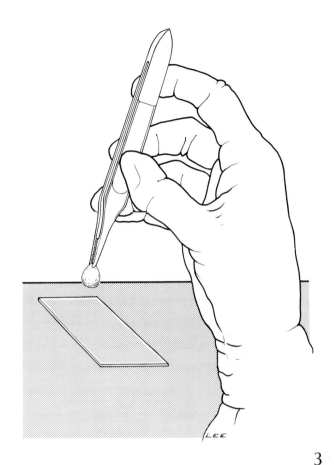

3

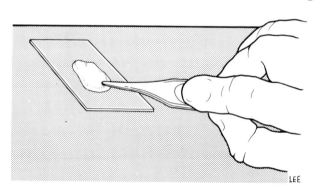

4

Table 1 Surgical specimens

Urgency	Fixation	Time received	Time reported
Very urgent	None (Frozen section)	Any	15 min
Urgent	Formalin	By 14.00, day 1	By noon, day 2
Non-urgent	Formalin	Fixed day 1, cut day 2	By 17.00, day 3
Non-urgent	No formalin (see p. 70)		

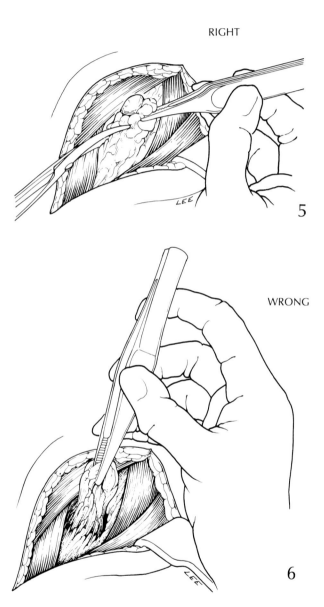

RIGHT

5

WRONG

6

5 & 6

Lymph nodes

Nodes should be carefully dissected, handling the surrounding tissues *not* the specimen, and removed entire. Diagnosis is frequently difficult and may be impossible if surgical artefacts are introduced by taking out the node piecemeal, which makes assessment of the architecture difficult or impossible, and by pulling during removal, which turns the nuclei into long thin strings.

7, 8 & 9

Request form

Identification   Inadequate and/or illegible documentation is very common and very dangerous. Most histopathology files contain upwards of 100 000 reports, so the possibilities for error are considerable.

Indicate previous biopsy   This contributes to the useful reporting of the current biopsy. Provide the surgical report number if possible.

Indicate clinical problem   With extra information the report can be more efficient and helpful.

Indicate important site on specimen   Mark by a suture if necessary. Put the relevant question on the form.

Prevention of infection   Any known or probable infection hazard must be clearly stated.

WRONG

Histopathology, St. Mary's Hospital, London W2.	
Surname : SMITH	Age :
Forenames :	Sex :
Hospital number :	Ward :
Consultant : Mr~~~~~	
Site of specimen : Large Gut	
Previous biopsy :	
Clinical summary : Backache	

7

RIGHT

Histopathology, St. Mary's Hospital, London W2.	
Surname : SMITH	Age : 56
Forenames : JOHN HENRY	Sex : M
Hospital number : 801630	Ward : ALBERT
Consultant : MR. BROOKS	
Site of specimen : RECTO-SIGMOID	
Previous biopsy : RECTAL. S.D. 3197-80	
Clinical summary : Carcinoma of Rectum Please check adhesion at stitch.	

8

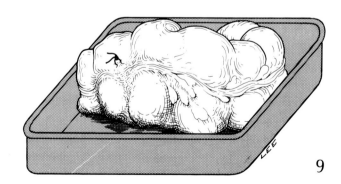

9

Safety

The 'Code of Practice for the Prevention of Infection in Clinical Laboratories and Post-Mortem Rooms' (HMSO, 1978) specifies precautions to be taken in respect of possible infection.

10

Essentially, laboratories *must* be warned of known or probable infection hazards in a specimen before the specimen is handled.

Few laboratories are able to cope with the most dangerous (Category A) infections (e.g. Lassa fever, rabies, smallpox), and the major problem is with Category B specimens (notably specimens *known or suspected* to contain TB or hepatitis B). Frozen sections of unfixed material must not be cut on Category A or Category B specimens, and the clinician requesting a frozen section has an obligation to inform the laboratory of any possible risk at the time of the request.

Histopathology, St. Mary's Hospital, London W2.	
Surname : SMITH	Age : 56
Forenames : JOHN HENRY	Sex : M
Hospital number : 801630	Ward : ALBERT
Consultant : MR. BROOKS	
Site of specimen : Lymph node - neck	
Previous biopsy : NONE	
Clinical summary : ?T.B. T.B.	

10

11

The other main requirement is that contaminated forms and containers with contaminated external surfaces (from any patient) must not be sent to the laboratory.

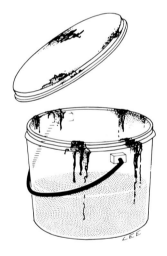

11

Bacteriology

Table 2 shows the main bacterial species associated with infection in different sites. Of those listed, the most difficult to isolate are:

1. anaerobes – killed by exposure to air;
2. *Haemophilus influenzae* and gonococci – strict growth requirements;
3. mycobacteria – often very scanty, most species slow growing.

Table 2

Site	Main organisms causing infection
Gastrointestinal Biliary Intra-abdominal	Sporing/non-sporing anaerobes, enterococci, Pseudomonads, coliform bacilli
Female genital tract	Sporing/non-sporing anaerobes, haemolytic streptococci, gonococci, coliform bacilli
Bone/joint	Staphylococci, streptococci, pneumococci, *H. influenzae*, mycobacteria
Respiratory tract	Pneumococci, *H. influenzae*, mycobacteria, non-sporing anaerobes
Skin/lymph node	Staphylococci, streptococci, mycobacteria
Central nervous system including cerebral abscesses	Streptococci, pneumococci, meningococci, staphylococci, non-sporing anaerobes, mycobacteria
Urinary tract	Coliform bacilli, Pseudomonads, enterococci, staphylococci
Blood	Any of the above (except mycobacteria) and Candida *sp.*

The key to a good yield from bacteriological investigation is the quality of the specimen which can be ensured by the following.

1. Sufficient quantity of a representative sample as free as possible from extraneous contamination.
2. Rapid delivery to the laboratory.
3. A suitable container. No preservative or fixative should be used.
4. Properly completed request forms with *relevant* clinical details.

Specimens

Tissue

Place in a sterile glass or plastic container. No fixative or preservative should be added. When available, 'gassed out' tubes or vials may be used if anaerobes are thought to be implicated.

Pus/aspirate

As above. If the sample has been taken into a syringe this can be sent directly to the laboratory with the needle still attached. The point should be embedded in a cork.

If there is insufficient material to be aspirated directly the site can be irrigated with a little sterile saline and this sent to the laboratory instead.

Swabs

Swabs should only be used where no other type of sample can be obtained.

Blood

Where serious sepsis is suspected blood cultures should always be taken.

N.B. Only tissue, pus and aspirates are suitable for anaerobic culture.

Acknowledgement

The section on Bacteriology in this chapter has been contributed by Dr C. S. F. Easmon, MD, PhD, MRCPath, Reader, Department of Bacteriology, St Mary's Hospital, London.

The general therapy of malignant disease

Spencer Raab MD
Division of Hematology/Oncology, Department of Internal Medicine,
East Carolina University, Greenville, North Carolina

Mary Raab MD
Division of Hematology/Oncology, Department of Internal Medicine,
East Carolina University, Greenville, North Carolina

Introduction

Although surgery remains the most effective curative therapy for localized malignant disease, it still has many failures; only about one-third of all patients whose tumours have not grossly metastasized are cured by surgery alone. For example, at least two-thirds of patients with breast cancer will have micrometastases at the time of surgery and eventually die. In consequence, to do justice to his patients the surgeon must understand that the treatment of cancer is rightly a multidisciplinary undertaking. Modes of therapy are constantly changing. Familiar techniques are being supplanted or augmented by newer methods. The surgeon should secure the most up-to-date information from his own discipline, and those of radiology, immunology and medical oncology, so as to offer the most effective forms of treatment.

As Lane[1] has wisely cautioned, the chemotherapy of any form of cancer must not be considered to be 'established' or 'conventional'; the field is constantly changing. Administration of chemotherapeutic and hormonal agents should be carried out by a clinical oncologist, whether internist, paediatrician or surgeon, who has the knowledge to deal with this relatively new form of therapy and its consequences.

Sources of information

Cooperation between the various therapists in the field has created regional, national and international study groups and information agencies; numerous protocols with detailed technical instructions and dosages now exist to promulgate new knowledge and clearly to delineate programmes of treatment and follow-up. The surgeon should avail himself of compilations of the current literature before undertaking the treatment of any cancer. There are four main sources.

1. The Cancer Information Clearinghouse of the National Cancer Institute, 9000 Rockville Pike, Bethesda, MD 20205, USA, tel: (301) 496 4070 – collects and disseminates information on cancer materials, programmes, and resources from thousands of independent groups, institutions and organizations.
2. *The Directory of Cancer Research Information Sources*, from the US Department of Health and Human Resources (formerly Health, Education and Welfare), Public Health Service, National Institutes of Health and National Cancer Institute – aims to provide cancer researchers with a single-volume listing of most of the available cancer information sources from around the world.
3. L'Union Internationale Contre Cancer (UICC), 3 rue de Conseil-General, Geneva 1205, Switzerland, tel: (022) 20-18-11.
4. The International Cancer Research Data Bank (ICRDB) of the National Cancer Institute provides data bases. This service is available through more than 1200 health sciences and hospital libraries throughout the United States, and in Australia, Brazil, Canada, France, Germany, Iran, Italy, Japan, Mexico, Sweden, Switzerland, South Africa and the United Kingdom. A search can be

made through the literature for any specified time period, in English or any one of several other languages, for a specific type of tumour. Information about this resource and others may be obtained from the National Cancer Institute, Blair Building, Room 114, 8300 Colesville Road, Silver Spring, MD 20910, USA, tel: (303) 427 8759, or from MEDLARS Management Section, National Library of Medicine, 8600 Rockville Pike, Bethesda, MD 20209, USA, tel: (800) 638 8480 or (301) 496 6193.

Evaluation

It goes without saying that an unequivocal tissue diagnosis must be obtained before any therapy. When this has been done, many malignancies can be 'staged' to quantify the extent and to determine the location of the cancer. Each disease category may requires different procedures for staging. Unfortunately, no all-inclusive international standards for tumour staging exist, but efforts to arrive at such standards continue. Pool documents are useful, such as The International Classification of Diseases, The International Classification of Diseases for Oncology and The International Histological Classification of Tumours, all from WHO. The UICC classification, entitled *Tumours, Nodes, Metastases* (TNM), is available from that organization. All these offer sufficient guidance so that the surgeon may confidently proceed to a decision about treatment.

Staging procedures may be divided into two categories.

1. Non-surgical, which may include lymphangiography, arteriography, bone-marrow aspiration, CT scan, intravenous pyelogram, chest radiography, liver scan, isotopic scans of various other organs, and ultrasound studies.
2. Surgical, including procedures ranging from needle biopsy to major exploration. *Table 1* lists some surgical staging procedures.

In many cases, the non-invasive study suffices to establish the extent of the disease. At other times, studies will raise questions or uncover new lesions, and the surgeon may need to perform further surgery or biopsy.

Once staging is established, the choice of therapy must be undertaken. Those lesions potentially amenable to cure by surgery alone should be identified; yet even after so-called 'curative' operations, patients may later develop local recurrence or widespread disease because micrometastases are present at the time of surgery. Chemotherapy given at this stage to patients who would otherwise have a high risk of recurrence *may* reduce the likelihood that the disease will later become widely disseminated, or alter the time of presentation of such dissemination.

In identifying the tumour and staging its spread, it is essential for the physician to evaluate the patient's physical, emotional, social and financial status before proceeding with therapy. What may be ideal treatment for a young, intelligent executive may be totally inappropriate for an elderly, isolated patient with heart disease.

Table 1 Examples of surgical staging procedures (adapted from Rubin[2])

Tumour	Procedures
Breast cancer	Excision of axillary contents Needle biopsies of metastases
Oesophageal cancer	Oesophagoscopy with biopsy Exploratory laparotomy for tumours in the lower third
Hodgkin's disease and some non-Hodgkin's lymphomas	Tumour biopsy Exploratory laparotomy with liver and node biopsies, splenectomy
Lung tumours	Bronchoscopy with brushings Blind mucosal biopsies Node biopsy Mediastinoscopy Thoracotomy
Melanoma of the leg	Femoral and iliac node biopsies
Metastatic cervical lymph nodes, primary unknown	Node and blind mucosal biopsies
Selected cases of cervical, prostatic, bladder tumours	Node biopsy
Testicular tumours	Exploratory laparotomy

Chemotherapy

In the past, chemotherapy has been resorted to only when surgery has failed; yet because this systemic form of treatment has the potential for destroying malignant cells, whatever their location, it should be considered for inclusion in the first stages of treatment.

There are two general categories in which chemotherapy is administered.

1. Chemotherapy given alone, either primarily or for the treatment of advanced or disseminated disease.
2. Adjuvant chemotherapy, administered either before or after surgical treatment.

Chemotherapy alone

There are a small number of malignancies that may be cured by chemotherapy (*Table 2*). These include Burkitt's lymphoma, choriocarcinoma in women, Hodgkins' disease and acute lymphoblastic leukaemia in children. The surgeon's role is to recognize their existence, so that when he makes the diagnosis, either clinically or, as may often be the case, by biopsy of a mass or lymph node, he will refrain from further surgical intervention and either undertake chemotherapy himself or, more usually and appropriately, ensure that this is done by the best qualified person.

Other patients with disseminated cancers, such as breast or prostate, though incurable, may expect longer life because of chemotherapeutic treatment.

Adjuvant therapy

Cure rates or disease-free survivals in patients with some solid tumours have increased with integration of chemotherapy into modalities for primary treatment. This is particularly true of embryonal tumours (e.g. Wilms' tumour), osteogenic sarcoma and testicular tumours. All such patients should be referred to major centres where the best current chemotherapy can be provided and the toxic effects minimized. As advances take place, more and more patients will undergo such combined approaches.

Adjuvant chemotherapy can be undertaken either preoperatively or postoperatively. Consultation between surgeon and oncologist is indicated before an approach is selected. Chemotherapy given before surgery may shrink a tumour mass quite dramatically, thus affording the surgeon a clearer view of the operative field, minimizing blood loss and reducing significantly the bulk of the lesion to be resected. Preoperative agents most commonly used at present are methotrexate, *cis*-platinum and bleomycin.

Choice of regimen

The surgeon should rarely agree to a chemotherapeutic programme which is likely to be of little ultimate value. The risks and morbidity associated with chemotherapy are

Table 2 Results of chemotherapy in disseminated cancers (from J. Chamberlain, MD*)

Potential cure	Extended survival or useful palliation	Refractory
Acute lymphoblastic leukaemia	Acute myelogenous leukaemia	Bladder cancers
Hodgkins' disease	Chronic myelogenous leukaemia	Bronchogenic cancer
Histiocytic lymphoma	Lymphocytic lymphoma	Oesophageal cancer
Burkitt's lymphoma	Plasma cell dyscrasias	Hepatic cancer
Trophoblastic tumours	Chronic lymphatic leukaemia	Pancreatic cancer
Testicular tumours	Small cell cancer of lung	Stomach cancer
Ewing's sarcoma	Ovarian cancer	Renal cancer
Rhabdomyosarcoma	Soft-tissue sarcomas	Melanoma
Wilms' tumour	Neuroblastoma	Cancer of uterine cervix
Retinoblastoma	Follicular thyroid cancer	
	Breast cancer	
	Osteogenic sarcoma	
	Colon cancer	
	Endometrial cancer	
	Thyroid cancer	
	Adrenal cortical cancer	
	Head and neck cancers	
	Prostate cancer	

* Division of Hematology-Oncology, Department of Medicine, School of Medicine, East Carolina University, Greenville, NC

too great for it to be used merely as a sop. Tumours which have been shown to be relatively unresponsive to chemotherapy should not be treated just to give the patient the feeling that something is being done for him unless there is real hope of cure or palliation. For example, gastric carcinoma, carcinoma of the cervix, melanomas and most lung tumours have not responded significantly to chemotherapy, nor have cancers of the bladder, oesophagus, liver or pancreas, although clinical trials for some of these are still going on as newer chemotherapeutic agents are found.

It is of critical importance in beginning a chemotherapeutic regimen to take into acount all variables likely to affect the patient's response to treatment. Thus, in breast cancer there is now good evidence that the outcome of adjuvant therapy aimed at cure is influenced by: menstrual status (premenopausal doing better than postmenopausal patients); oestrogen-receptor content (receptor-positive doing better than receptor-negative); degree of differentiation on histological examination (perhaps correlated with receptor status); duration of time to first recurrence (the shorter the interval, the poorer the response).

Antitumour agents may be used singly, but are now generally given in combination, which seems to offer advantages: antitumour effects may be additive, with no additive toxicity to the patient; and tumour cells may undergo cell death under attack by several agents, when they might repair or compensate for damage done to them by one agent alone.

Drugs that are toxic to cancer cells are also toxic to the non-cancerous cells. The therapist must determine, as far as possible, the patient's potential tolerance for the rigorous regimens involved and the often unpleasant effects of chemotherapy. Antitumour agents can cause damage to the liver, kidney, pancreas, nervous system, lung, bladder and heart; other effects that may occur are bone-marrow depression, hair loss, and local allergic reactions. Fortunately, most of these are reversible if the responsible drug is stopped soon enough.

Table 3 Common chemotherapeutic agents (from American Cancer Society[3])

Common name	Chemical name	Trade or other name
Alkylating agents		
Nitrogen mustard	Mechlorethamine	Mustargen
Melphalan (L-PAM)	L-phenylalanine mustard	Alkeran
Cytoxan	Cyclophosphamide	Cytoxan
Chlorambucil	Chlorambucil	Leukeran
Myleran	Busulfan	Myleran
Thiotepa	Triethylenethiophosphoramide	
Antimetabolites		
Methotrexate	Amethopteran	Methotrexate
5-FU	5-Fluorouracil	
5-FUDR	5-Floxuridine	
Ara-C	Cytosine arabinoside	Cytosar
6-TG	6-Thioguanine	
6-MP	6-Mercaptopurine	
Vinca alkaloids		
Vincristine		Oncovin
Vinblastine	Vincaleukoblastine	Velban
Antibiotics		
Adriamycin	Doxorubicin hydrochloride	Adriamycin
Daunomycin	Daunomycin	
Bleomycin	Bleomycin	Blenoxane
Mithramycin	Mithramycin	Mithracin
Mitomycin C	Mitomycin C	Mutamycin
Actinomycin D	Dactinomycin	Cosmegen
Streptozotocin	Streptozotocin	
Streptonigrin	Streptonigrin	
Miscellaneous		
BCNU	Bis-chloroethyl nitrosourea	Carmustine
CCNU	Cyclohexyl-chloroethyl nitrosourea	Lomustine
Methyl-CCNU		
DTIC	Dimethyl-trianzeno-imidazole carboximide	Dacarbazine
Procarbazine		Matulane
L-Asparaginase		
Cis-platinum	Cis-dichlorodiamminoplatinum	
Hydroxyurea	Hydroxyurea	Hydrea
o,p'-DDD	Orthopara'-DDD	Lysodren

Available agents

The main general categories of antitumour drugs are the alkylating agents, antimetabolites, vinca alkaloids, and antibiotics, as well as some other miscellaneous compounds. *Table 3* lists some of the better-known drugs presently in use for cancer chemotherapy.

Irradiation

As with chemotherapy, radiation may be used alone or in combination – with either surgery or chemotherapy. All the caveats about chemotherapy apply equally to radiation. Apart from its primary use in lymphomas, and by some in oesophageal carcinoma, it is at present chiefly employed in the therapy of those tumours surgeons commonly encounter, as follows: preoperatively to shrink bulky lesions; postoperatively to reduce the risk of local recurrence (e.g. in node-positive patients after simple mastectomy or lesser procedures for breast cancer, and after excision of osteogenic sarcomas); in combination with chemotherapy for lesions unsuitable for radical excision (e.g. embryonal rhabdomyosarcoma). Radiotherapy in skilled hands has also a definite role in the palliation of localized lesions which are painful (e.g. breast-tumour deposits in the spine) or are ulcerating.

Hormone therapy

The demonstration that hormonal manipulation can provide long-term control of endocrine-dependent tumours was a milestone in oncology; today, hormone therapy and endocrine ablation continue to be highly effective approaches to sensitive cancers of the breast and prostate, producing good results in appropriate patients, with minimal morbidity. In other circumstances, not surprisingly, they have been less effective.

The treatment of breast cancer offers an excellent example of the general approaches used in hormone therapy. Most important is the initial determination of the tumour's potential sensitivity to endocrine manipulation. The history, pattern of spread and degree of differentiation can all provide some clues, but the most reliable test is the determination of the presence or absence of oestrogen-receptor sites on the tumour.

The effectiveness of adjuvant endocrine therapy *for cure* (or better, increasing the disease-free survival time) in breast cancer is uncertain. The early results of oöphorectomy in premenopausal women were encouraging, but have not stood up to 5-year analysis. More recently, the oestrogen-receptor *tamoxifen* has been thought to show promise, but further experience is required to confirm this.

A larger place has been established for hormonal manipulation in arresting the progression of disseminated disease. In the premenopausal and up to one year post-menopausal time band (vaginal smears are useful in border line instances) surgical oöphorectomy – which is to be marginally preferred to irradiation – has been the front line of therapy, but ovarian suppression by *aminoglutethimide* may supplant the operative procedure. More heroic endocrine ablation, such as adrenalectomy or hypophysectomy, is now rarely indicated, though transnasal hypophysectomy can dramatically relieve pain from bony metastases by a mechanism that may or may not be endocrine. In postmenopausal patients, somewhat paradoxically, either oestrogens in the form of the synthetic, stilboestrol, or tamoxifen (which is preferred because of its lack of effect on smooth muscle) may be effective. There is now little place for other forms of endocrine therapy – progestogens or androgens.

The therapy of prostatic adenocarcinoma follows somewhat similar lines to that for breast cancer.

References

1. Lane, M. Chemotherapy of cancer. In del Regato, J. A., Spjut, H. J., eds. Cancer, 5th ed., pp. 105–130. St Louis: C. V. Mosby, 1977

2. Rubin, P. (ed.) Clinical oncology for medical students and physicians, 5th ed. New York: American Cancer Society, 1978

3. American Cancer Society. Cancer: a manual for practitioners, 5th ed. Boston: American Cancer Society, 1978

Design and safety in the operating suite

Major General W. J. Watson MBE, QHP, FACMA, RAAMC
Director General, Army Health Services, Canberra

J. F. Mainland FFARACS, BSc
Associate Professor (Anaesthesia), Monash University, Alfred Hospital, Melbourne

Hugh Dudley ChM, FRCS(Ed.), FRACS, FRCS
Professor of Surgery, St Mary's Hospital, London

Introduction

Definitions

Europeans, and particularly those in Britain, still refer to the place where the operation is done as the 'theatre' and in consequence the overall area as the 'operating theatre suite'. Those in North America prefer the less thespian 'operating room' and often use this or its abbreviation 'OR' for the suite.

History

The operating environment has evolved from room and amphitheatre to a complex of areas designed to see the patient through the whole of the surgical procedure, usually now including the immediate (recovery) postoperative phase. The architectural solutions are many and often dictated by cost, special needs, a predetermined envelope for a building and, let it be admitted, personal whims of both users and designers. Interested readers are referred to Pütsep's comprehensive text[1].

During the first 20 years after the Second World War, operating suite design in the Western World went through a period of analysis and elaboration which was without equal in surgical history. A vast amount of effort was concentrated on maximizing safety through design, and on seeking flow patterns for goods, operating team and patients which would economize in time and movement. One of the chief emphases was on physical isolation of the whole suite and particularly the operating room and its adjacent areas from the external world by the use of complex zoning arrangements in an attempt to sustain sterility of air. However, the cost and complexity of these arrangements has made them less easily achieved in surgery than in industry (where 'clean rooms' for the assembly of complicated electronic and micro-engineering equipment are a commonplace); furthermore, there is a paucity of convincing evidence that large gains can be achieved in terms of reduction of airborne sepsis for the majority of procedures merely by whole-hearted physical isolation. This is not to countenance sloppy physical circumstances. Clean, logically designed suites will always be better in this respect than dirty and messy ones. However, human factors leading to sepsis are only partly mitigated by design and are more dependent upon high standards of hygiene and operating room technique. Design of course can and does contribute to good behaviour. Finally, in many procedures endogenous infection is of greater importance than exogenous.

Overall layout

1

Relationships and patient flow

In circumstances where a continuous if variable flow of casualties or other emergencies has to be planned for, it is wise to try and arrange a layout which corresponds to the needs of triage (untreatable, urgent salvage required, minor treatment only). The pattern is illustrated (based on 1st Australian Field Hospital Vietnam) and can be achieved in either a permanent design or by improvization in mobile or temporary premises.

   When a general purpose operating suite is being incorporated into a hospital design the same flow patterns prevail but usually have to be modified by other planning needs such as the convenient siting of a radiodiagnostic department.

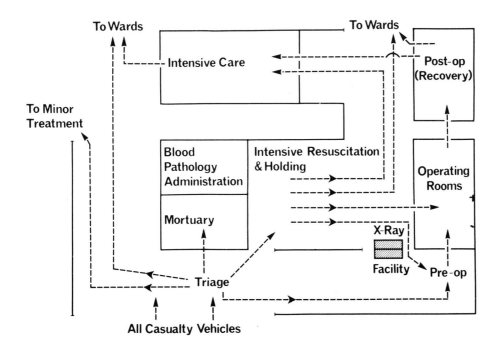

1

Interrelations of operating rooms and ancillary areas

Individual structural constraints will usually govern the actual layout of operating room complexes, but it is conventional to build a module of operating room (usually no smaller than 6 × 6m and larger for procedures which require supporting equipment such as a pump-oxygenator), anaesthetic room and supply/setting up/disposal area. The last may be shared with an adjacent module and its design will be somewhat dependent upon the system of instrument and materials handling chosen (*see* p. 88).

2

A typical modular design is illustrated. The relationship of these modules to the rest of the operating suite is less critical but an endeavour should be made to minimize distances which have to be travelled by personnel.

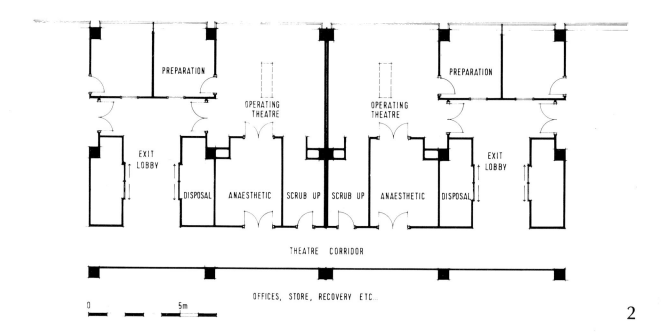

2

3

Constraints on entry

It is difficult to demonstrate that a physical barrier to entry into the suite is of importance. However, it is rational as far as possible to limit entry, if only to preserve relative peace and quiet and to reduce slightly the statistical chance that one heavily infected individual may disastrously contaminate the suite. The barrier need not be complex and the amount of changing done there can vary. Overshoes at least should be put on and preferably the trolley carrying the patient and its coverings changed. Similar barriers should govern the entry of staff, though complex showering arrangements are not needed and indeed may lead to a temporarily increased dissemination of bacteria from the skin.

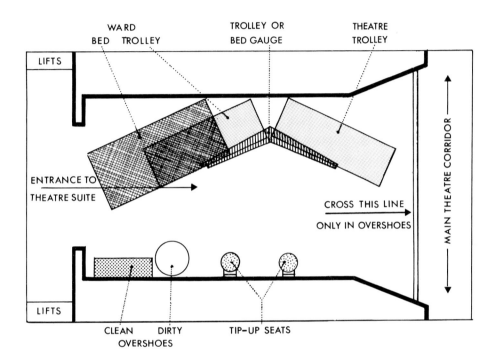

3

4a & b

Air sterilization

The conventional practice is to use the vertical piston displacement effect designed by Blowers[2], in which air is released by weighted flap vents in the lower parts of the walls (a). When other temporary air escape occurs (e.g. a door opening), these vents close (b), so maintaining a positive pressure in the theatre. With an air change rate of 20/h such ventilation preserves a reasonably low bacterial count in the air around the operating environment. A turbulent air flow on the same principle may well be just as satisfactory.

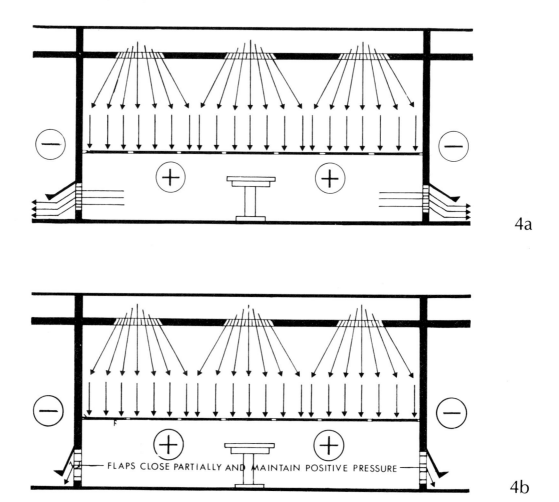

4a

FLAPS CLOSE PARTIALLY AND MAINTAIN POSITIVE PRESSURE

4b

5a & b

The provision of a near total air sterilization is of greatest importance when the only major residual problem in wound sepsis is airborne, either from without or from the theatre team. Such circumstances occur in replacement of joints and other major prosthetic insertions. Current practice is to ensure the micro-environment around the operating field by the use of ventilated enclosures[3]. Either vertical or horizontal air flow may be used, though general surgical practice favours the latter (a) in that industrial units are available and can be readily adapted to existing operating rooms. They are of such a size that the team can operate within them, but packaged instruments and other material are held without and inserted only as necessary. Smaller enclosures (b) may be used for specific procedures such as hip replacement and the ultimate in refinement, if not in ease of operation, is the exclusion of the surgeon's and his assistant's body from the field so that the procedure is essentially done in a sterile enclosure comparable to that used for germ-free animals[4].

These enclosures are of course much easier to maintain sterile for airborne organisms than are either the operating room as a whole or the whole suite. However, though such an approach is rational, particularly when the outcome of sepsis is so disastrous, the evaluation of reduction in incidence is extremely difficult and 'hard' data to this effect have not been conspicuous. We imply by the last statement that surgeons should not feel totally debarred from, say, complex orthopaedic procedures merely because these facilities are unavailable. Good tissue technique, high standards of personal and environmental cleanliness, the observation of basic rules of sterility, all remain as important as ever. Design can best contribute to these by providing simple, uncluttered spaces which are lined with impervious material, easily washed down and serviced. The general flow of ventilation should, as far as possible, be from the operating room outwards and, if laminar flow is not available, piston-type downward displacement at 20 changes an hour is the next best option.

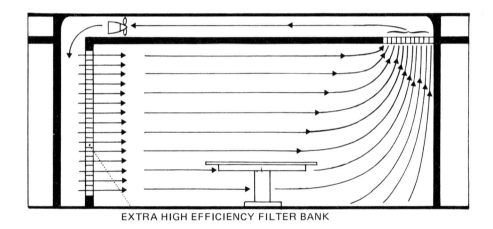

EXTRA HIGH EFFICIENCY FILTER BANK   5a

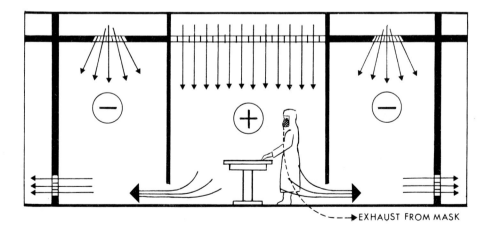

EXHAUST FROM MASK   5b

Instrument and materials handling

The choices theoretically available, with their various advantages and disadvantages, are shown in *Table 1*. The choice between them or any of their modifications will be determined by the purpose and size of the organization into which they are to be introduced. A small hospital in a developing country will choose one approach, a major metropolitan institution in the Western World another. Generalization is impossible as well as undesirable.

Table 1

System description	Instruments	Sutures	Soft goods	Advantages	Disadvantages
Conventional/local	Circulate locally. Steam or hot water sterilization. Hand or ultrasonic cleaning.	Usually prepacked but non-absorbable. May be sterilized on site.	Prepacked in suite or elsewhere (CSSD)*. Sterilized in suite or elsewhere.	Few instrument sets required. Personal supervision. Cheap.	Labour intensive. Instrument care usually not good. Creates noise and movement adjacent to theatre.
Theatre Service and Supply Unit (TSSU)	Sterilized supply, serviced for a suite of theatres.	Prepackaged. Presterilized.	Prepackaged and sterilized in unit or in CSSD.	Size creates efficiency and economy. Purchasing policies uniform. Instrument care possibly improved.	Requires uniformity. Failure of system may immobilize many theatres. Impersonal.
Theatre Supply	Complete operation packs plus or minus soft goods supplied from central source.			Personal wants of surgeons catered for. Good control of instruments. High standards. Ideal where repetitive procedures are common.	Probably costly. Many instruments required. Breakdown disastrous. Possibly inflexible for unexpected.

* Central Sterile Supply Department

Temperature and humidity

The air flow and conditions produced for purposes of bacterial cleanliness are in effect air conditioning and provide comfort conditions for (usually) lightly clad theatre staff in the temperature range 19–24 °C (66–75 °F) but usually nearer the lower end of these values and with a relative humidity of less than 50 per cent. These figures are less satisfactory for the naked anaesthetized (and therefore vasodilated) patient. Heat loss in excess of production – and therefore body cooling – occurs in such circumstances, particularly in prolonged operations with wide openings into body cavities and in neonates who have a large surface area relative to their heat-producing mass. Design and use must recognize these facts. Protection from hypothermia may be possible by adjusting the environment to the upper range of the comfort zone or by local heating (electric or water circulation under blankets, but *see* 'Lighting') with the addition of heat-preserving coverings for those parts of the body outside the operating field (lightweight aluminium foil blankets).

6

Design of service delivery systems

The design of anaesthetic and other service delivery systems has also undergone considerable evolution. Gone from new suites are trailing cables and pipes. Ceiling-mounted pendants or wall-supported cantilevers are integrated sources of supply for all piped gases, power and suction. Originally, remote lines for monitoring were also channelled through the same route to distant equipment, but with rare exceptions this has given way to local small-scale instruments as the bulk of the electronic equipment has lessened. Fixed plinth systems for operating tables are excellent but a little inflexible and most surgeons favour mobile tables.

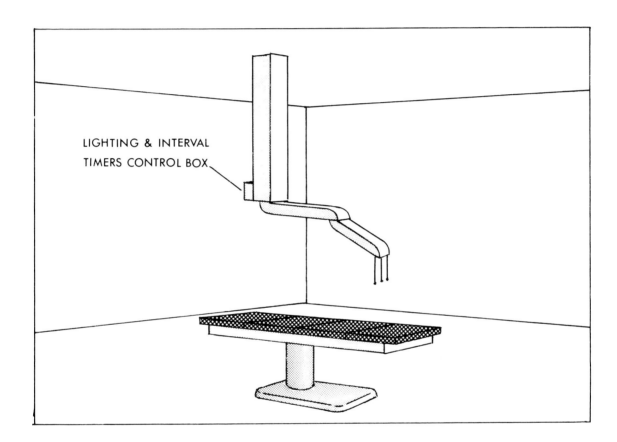

LIGHTING & INTERVAL
TIMERS CONTROL BOX

6

Lighting

Most surgeons know little about lighting except how to complain when it is inadequate. They also tend to forget that the high intensity light they demand in the operating field (which permits a small iris diameter and therefore very precise focussing) may not be associated with similar qualities in the peripheral zones where other staff have to work. This problem is particularly severe for a scrub nurse (theatre sister) whose eyes are constantly switching from the operating zone itself to her instrument table. Also, peripheral lighting has to be of a standard to allow meticulous cleaning of the room.

The problem is compounded by the complex terms of measurement used in lighting engineering. In the Système International (SI) the unit is the lux (lx) which is 1 lumen per m², the lumen in turn being defined in terms of the base measurement candela which is a measure of luminous intensity derived from a standard source (the old foot-candle is approximately 11 lx).

7

Recent draft standards from Australia[5, 6] recommend, after careful consideration, that a clear distinction should be made between *service illuminance* – of the room as a whole – and light for the field provided by a *surgical luminaire* – the operating lamp itself in whatever form.

For service illuminance three levels are proposed at 1 m from the floor.

1. 15–20 lx to permit safe movement during procedures which require reduced illumination.
2. 200–800 lx to give a satisfactory working environment and gradation of brightness from the high intensity of the operating field.
3. 1200 lx for adequate inspection, maintenance and cleaning.

For the surgical luminaire a 'light patch' of between 25 and 40 cm in diameter is required in which the illumination should be 20 000 lx but shading off at the edges.

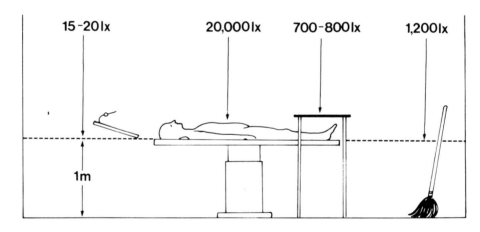

7

SPECIAL HAZARDS

Two major hazards exist: electrical to both patients and staff, and chemical to staff.

Electrical hazards*

Hazards related to electrical equipment are: (1) electrical power failure; (2) fires and explosions; (3) burns; (4) electrocution and shocks; (5) electrical interference.

Electrical power failure

The complex functions of a modern operating suite are largely dependent upon the safe continuous supply of electric power from the mains.

As a minimum, provision must be made for failure of mains power by having battery power available to both general and operating lights, plus an alternative to mains power or a gas source available to generate suction.

Although an automatic-start diesel alternator may appear the ultimate in supply of standby power, it is not without its own problems. These relate not so much to the source itself as to the simply inverse relationship between complexity and reliability. Standby power sources for operating suites must be rigidly maintained and the services of experienced engineering staff available 24 h a day.

While the design of main switch rooms in hospitals revolves around their safety in relation to the staff operating them, it is imperative that access to these vital areas be unavailable to the irresponsible. Furthermore, the operation of large installations often depends on battery-powered relays to switch over from mains power to standby power. Good design must include both automatic change-over *and* manual change-over to allow for the rare event of malfunction of relays and their associated circuits.

Fires and explosions

Because it is very difficult to exclude all sources of ignition, fires and explosions may occur in operating rooms. In the main, diathermy (electrocautery) is a necessary part of the surgeon's armamentarium. Many hospitals have now sought the cooperation of their anaesthetic staff who have, after serious consideration, agreed not to use flammable anaesthetic agents. This wise decision alters not only safety in operating rooms but also their design. For hospitals in which staff have agreed to act in this way, it is now possible to design operating theatres without expensive conductive flooring. Furthermore, relative humidity of the air supplied to the operating rooms can be dropped to a level similar to that experienced in non-medical establishments. This change alone produces tremendous alterations in the design of air conditioning systems for operating theatres, as well as a very big saving in energy.

---

* The European term 'earth' and the American 'ground' are used interchangeably

If flammable anaesthetic agents are used then it is imperative that the appropriate code is followed[7,8,9]. Such codes ensure that:

8a & b

1. Electrostatic discharges from clothing and bodies are minimal or non-existent. This condition is achieved by the use of a humidified atmosphere (e.g. 55 per cent relative humidity) to reduce static build-up and a safe conductive pathway for static electricity to leak away through to a floor of relatively low resistance. The latter is achieved by connecting equipment and people to the floor by conductive material such as carbon-containing rubber wheels and shoe soles. Likewise, all items in contact with the patient are rendered conductive to allow any electrostatic charge also to leak away.

2. 'Spark-over' from switches, plugs and contacts does not occur in any area that contains a flammable and/or explosive mixture of anaesthetic gas or vapour. Though appropriate electrical solutions *can* be found for switches and plugs, this last condition does mean that surgical diathermy and a flammable anaesthetic agent are incompatible and must never be used together.

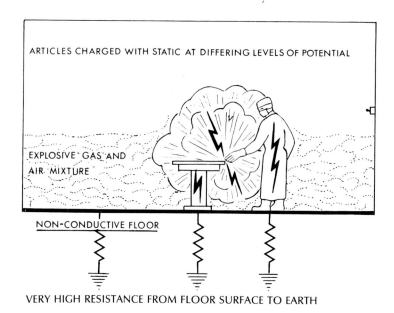

ARTICLES CHARGED WITH STATIC AT DIFFERING LEVELS OF POTENTIAL

EXPLOSIVE GAS AND AIR MIXTURE

NON-CONDUCTIVE FLOOR

VERY HIGH RESISTANCE FROM FLOOR SURFACE TO EARTH   8a

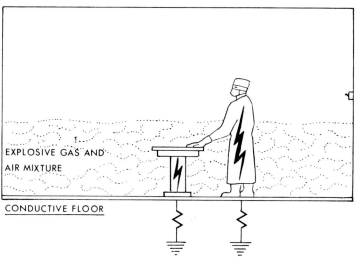

EXPLOSIVE GAS AND AIR MIXTURE

CONDUCTIVE FLOOR

LEAKAGE OF STATIC BUILD-UP TO EARTH VIA CONDUCTIVE FLOORING   8b

Burns

The use of flammable solutions for skin preparation when diathermy is to be used constitutes a risk of burns to the patient. The exclusion of one or other of this incompatible combination is essential to safe patient care.

Radiant heat may also cause burns so that the operating light must carry a heat filter.

Warming blankets used to prevent hypothermia during prolonged procedures and in operations on neonates and infants may be directly heated electrically or indirectly by way of circulated water. In either case it is imperative that both the patient's temperature and the temperature of the blanket in contact with the patient be monitored. Care is required with both types of warming blankets to see that electrical isolation is adequate as well as to ensure that an unsafe return pathway for diathermy current is not provided in the event of a fault occurring in an unisolated diathermy system. Any blanket must be smoothly applied so as to avoid 'hot spots' of contact with the patient.

A more common risk of burning to patients occurs when faulty diathermy and an unisolated electrocardiograph are used together. In such circumstances a considerable current density may build up across an ECG lead which acts as the 'return' for the diathermy instead of the normal plate.

Care in the application of the leads and plates of these pieces of equipment is imperative. *Ideally clinicians should use electrical equipment that has been specifically designed for full isolation from earth.* In this way currents from diathermy will no longer cause burning at ECG electrode sites or sites of patient contact with metal of the operating table.

9

Electrocution and shocks

The problem of electrocution and shocks applies to both patients and staff. All accidents are the consequence of the body acting as a connector between a source of high potential and a return or earth (ground) wire. Current can then be injected into the body. Electrocution death results when ventricular fibrillation occurs. Shocks are commonly divided into two types both of which can be lethal under given circumstances: (1) macroshock, where the current is above the threshold of perception; (2) microshock, where current is below the threshold of perception.

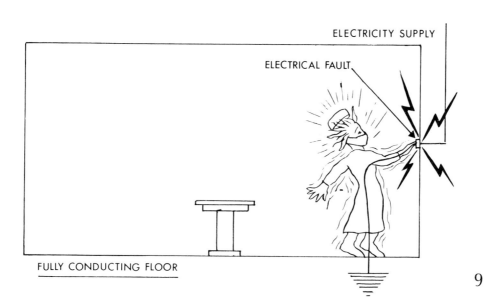

ELECTRICITY SUPPLY

ELECTRICAL FAULT

FULLY CONDUCTING FLOOR

9

Macroshock

The prevention of macroshock to patients or staff is achieved in three ways.

Impeccable maintenance of the electrical installation and electrical equipment   It is essential that periodic inspections and leakage current measurements be carried out on all equipment to be used on patients. Of particular importance is a check of patient circuit leads to ensure that a device, such as an electrocardiograph, does not in itself inject current into a patient. Faults in extension leads constitute the commonest cause of electrocution inside and outside hospitals. For this reason their maintenance is vital to the safety of both patients and staff.

Some consider that it is not possible to achieve maintenance standards of sufficiently high quality to view this method *alone* as even practical.

Core balance earth-leakage devices   These devices placed between the mains supply and the appliance in use are capable of disconnecting the supply of power in such a short time that electrocution of the patient or staff is not physiologically possible should a fault in the appliance develop. They are not suitable where cessation of electric power cannot be tolerated for even a short time.

Isolated supply   This type of electrocution protection involves the use of a transformer between the mains supply and the appliance in use. The transformer isolates the active wires of the main electrical supply from earth so that contact with one active wire and earth does not result in electrocution. The magnitude of any fault current will be limited by this type of protection. The isolated electrical system is best fitted with an alarm that is actuated in the event of a fault occurring within the system. Supply of power is thus maintained.

Both the core balance earth-leakage device and the isolated supply system can be designed for installation into an electrical system or can be used as portable units whenever an electrical appliance is used in the suite. Incorporation by design is preferable.

The electrical installation for an operating suite cannot be designed to protect staff from electrocution by a defibrillator. That electrical hazard must be overcome by design of the instrument, good maintenance and a safe routine in the manner in which the defibrillator is used.

Microshock

The patient with an exteriorized electrically conductive pathway directly to the heart by way of an external pacemaker, wire or cardiac catheter may suffer microshock or electrocution death if currents in excess of $100\,\mu A$[10] are allowed to pass to the heart via these exteriorized pathways. Such minute currents may pass if the catheter or wire is in contact with a piece of equipment which is supposedly earthed but which is in fact part of a ground loop, and so carrying current. These currents can result from two or more pieces of equipment which are assumed to be at the same potential, but are not so because of inadequate earthing. The solution to the risk lies in the design of the electrical systems for operating theatres.

By the installation of an equipotential earth system   Details of such design are available from electrical codes for countries that have specified standards for electromedical treatment areas in hospitals[9]. The use of such an equipotential earth system means that any circuit or electrical conductor that may touch the patient will itself be kept substantially at the same potential so that no current will flow between any patient circuit, earth and any other conductor likely to touch or be touched by the patient.

By limiting any fault current that can flow through the equipotential earth system   This can be achieved by:

1. the use of a core balance earth leakage protection device that will limit the *duration* of the fault current;
2. the use of an isolation transformer that will limit the *magnitude* of the fault current.

Electrical interference

Only rarely do signals from mains-carried interference constitute a problem in operating rooms provided circuits to them are kept separate from other power circuits outside the operating suite. However, interaction between electrical devices within operating rooms is seen and an example is interference to the ECG signal from surgical diathermy. It is of practical interest to see engineering development now producing diathermy equipment that does not interfere with the ECG signal. Similarly, ECG monitors using satisfactory filters can reduce considerably interference from diathermy equipment.

Although interference of cardiac pacemaker function by diathermy can occur, their mutual use should not automatically be disqualified. To obviate the problem a few basic rules must be adhered to.

1. The diathermy leads must be positioned so that the electromagnetic field induced by the current flowing through them is as far from the cardiac pacemaker lead(s) as possible.
2. The pulse and ECG must be continuously monitored throughout the procedure.
3. A defibrillator and a spare external pacemaker with percutaneous electrodes must be available in the operating room preoperatively.
4. Special care needs to be taken when a demand (non-fixed rate) type pacemaker is in use.

Chemical hazards

It can be shown that in the absence of satisfactory venting of spilt anaesthetic gases and vapours, the tissues of people working regularly in theatres come into equilibration with the contaminating gases and vapours. Many studies have now been carried out to correlate this fact with a harmful, or significant morbidity result, so far without success. Suggested complaints and conditions not yet proven as statistically significant are:

headache[12]
irritability[12]
gastrointestinal upsets[12]
bronchitis[12]
death[13]
spontaneous abortion[12, 14, 15, 16]

tumours of the reticulo-endothelial system[13]
suicide[13]
congenital abnormalities[14, 16, 17]
infertility[15]

Until it can be shown[18] that the cause of these conditions is or is not related to the inhalation of spilt anaesthetic gases and vapours, it is good practice to exhaust the spilt agents outside the operating suite.

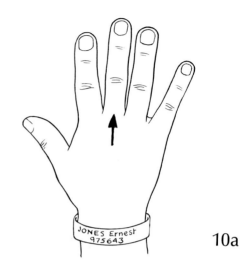

10a

Other hazards

10a & b

Identification of patient and operation site

Identification bracelets are commonly used but are only as good as those who are prepared to read and check them. Operation sites – where there is laterality – should be marked with a cross and digits with an arrow, but again this in no way absolves the surgeon from a personal and final check with the patient before anaesthesia is induced.

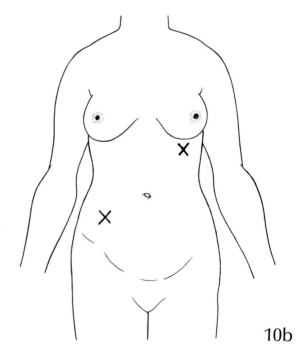

10b

11a–f

Pressure injuries

Foam rubber padding should protect any bony prominence. Sites particularly susceptible to injury are shown. Sudden use of steep Trendelenburg may shift the body on the arms so as to stretch the brachial plexus or impact it against shoulder supports or the head of the humerus if that is thrown forward by full external rotation of the shoulder joint.

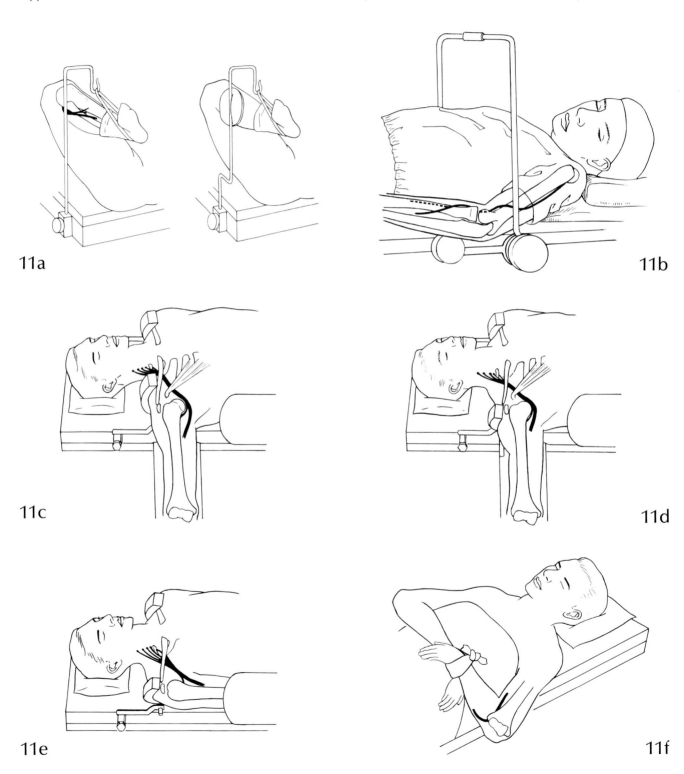

11a

11b

11c

11d

11e

11f

Strains

Unusual positions maintained for many hours may cause ligamentous strain, as may asymmetrical movement of limbs such as lifting a single limb into the lithotomy position, particularly if full relaxant anaesthesia permits an unusual degree of mobility.

Acknowledgement

Illustrations 1 and *3–10* have been adapted from *Safety in the Operating Theatre* (Edited by J. F. Mainland and Hugh Dudley, 1976) by kind permission of the publishers Edward Arnold (Australia) Pty Ltd, Melbourne. *Illustration 2* was kindly supplied by Mr John Weeks, and Illustration 11 has been adapted from Canadian Anaesthesia Society Journal 1969; 11: 514

References

1. Pütsep, E. Modern hospital: international planning practices. London: Lloyd Luke, 1979

2. Blowers, R., Craw, B. Ventilation of operating theatres. Journal of Hygiene 1960; 58: 427–448

3. Charnley, J. Theatre design. In: Karran, S., ed. Controversies in surgical sepsis, p. 3. Eastbourne and New York: Praeger, 1980

4. Joffe, S. N., Thomson, W. O., McGavigan, J., Trexler, P. C. A closed system surgical isolator for major elective abdominal operations. World Journal of Surgery 1978; 2: 123–130

5. Standards Association of Australia. Surgical Luminaires. AS 2501, 1981. Sydney: Standards Association of Australia, 1981

6. Standards Association of Australia. The lighting of operating rooms. AS 2502, 1981

7. British Standards Institution. Code of practice for selection, installation and maintenance of electrical apparatus for use in potentially explosive atmosphere (other than mining applications or explosive processing and manufacture). BS5345, Parts 1, 3, 4, 6, 7, 1976–1979

8. National Fire Protection Association. Inhalation anesthetics. NFPA56A, 1973. New York: National Fire Protection Association, 1973

9. Standards Association of Australia. Rules for minimising hazards arising from the use of flammable medical agents and non-flammable medical gases. AS1169, 1973

10. Watson, A. B., Wright, J. S., Loughman, J. Electrical threshold for ventricular fibrillation in man. Medical Journal of Australia 1973; 1: 1179–1182

11. Standards Association of Australia. Rules for electrical wiring and equipment in electro-medical treatment areas of hospitals. AS3003, 1976

12. Vaisman, A. I. Usloviia truda v operatisionnykh i ikh vliianie na zdorov's anesteziologov. Eksperimentalnaya khirurgiya i anesteziologiya 1967; 12: 44–49

13. Bruce, D. L., Eide, K. A., Linde, H. W., Eckenhoff, J. E. Causes of death amongst anaesthesiologists: a 20 year survey. Anaesthesiology 1968; 29: 565–569

14. Askrog, V. S., Harvald, B. Teratogen effect of inhalations. Anaestetika Nordisk Medicin 1970; 83: 498–500

15. Cohen, E. N., Belville, J. W., Brown, B. W. Anaesthesia, pregnancy and miscarriage. Anaesthesiology 1971; 35: 343–347

16. Knill-Jones, R. P., Rodrigues, L. V., Moir, D. D., Spence, A. A. Anaesthetic practice and pregnancy. Controlled survey of women anaesthetists in the United Kingdom. Lancet 1972; 1: 1326–1328

17. Fink, B. R., Shepherd, T. H., Blandau, R. J. Teratogenic activity of nitrous oxide. Nature 1967; 214: 146–148

18. Editorial. Harmful pollution by anaesthetic gases? Lancet 1972; 2: 519–521

Illustrations by Gillian Lee, Michael Courtney and Geoff Lyth

Operative techniques

Hugh Dudley   ChM, FRCS(Ed.), FRACS, FRCS
Professor of Surgery, St Mary's Hospital, London

Walter J. Pories   MD, FACS
Professor and Chairman, Department of Surgery, School of Medicine,
East Carolina University, Greenville, North Carolina

Introduction

Every surgeon is an individualist and every surgical team has its own particular way of doing things. There is sufficient scope for difference in the craft of surgery to make these statements appropriate. All that this section sets out to do is to provide some general rules about operating room layout and the techniques of handling common surgical instruments against which surgeons can study, assess and possibly modify their own practice.

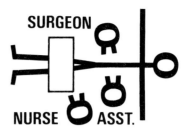

1a

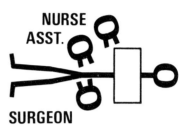

1b

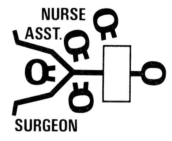

1c

Operative dispositions

1a, b & c

Operating team dispositions

Where, as is most often the case, there is a scrub nurse
and a surgeon as the basic team, the principle of 'right
hand to right hand' should be followed. This means that
for, say an upper abdominal procedure, the arrangement
is as in *Illustration 1a* and for a lower abdominal procedure
as in *Illustration 1b*. Note that as in *Illustration 1b* this
means that the instrument table will be over the patient's
head and shoulders for a pelvic procedure done by a
right-handed surgeon. It is often helpful to set up the
patient for a lower abdominal procedure as shown in
Illustration 1c – the lithotomy-Trendelenburg position –
even if a perineal procedure is not initially contemplated.
First, it allows manipulations per rectum such as wash-
outs; second, it permits a perineal operation to be done
if occasion arises; third, a second assistant can stand
between the patient's legs. Similar dispositions can be
worked out for operations on the chest and head and
neck.

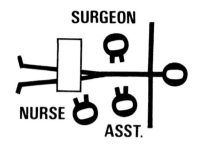

2a

2a, b & c

Visibility

At all times the scrub nurse should be able to see the operating field. Intelligent anticipation of the sequence of an operation is based on such visibility. For abdominal surgery an eccentric position for the instrument table (*Illustration 2a*), rather than that shown in *Illustrations 1a* and *b*, helps, but even so the nurse is likely to be at a greater distance from the site of the operation than is the surgeon. Consequently, if she is to see she must be at a slightly higher level (*Illustrations 2b* and *c*). This also facilitates drop passage of instruments (*see next page*).

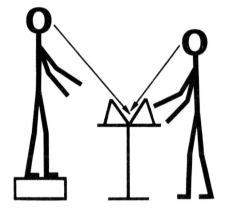

2b

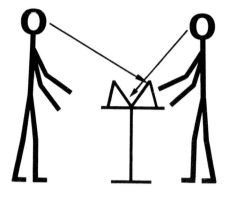

2c

3

Instrument zones

The general arrangement for all procedures should be: an in-use zone (for an abdominal procedure the field and its immediate vicinity) in which instruments are either in use or are discarded; a ready-use zone – usually an instrument stand or table; and a back-up zone that contains reserves. The last may be a completely packaged supply system rather than a layout. The contents of each zone will be determined by the instrument supply system and the individual procedure. The back-up zone is often heavily overloaded if it is a layout as distinct from specially designed trays, and operating room staff should be encouraged to prune this as much as possible.

The ready-use zone in which nursing staff handle instruments and sutures often suffers in terms of illumination by comparison with the operating field. This makes increasing demands on the visual acuity of nursing staff; a high standard of illumination is called for and can be achieved (*see p. 90*).

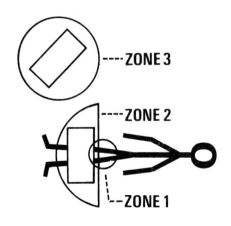

3

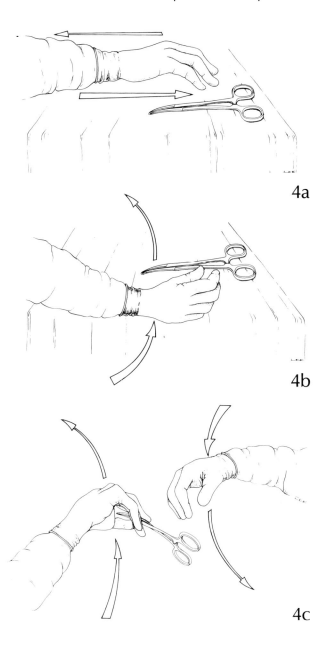

4a

4b

4c

4a, b & c

Interaction between scrub nurse and surgeon

Good surgical practice is based on a smooth flowing sequence of movements by the surgeon, the scrub nurse and by both in relation to each other. To and fro 'grab' movements (*Illustration 4a*) require acceleration and deceleration of the hand-arm complex and thus tend to be imprecise. By contrast, ballistic movements (*Illustration 4b*) in which the hand moves in an arc are associated with smooth changes in pace. Double ballistic movements in opposite directions (*Illustration 4c*) permit interchanges of instruments most elegantly and efficiently between scrub nurse and surgeon. Note that it is essential that the scrub nurse holds the instrument in such a way that its handles are clear for the surgeon to grasp. Curved instruments – which are the rule – must be adjusted in their delivery so that they follow the curve of the right or left hand.

5

'Drop passages'

Some instruments such as dissecting forceps are taken into the hand in particular ways which require the surgeon to have access to the whole instrument. To achieve this, the scrub nurse needs to keep the instrument vertical while the surgeon's hand sweeps the instrument away. This is most easily achieved if the scrub nurse is at a slightly higher level than is the surgeon – the instrument drops to his level as it is passed.

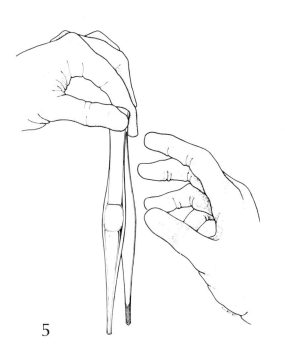

5

Basic instruments and techniques

Dissecting forceps

6

It is remarkable how a few basic instruments have stood the test of time. The top end spring tweezer, the basis of the dissecting forceps, goes back at least 3000 years. It is *normally open* and graded pressure using the triangular grip of Vanghetti allows very precise closure and by its opposition of forces reduces tremor at the tips.

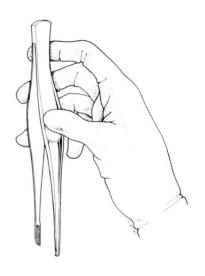

6

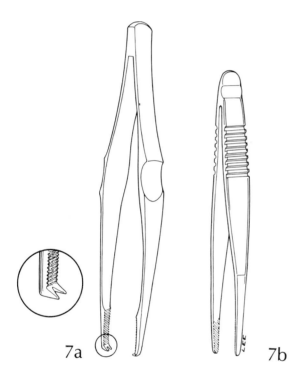

7a   7b

7a & b

There are two main types: (*a*) toothed for grasping tissues which contain large amounts of collagen and thus have strong tear resistance; and (*b*) plain which exert their grip over a wide area and thus are relatively less likely to do damage. There are many varieties of both and little to judge in terms of performance, though in this as in many other areas, the surgeon will soon develop his special like or prejudice. Either type may be 'bridged' so that the grasp of a needle is facilitated (the toothed forceps in (*a*) has this construction) as is described on p. 117).

8

One of the greatest conveniences of the dissecting forceps is that it can be stored in the palm of the hand between the fourth and fifth fingers and the hypothenar eminence.

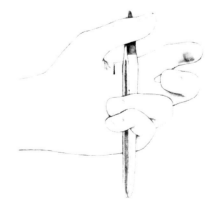

8

Ringed instruments

9a–d

Ringed instruments may either be simple crossovers such as a scissors or incorporate a fixing ratchet (usually ascribed to Spencer Wells) which locks them in position. Most surgeons will favour curved instruments for these are an extension of the curved ballistic orientation of the hand (a). It follows that the instrument must be presented to the surgeon appropriately aligned to the hand. Such instruments usually have their point applied to the tissues, either to grasp or cut, and this is best achieved using the thumb and a combination of third and fourth fingers for grasping and the index finger to orientate the tip (b) – again a triangular grip. Such instruments will normally be used with the hand in supination (c) because pronation (d) obscures the operator's view.

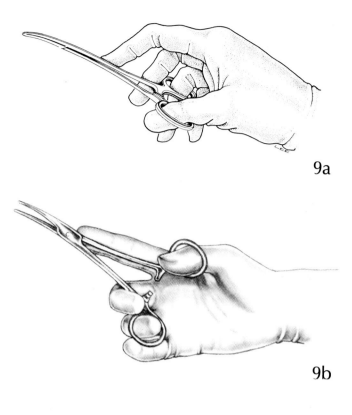

9a

9b

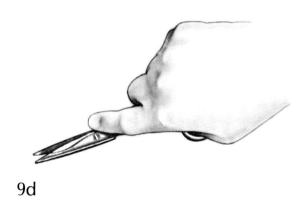

9d

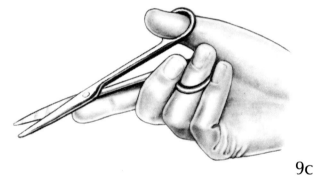

9c

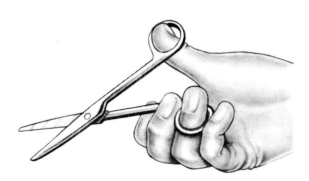

10

10

Scissors work because of the angular apposition of their blades. To achieve this the right-handed surgeon pushes up with the thumb and pulls down with the ring and middle finger. Again this action is facilitated by full supination. A left-handed surgeon has to make the reverse movements which accounts for his potential awkwardness, particularly when beginning his training. However, with suitable initial conscious instruction the use of a scissors in the left hand soon becomes second nature, whatever the initial 'handedness' of the individual.

11

Ringed instruments may be palmed in the same way as dissecting forceps.

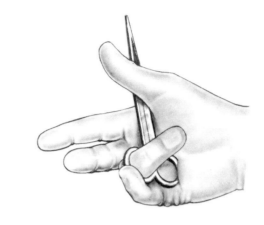

11

12

Assistants will often turn a scissors even further back on the fourth finger so that the blades lie in line with the forearm. This is tidy, but flexibility in terms of bringing the instrument into use is lost.

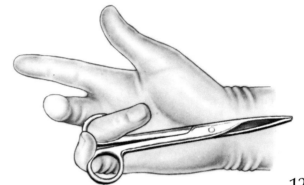

12

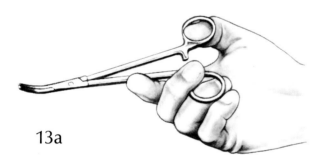

13a

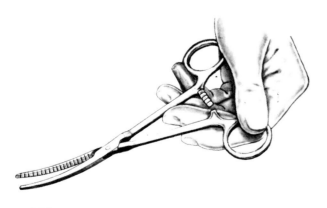

13b

13a & b

Removing ratchet instruments

The temptation is to remove these forceps in the same way as they are applied, by inserting the fingers into the rings. This is not necessary – the techniques shown permit the hand to be kept supine and, as practical experience will attest, full control to be maintained over the tips.

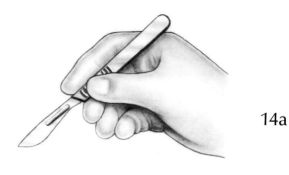

14a

14a, b & c

Handling the knife

Knife blades are a compromise between stabber and shearer because in many procedures a little of both is required. Two grips are available – (a) the pen grip which permits fine angulation and (b and c) the 'stroke' grip which allows the knife to be used with some force. The pen grip is suitable for fine dissection, but cannot properly incise (say) the abdominal wall. It is to be noted that passage of the knife from scrub nurse to surgeon should again be by the 'drop passage' or else the scrub nurse can be injured by the surgeon drawing the knife down out of her hand.

Dissection

The basis of soft tissue dissection is that tissues are placed in tension – one cannot dissect a jelly. This may be achieved by either of two ways.

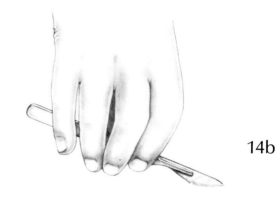

14b

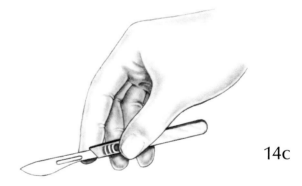

14c

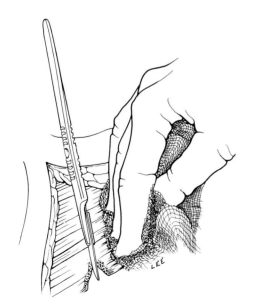

15

15

1. Displacing the tissues with one hand while using a sharp instrument with the other. The illustration shows a fascial plane being dealt with but the principle is equally applicable to say the dissection of the fatty contents of the axilla off the axillary vascular pedicle (*see* p. 271).

16a, b & c

2. Lifting the tissues with dissecting forceps in the left hand while using a sharp instrument, usually scissors but sometimes a knife, with the right. Such dissection may be sharp (*a*) or blunt (*b* and *c*) in which the scissors are used to prise the tissues apart by opening the blades.

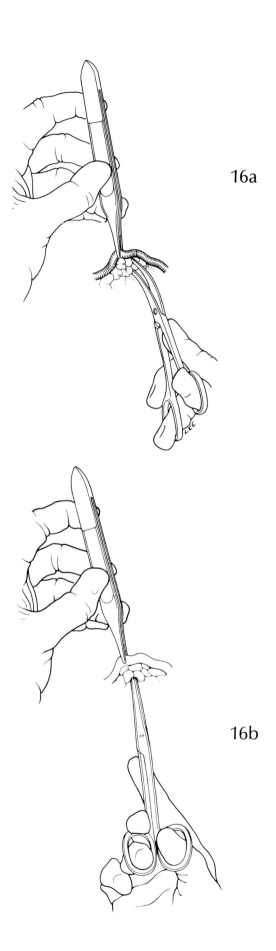

16a

16b

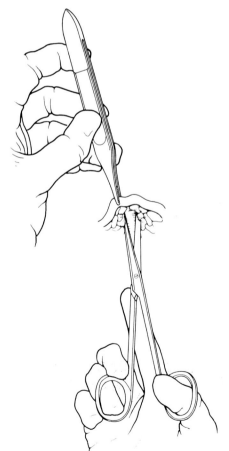

16c

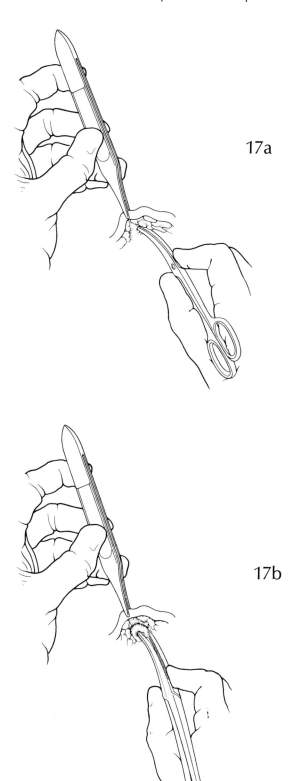

17a

17b

17a & b

Other techniques of blunt dissection may use the tip of an instrument such as scissors or artery forceps to push tissues to one side (a), or a pledget (Lahey; 'newt'; dab) for the same purpose (b).

Dissection styles differ with surgical cultures. Blunt dissection is usually safer unless the surgeon has a very delicate touch and great anatomical familiarity with the region. Sharp dissection is more precise, less traumatic and, in the last analysis, has elegance.

Haemostasis

18

Pressure and traction

Pressure is the simplest and perhaps the most effective technique for controlling haemorrhage. Even large vessels will frequently stop bleeding if pressure is maintained evenly and long enough. A minimum of 5 min is required; 10 is even better. The pressure must be timed by the clock as it is hard to gauge time accurately in an emergency. A combination of pressure and traction are the assistant's best surgical tools. A firm continued pull exposes tissue, controls ooze and provides stability for the surgeon.

19

Packing

Although haemostasis is best achieved by ligation or cauterization of individual vessels, there are times when such precise control is not possible. Such challenges arise, for example, when diffuse pelvic venous bleeding follows an abdominoperineal resection, when drainage of an abscess is followed by a continuous ooze, or in situations where the patient's condition is too serious to allow further dissection and additional blood loss. Packing is an effective approach in such situations. The space is tightly filled with dry gauze rolls, in a manner which allows a tail of each bandage to protrude. The packs can usually be removed after 48 h. This technique is used less frequently today, because the new haemostatic agents, such as absorbable gauze (Surgicel) and collagen generally control such situations more safely and more effectively.

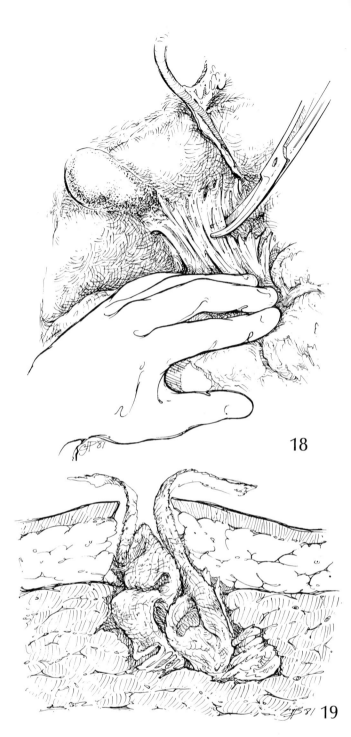

18

19

20

Clamp and twist

Clamping and twisting of small bleeding vessels is a useful technique in the emergency room or during a minor surgical procedure when no assistant is available for ligature. The technique is simple, but it must be performed precisely to be effective. The vessel must be clamped cleanly and twisted two or three times before release. Inclusion of nearby fat, skin or fascia interferes with the method and must be avoided.

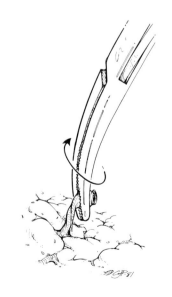

20

Clamp and ligature

The clamp and ligature remain the mainstays of modern surgical technique. Although many types of clamps and ligatures are available, the principles of the technique remain constant.

21

1. The vessel should be grasped cleanly with the tip of the clamp, avoiding the inclusion of other tissues.
2. When the clamp is held for ligature, it should be handled gently, because one may easily shear off the vessel, especially in inflamed tissues. The ligature can be managed more easily if the tip of the clamp is pointed gently upward.

22

3. The clamp should be removed slowly so that the ligature can be tightened while the vessel is still under control and so that the tissues can be gathered by the tie without being torn.
4. The ligature should be tightened against itself, rather than off at an angle.
5. Small ligatures usually suffice; it is unusual to require anything larger than a 3/0 suture.
6. Ligatures should be snug but not forced down too tightly; vessels are easily cut.

23a, b & c

Clamping with double ligature

It is often wise to secure a large or critical vessel with a double ligature. The two-clamp technique assures control of the vessel while the ligature is being applied and facilitates separation between the two ties. After two gently curved clamps are applied in parallel fashion, the first ligature is applied below the paired clamps, and, as the knot is tightened, the lower clamp is removed. The remaining clamp is then handled in the usual manner, leaving the vascular stump with two ties 1 mm apart.

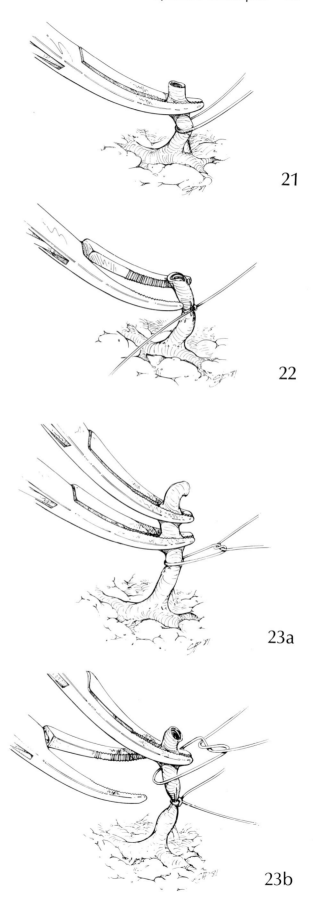

21

22

23a

23b

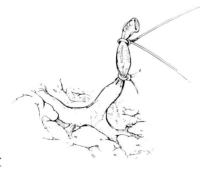

23c

24a–e

Ligature in continuity

Ligature in continuity is another way to provide additional safety in haemostasis and is therefore useful in the management of larger vessels. Following dissection of the vessel so that an adequate length of vessel is exposed, two ties are pulled through and ligated as far apart as is reasonably possible. The division is begun with a small initial cut to ensure that flow has been fully controlled and is then completed if the field remains dry. Occasionally, it may be wise to ligate each vessel twice before division; if so, a second tie may be placed immediately over the first and tightened down, the 'tie on tie, but not knot on knot' technique.

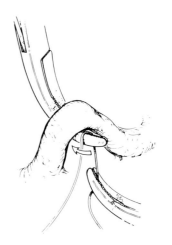

24a

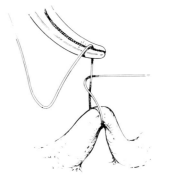

24b

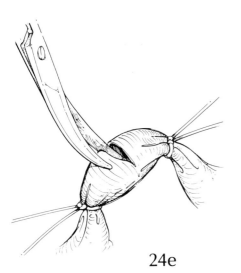

24e

24d

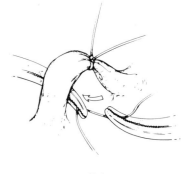

24c

25a, b & c

Suture ligature

Additional security may be obtained by the suture ligature, which prevents slipping of the tie in a layer of friable vessel. After the vessel has been doubly ligated, it is transfixed with a swaged-on suture which is then looped around the vessel before it is tied.

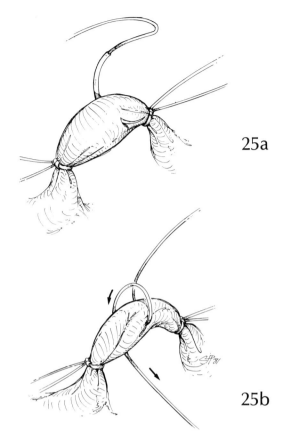

25a

25b

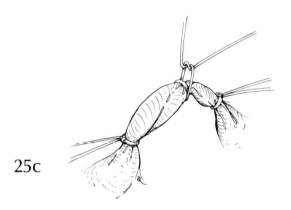

25c

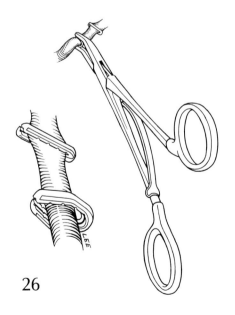

26

26

Clips

As an alternative to ligature, fine clips may be used, applied with special forceps. The vessel must be completely cleared of adventitious tissue. It is not advisable to use these clips where further dissection is to be undertaken because they are quite easily entangled in gauze and pulled off.

27

Ligature or embolization of 'feeding' vessels

Occasionally, diffuse bleeding in such areas as the pelvis can be almost impossible to control by local measures. In such cases, as in severe pelvic fractures, ligature of the proximal feeding vessels, in this case the internal iliac arteries, can be most helpful. More recently, embolization of such vessels with wire springs or absorbable gelatin sponge (Gelfoam) by percutaneous catheter fluoroscopic approaches has proven to be equally effective in appropriate cases.

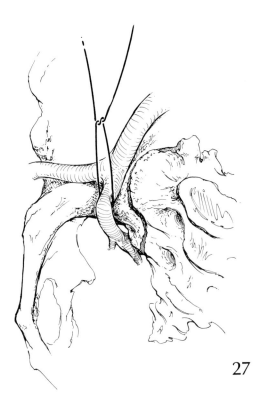

27

Emergency repair of injured vessels

When critical vessels are injured, ligature may not be safe, and repair may be needed instead. Details of the various vascular surgical techniques are presented in the *Vascular Surgery* volume, but it is appropriate to give the basic principles here.

Control of proximal and distal flow

28

This can be achieved by a number of techniques, varying from finger pressure and vessel loops to vascular clamps. A particularly useful instrument for control of large vessels in emergency situations is the 'sponge on two sticks', consisting of a tightly folded 10 × 20 cm (4 × 8 inch) sponge held by two sponge sticks. The instrument is quickly assembled from universally available items, allows application of firm pressure, takes up little room in the operative field, does not damage the vessel, and is easily held by the assistant.

28

29

When dissection of the vessel is difficult or injudicious, a balloon catheter may also be used to provide vascular control. A Foley catheter with a 5 ml bag is just about the size needed for control of the aorta or vena cava, and Fogarty catheters in various sizes suffice for most smaller vessels.

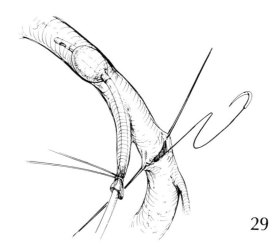

29

Avoidance of occluding clot

A vascular repair is useful only if it restores flow. The two ends of the vessel should therefore be vigorously flushed of clots, and, if flow is not good, an embolectomy catheter should be passed. Flow is often hard to judge; in questionable cases, intraoperative angiography is strongly recommended.

Whether heparin is useful in such cases remains a disputed point. Most surgeons use it, at doses of 5000–10 000 u, but there are many reports of extensive vascular procedures without anticoagulants. If they are used, however, reversal with protamine is advised, to avoid postoperative haemorrhage.

Gentle handling of vascular tissues

Vascular tissues are delicate and repay the surgeon for clumsiness and rough technique by clotting and developing atherosclerosis later at the areas of intimal injury. Even in emergencies, the surgeon is cautioned to use special vascular clamps and gentle techniques.

Fine suture material

Alexis Carrel pointed out long ago that fine needles and sutures are essential for excellent vascular repair. His principle still applies. Fine tapered needles are used, swaged onto monofilament polypropylene sutures, varying from 6/0 to 3/0, depending upon the size of the vessels.

Protection from infection

Vascular suture lines are vulnerable to infection and do not stand up well under infection. At best, the vessels thrombose; at worst, the anastomoses break down, resulting in serious or fatal haemorrhage. Infection is best minimized in vascular emergencies by the following measures.

Careful asepsis and debridement
Avoidance of vascular synthetic prostheses
Coverage with viable tissues
Antibiotic administration at the time of repair and for at least 48 h thereafter; a cephalosporin is most suitable

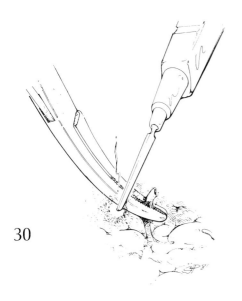

30

30

Cautery

The cautery, previously discredited as an instrument which produced too much gangrene and encouraged infection, is widely used today. Both monopolar and bipolar instruments are available. The cautery, like ligature techniques, works best when it is precisely directed at a cleanly grasped vessel and used in brief spurts. When it is used to cut skin and to burn large areas of tissue indiscriminately, however, it will leave large areas of necrosis likely to interfere with healing and support infection.

Haemostatic agents

A variety of haemostatic agents is now available for use in the operating room.

31a & b

Haemostatic cellulose gauze

Surgicel and Oxycel are gauzelike materials made of cellulose which have proved over the last decade to be particularly effective in vascular surgery. Surgicel can be applied directly to suture lines and held in place with gentle pressure for about 5 min. One of its great advantages is that it can be left in place. It appears to have considerable anti-infective properties.

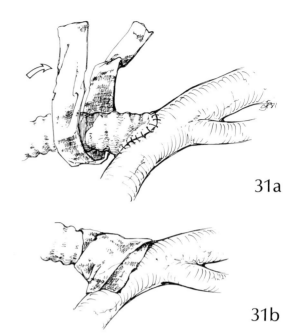

31a

31b

32

Gelatin sponge with thrombin

Pledgets of gelatin prepared to spongelike consistency and soaked in a solution of thrombin (Gelfoam) can be an effective haemostatic agent, especially in small areas of ooze, as in brain surgery. It has not been proven to be as useful in vascular surgery or most general surgery.

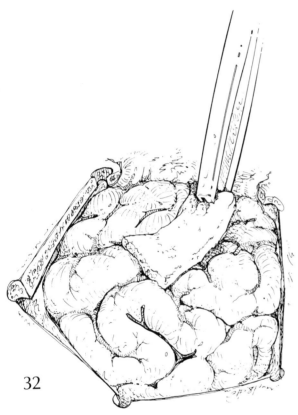

32

33

Fibrillary collagen

Avitene is a powdery, fluffy and effective haemostatic agent prepared from collagen. It is particularly useful for controlling haemorrhage from capsular injuries of the liver, spleen and kidney. The powder is difficult to handle because it sticks to gloves and instruments as well as to tissues. It must therefore be applied with clean forceps and held in place with a clean, dry sponge. Temporary occlusion of inflow to the injured organ during the application of the Avitene can be helpful if the bleeding is brisk.

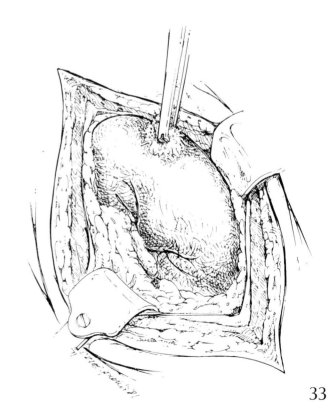

33

34

Bone wax and other materials

Bleeding from bony surfaces, such as occurs with a sternotomy, is best handled by the application of small pledgets of beeswax into the oozing interstices. Alternatively and preferably, a fibrin preparation made from whole blood has the same effects. The excess can be wiped away easily; the small amount left in the bone is well tolerated.

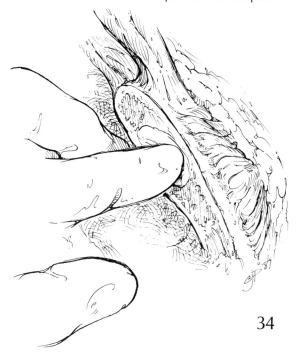

34

Percutaneous catheter embolization

Embolization by the new percutaneous radiographic catheter techniques is not a procedure generally performed by surgeons, but it is so useful that it is included here for completeness. The authors have experience of its effective use in massive haemorrhage from the colon, duodenum and pelvic fractures. Angiographers have reported good results with autogenous clots, Gelfoam, Oxycel, Ivalon, Silastic and metal spheres, autogenous fat and muscle, isobutyl 2-cyanoanalate, silicone rubber, sclerosing agents, wool coil occluders and balloon catheters.

35 & 36

The illustrations show the pre- and postembolization films of a man aged 71 years with massive bleeding from a fistula between the superior mesenteric artery and vein following drainage of an abscess. The bleeding was controlled, and the patient recovered uneventfully. The reader is directed to the excellent review by Johnsrude and Jackson[1] for further information about this new approach.

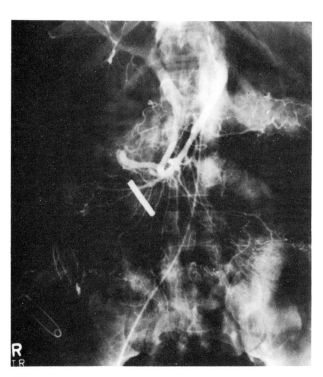

35

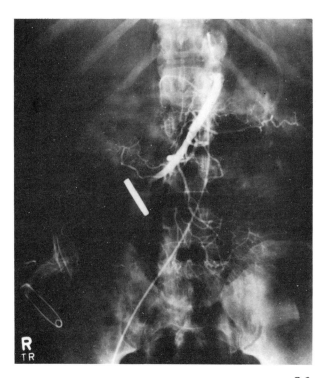

36

Sewing

Opinion is divided on the use of the hand or of a needle holder. Obviously the dictates of fine work require a needle holder to carry the small needles involved and this is seen at its acme in microsurgical work. However, many would argue that to hold the needle in the hand permits more accurate placement of the point. The problem remains unresolved, but clearly there are many circumstances in which only a needle holder will suffice.

37a & b

Hand sewing

Two forms are seen: (a) a curved needle which is used like any curved instrument along the ballistic trajectory of the hand and predominantly *towards* the surgeon; (b) a straight needle pointed away from the operator and held in a pinch or driving grip. The latter is more applicable to structures which are on or can be brought to the surface. Both techniques are precise, but obviously the size of the hand limits the fine nature of the work. Hand sewing is particularly suitable for the insertion of continuous sutures in, say, the abdominal wall or skin. Precise work on viscera, vessels or nerves usually calls for small sutures inserted with a needle holder.

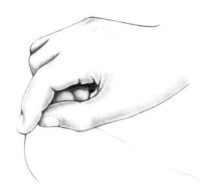

37a

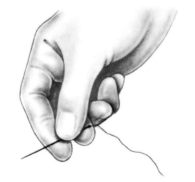

37b

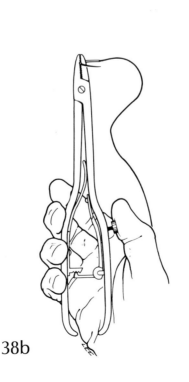

38a

38b

Needle holder sewing

38a & b

Conventional needle holders follow the ratchet principle, presumably because the surgeon is most familiar with it. However, they are most commonly used in the palm of the hand, the ratchet being swung on and off by gentle pressure (a). This is mechanically effective but does require angular motion. For this reason many 'spring-loaded' needle holders have been devised, prominent amongst which is Hegar's (b). However, perhaps because of the surgeon's adaptive dexterity, none is commonly used except in microsurgery.

39a, b & c

The tissue is grasped with the appropriate dissecting forceps (a) to provide counter pressure against which the needle can be thrust. Then either the needle holder is transposed to draw out the emerging end of the needle (b) or this is achieved with the dissecting forceps (c). Both techniques are useful in specific circumstances, but in either event it is important to impart a rotary movement to the needle so as not to tear the tissues with its haft.

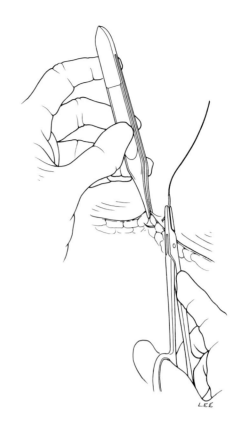

39a

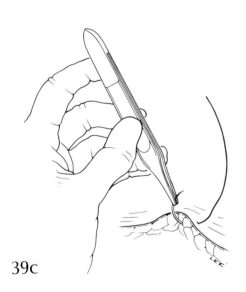

39c

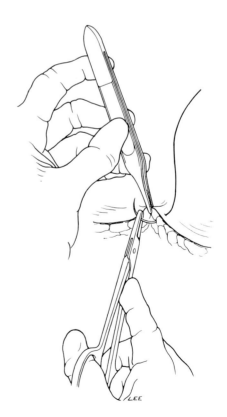

39b

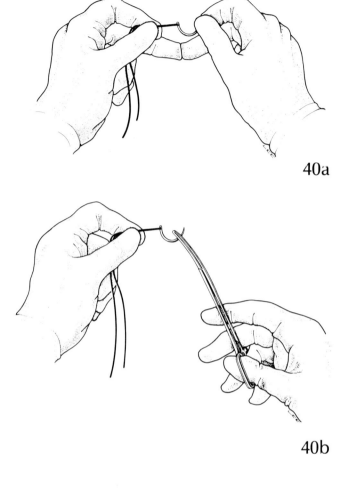

40a

40b

40a & b

When fine interrupted sutures are to be inserted in large numbers, the surgeon, armed with a needle holder, can accept these from the scrub nurse one at a time – either from between the fingers (a) or if she holds them in a forceps (b). As he uses the needle he can conveniently discard it into a small dish from which all can be retrieved and counted.

Reference

1. Johnsrude, I. S., Jackson, D. C. A practical approach to angiography. Boston: Little, Brown & Co., 1979

Ligatures and suture materials

C. R. Kapadia, MB, FRCS
Lecturer in Surgery, Academic Surgical Unit, St Mary's Hospital Medical School, London

Fundamentals

Though surgeons choose suture materials for individual tasks largely on the basis of pragmatics and tradition, some fundamentals can be stated with varying degrees of confidence.

Tissues that are mainly formed of collagen – fascia, aponeurosis and tendon – heal slowly, so that only about half of the original tensile strength has been recovered at 3 months. Thus, absorbable sutures whether natural (catgut), synthetic (braids of polyglycolic acid: Dexon; Vicryl) or, more recently, monofilament polydioxanone (PDS) do not persist long enough for adequate structural integrity to be restored. However, the healing curve (which reflects the laying down of collagen) is initially steep so that fascial or aponeurotic wounds closed with absorbable sutures (particularly synthetics) may have just enough strength to resist disruption (*Figure 1*). This is the less likely if there are distractive forces such as occur in an abdominal wound (*see below*).

By contrast, tissues which do not contain much structural collagen develop this rapidly at the site of the wound so that – other things being equal (and sepsis and malnutrition may make this *not* the case) – the tensile strength at the suture line rapidly exceeds that of the wounded structure (*Figure 2*).

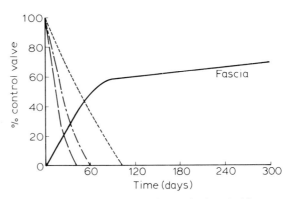

Figure 1. Healing curves of fascial wounds closed with monofilament polydioxanone (– – – –), polydioxanone/polyglycolic acid (– · – · –) and catgut (– – –)

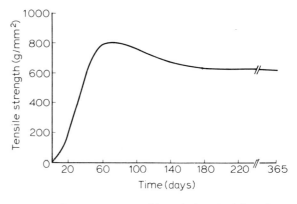

Figure 2. Healing curve in a small bowel where initial tensile strength is low (<400g/mm²)

Materials

Absorbables

Catgut, the conventional, natural, monofilament absorbable, provokes an inflammatory reaction which prolongs the preparative phase (that in which no increase in intrinsic tensile strength occurs) and is also synergistic with the common intestinal organisms in promoting wound sepsis. The comparative effects of some sutures on tissue reactivity and the ability to provoke sepsis are shown (*Figures 3* and *4*). Though synthetic absorbables do cause an inflammatory reaction, they do not promote wound sepsis and indeed polyglycolic acid may actually reduce it.

Non-absorbables

Non-absorbable sutures can be divided into natural and synthetic. Generally, the former results in more tissue reaction than the latter. Of the natural non-absorbables, cotton and linen are the most irritant; silk the least. Furthermore, their twisted or, preferably, braided structure does result in many nooks and crannies in which organisms can lurk, so that infection, once established, tends to persist until the suture material is discharged or removed.

Synthetic non-absorbables – stainless steel, nylon, polyester, polypropylene – may be provided either as monofilaments or as braids. All monofilaments provoke little or no reaction in the long term after an initial brief period of inflammatory cell infiltrate. Monofilament sutures have the advantage of not providing a nidus for the persistence of infection. However, most monofilaments handle less sympathetically than do braids.

Sutures must not only coapt wounds but also hold them so. Disruptive forces may be non-existent, moderate or severe. When disruptive forces are absent, it suffices that the suture lasts, or is left in, only until a good 'glue' holds the edges of the wound together. Such is the case with surface wounds which have been brought together by a longer lasting deep layer of stitches in the dermis. In this situation the wound edges can be approximated with skin sutures, clips or by 'sutureless closure' (e.g., Steri-strips, Op-Site – *see* p. 133) and these can be removed in 36–72 h. Where disruptive forces exist – and this is often the case in fascial layers such as the abdominal wall – the integrity of the wound is determined by three factors.

1. The absolute strength of the suture material which, for the purpose, may need to exceed that of the tissue to allow for the loss of strength at the knot.
2. The suture-tissue interface – the thicker the strand, the less the force per unit area at the interface and hence the less the tendency for 'cutting out' to occur.
3. The durability of the suture material, so that it provides support for as long as is required for intrinsic tissue strength to be restored.

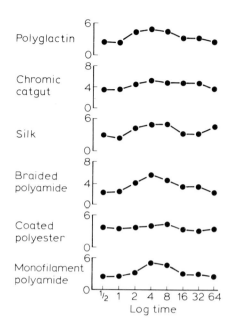

Figure 3. Time course and intensity of reaction to commonly used sutures

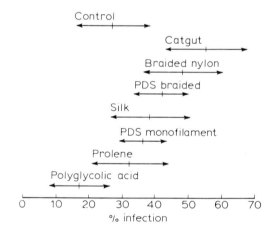

Figure 4. Effects of some sutures on incidence of experimental infection with mixed intestinal organisms. All sutures except polyglycolic acid are associated with some increase in infection

These factors, taken in conjunction with others, such as potential sepsis, make the use of non-absorbables – preferably synthetic monofilaments – the surgical *standard* for wound closure or reconstruction (e.g. tendons) whenever there are distractive forces. Thus, in closure of the abdominal wall, large bites which distribute force per unit area widely are preferred.

Table 1 Properties of common suture materials

Material	Nature	Type	Tissue response	Retention of tensile strength in vivo	Handleability	Potential advantages/ disadvantages
Catgut	Sheep submucosa	Absorbable	Inflammation more marked with plain catgut than chromic	Plain – 2/3 lost in 5–6 days Chromic – 2/3 lost in 10–15 days	Moderate	Unpredictable loss of tensile strength. Potentiation of sepsis, though this is limited by absorption. Variability of natural product
Reconstituted collagen	Sheep mucosa	Absorbable	Inflammation as with catgut	As for chromic catgut	Moderate	As for catgut, but more reliable product
Polyglycolic acid/polyglactic acid/polydioxanone	Synthetic polymer	Absorbable	Slight – absorbed with variable but muted inflammatory reaction	Variable – ½ lost in 15 days (braided). Monofilament loses strength much more slowly	Good – particularly in braided form	Predictable loss of tensile strength. Less potentiation of sepsis than catgut
Linen	Vegetable	Non-absorbable	Moderate inflammation	⅓ to ½ strength lost in 3–6 months	Very good	Cheap. Variability of supply and performance
Silk	Silk worm	Non-absorbable	Mild to moderate inflammation	½ strength lost in 2–12 months	Very good	Fairly cheap. Variability of supply. Cost likely to rise
Nylon	Synthetic polyamide	Non-absorbable	Minimal	⅔ strength retained up to 6 months	Poor in monofilament, good in braid	Knot slippage in monofilament
Polypropylene	Synthetic	Non-absorbable	Minimal	As for nylon	Superior to nylon in monofilament. Not available in braid	'Elastic' in its properties. Knot slippage. Can fracture in certain situations (artery)
Coated polyester	Synthetic (polytetrafluoroethylene coated braid)	Non-absorbable	Minimal to moderate	As for nylon	Good because of its combination of braid and monofilament coat	Knot slippage. Fracture of coat and increased inflammatory response
Stainless steel	Synthetic	Non-absorbable	Virtually nil	Theoretically indefinite, but monofilament shows fatigue fractures at 1 year	Poor in monofilament. Moderate in braided	Inertness. Troublesome knots and wound pain

The handling properties of sutures are of importance to the surgeon. In this respect braids are preferable to monofilaments. Attempts to combine the impervious qualities of the latter with the handling characteristics of the former by coating a braid with a film of inert plastic (e.g. polytetrafluoroethylene) have been promising but not entirely successful. A further property allied to handling characteristics is drag through the tissues: monofilaments are superior in this respect.

From the above considerations it is apparent that no single suture material could possibly satisfy the diverse criteria needed for suture materials in practice. The advantages and disadvantages of suture materials are shown in *Table 1*. However, opinion increasingly favours synthetic non-absorbable materials. The synthetic absorbables, polyglycolic acid, polyglactic acid and polydioxanone, are hydrolysed and absorbed in a more predictable fashion, unlike the absorption of catgut. Though associated with some inflammatory response, this is less than that obtained with catgut. Thus, they should be used in preference to catgut in situations where this material was previously used.

Technical aspects

It is now possible to produce suture material in a wide variety of sizes down to and beyond the visual acuity of the eye (*Table 2*). Such fine material has its place in the delicate coaptation of tissues subject to little disruptive force. For ordinary uses of macrosurgery, sutures ranging from 6/0 (1 metric) to 2 (6 metric) are adequate, the former being used for fine vessel anastomosis, the latter for the approximation of tissues such as the anterior abdominal wall where considerable distraction is foreseen.

Sutures may come in lengths or be ready swaged to a needle – the so-called atraumatic suture. Drag and tissue trauma are reduced by the latter and it should be only rarely that eyed needles are preferred. It must be admitted, however, that the exact benefit of the atraumatic needle in general surgical practice has never been established. The most we can say is that certain surgical procedures – e.g. vascular anastomosis and tendon repair – would be virtually impossible without them.

An addition to the armamentarium is the 'controlled release' suture, which will come off the needle when a quick jerk is applied between suture and needle – useful when multiple interrupted sutures are employed (e.g. in intestinal anastomoses).

Table 2

Metric number*	Former gauge	
	Catgut/collagen	Non-absorbables and synthetic absorbables
0.1	–	–
0.2	–	10/0
0.3	–	9/0
0.4	–	8/0 (virgin silk)
0.4	–	8/0
0.5	8/0	7/0
0.7	7/0	6/0
1	6/0	5/0
1.5	5/0	4/0
2	4/0	3/0
3	3/0	2/0
3.5	2/0	0
4	0	1
5	1	2
6	2	3 and 4
7	3	5
8	4	6

* Metric numbers – diameter of suture in tenths of a millimetre

1

Needles may be curved, J-shaped or straight; curved needles come in a wide range of diameters suitable for either hand-sewing or for use with needle holders. The needles themselves may either be round-bodied, taper-cut or cutting, the first being atraumatic, the last the most traumatic. Round-bodied needles are suitable for use in most general surgical situations, except the suture of tough, dense tissue, when a cutting needle is necessary.

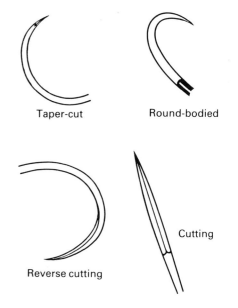

Taper-cut   Round-bodied

Reverse cutting   Cutting

1

Conclusions

Different surgeons will perform the same operations with sutures that differ widely in their properties and yet produce the same results. This is undoubtedly the consequence of Nature's ability to overcome many of our deficiencies and the relative margin of safety common to most suture material. However, the principles outlined can be used to provide a wise choice of the most appropriate suture material for any given surgical circumstance.

Further reading

The literature is very large but the following are useful further reading.

General

Hunt, T. K., Dunphy, J. E., eds. *Fundamentals of wound management*. New York: Appleton-Century-Crofts, 1979

Irvin, T. T. *Wound healing: principles and practice*. London and New York: Chapman and Hall, 1981

Specific

Healing in fascial layers

Douglas, D. M. The healing of aponeurotic incisions. British Journal of Surgery 1952–1953; 40: 79–84

Tissue responses

Fontaine, C. J., Dudley, H. A. F. Assessment of suture materials for intestinal use by an extramucosal implant technique and a quantitative histological evaluation. British Journal of Surgery 1978; 65: 288–290

Van Winkle, W., Hastings, J. C. Considerations in the choice of suture materials for various tissues. Surgery, Gynecology and Obstetrics 1972; 135: 113–126

Infection

Hunt, T. K., ed. *Wound healing and wound infection: theory and surgical practice*. New York: Appleton-Century-Crofts, 1980

McGeehan, D., Hunt, D., Chaudhuri, A., Rutter, P. An experimental study of the relationship between synergistic wound sepsis and suture materials. British Journal of Surgery 1980; 67: 636–638

Illustrations by Carol J. Pienta and Gillian Lee

Wound closure

Walter J. Pories MD, FACS
Professor and Chairman, Department of Surgery, School of Medicine,
East Carolina University, Greenville, North Carolina

Introduction

Good surgeons close wounds precisely. They recognize that careful reconstruction of the skin barrier protects against infection and deformity and that proper apposition of tissues is required for strong healing and avoidance of hernias, dehiscences and eviscerations.

Principles

Incisions

1

Good closures require proper incisions and elegant surgical techniques. The incision must be made cleanly and perpendicular to the skin.

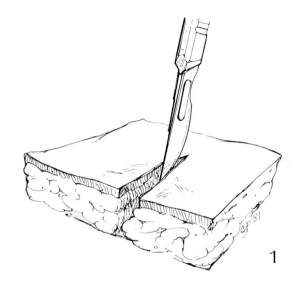

2

An incision which is made obliquely and in a jagged, erratic line will heal poorly, with a thick, irregular scar. Optimal incisions are easily made where the skin is taut, as on the extremities, chest and upper abdomen. Where skin is loose, as in the breast or around the navel, the skin must be stretched tight by traction as the incision is made.

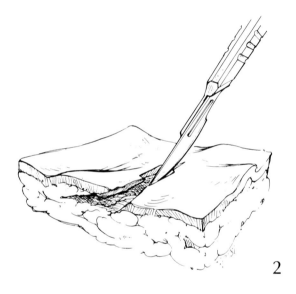

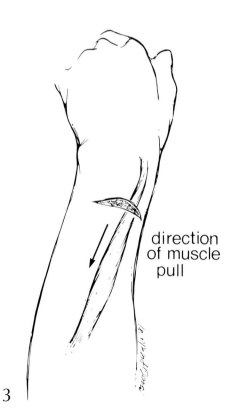

direction of muscle pull

3

Wounds heal better if they are made parallel to wrinkle lines and across the lines of muscle pull. Frequently such wounds approximate themselves; exercise and activity aid in keeping the wound edges together.

4

Wrinkle lines occur in all parts of the body. They are readily identified by pinching the skin and subcutaneous tissues. If the part to be incised is inflamed or distorted, examination of the normal limb or the mirror-image area of the head, neck or trunk in the same manner will serve as a guide. When the breast is examined in this way, for example, it is readily apparent that the most cosmetic incisions are circumareolar or within the submammary fold.

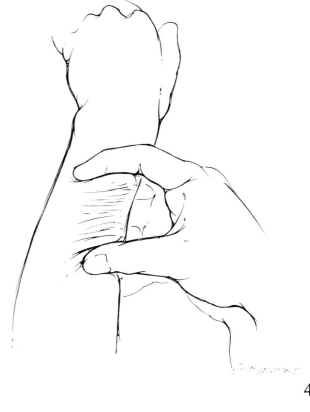

4

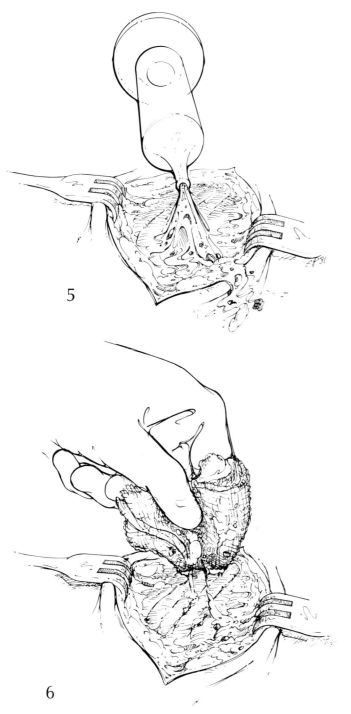

5

6

5 & 6

Irrigation

Irrigation is a mainstay of good wound closure. Washing the wound thoroughly with isotonic saline dilutes the bacterial population and removes pieces of dead fat, detritus and loose clot, each of which can serve as a nidus for infection. It is important to let the irrigation float these chunks off, or to pick them up with a sponge; simply sucking the pool of fluid just lets the fat and clots sink back down into the wound. Adding antibiotics (0.5 g kanamycin or neomycin per 1000 ml of solution) to the irrigating solution has proved helpful in contaminated cases.

Careful handling of tissues

7

Good wound closures require the approximation of normal tissues. Old scars should be excised, skin edges must not be burned by the cautery, the field should be dry, and foreign bodies, whether detritus, clot or suture material, should be kept to a minimum.

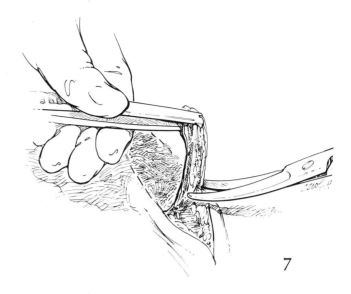

7

8

The tissues must be handled gently. Rough retraction with bruising and crushing from the carelessly placed clamp or too firmly squeezed forceps exacts a price in tissue damage, infection and ugly scarring. Wounds extending through several layers should be closed by reapproximating these layers as precisely as possible.

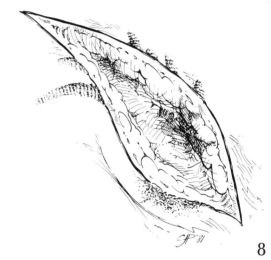

8

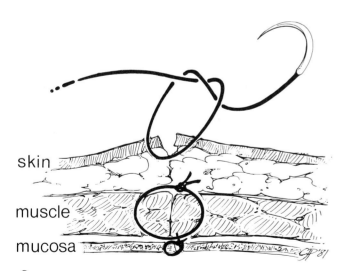

skin

muscle

mucosa

9

9

Suture technique

Sutures should approximate tissues, not strangle them. Knots should be tied gently and securely, both to avoid a noose effect and to ensure that the knots stay tied. We prefer an initial two granny knots to permit precise cinching of the knot, followed by a locking half-hitch which then squares the last knot. Other surgeons prefer three knots, with each of the latter two squaring the one preceding it. When monofilament material, which slips easily, is used, three surgeon's knots are preferable.

Types of closure

10

Primary closure

Tissues which are clean and free of infection can be approximated by primary closure. If the closure is well done, optimal healing and minimal scar formation follow.

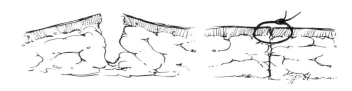

10

11

Secondary closure

Wounds allowed to granulate, either because of contamination, neglect or other reasons, are said to undergo secondary closure, or healing by second intention. The safety of this approach to infected wounds has been proven for centuries; its disadvantage is the long time required for healing and the heavy scarring which usually results.

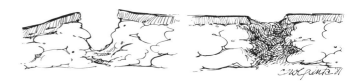

11

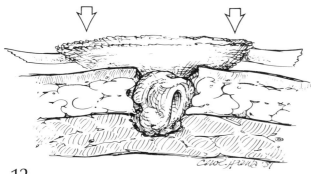

12

12 & 13

Delayed primary closure

Delayed primary closure offers the advantage of secondary closure without its disadvantages. This method is used for contaminated wounds such as those associated with emergency colon resections and war injuries. When the operation has been completed and all necrotic tissue and foreign matter have been removed, the wound is gently filled with fine mesh gauze and covered with a thick layer of gauze, secured with layers of tape to create an occlusive dressing. The dressing is not changed, unless the patient's condition worsens, for 4–5 days. At the end of that time, the dressing is removed under sterile precautions, preferably in the operating theatre. If the wound appears clean, the skin and underlying tissues can be closed securely. In most cases, the strength and cosmetic appearance of the wound will generally be as good as if the same tissues had been closed primarily after a clean operation. Delayed primary closure has saved many soldiers' lives; it is one of the major advances contributed by war surgery.

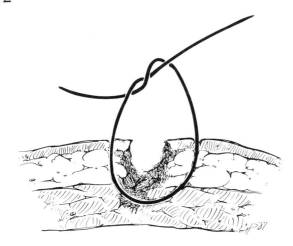

13

SELECTED SKIN CLOSURES

14

The *interrupted suture* remains the 'gold standard' for wound closure. If the sutures are precisely placed at the same level and the skin is gently reapproximated, optimal healing will take place, with minimal scar. For the best cosmetic result, in facial incisions or lacerations, for example, the sutures should be 1 mm apart and 1 mm from either edge; in other less noticeable areas, the stitches are usually 1 cm apart.

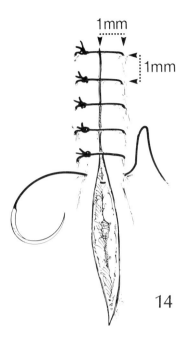

14

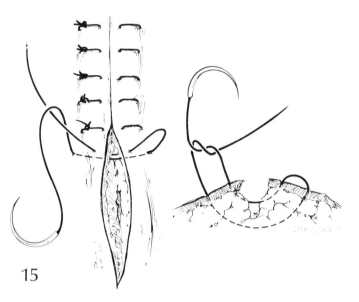

15

16

The *continuous overhand suture* is a rapid and efficient closure, but it is easily drawn too tight and tends to overlap. It is most useful where the skin is thick, as in the chest or back, or where rapid closure is desirable.

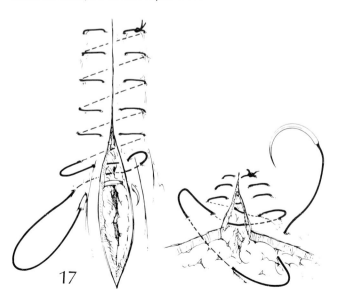

17

15

The *mattress suture* is most useful in areas where the skin is loose and overlap is likely to occur, as in the necks of aged patients, and for the beginning surgeon who has problems handling the over-and-over interrupted suture.

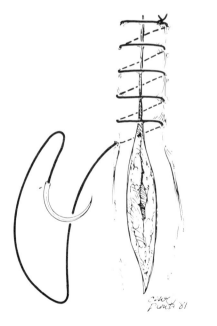

16

17

The *continuous mattress suture* is a useful and effective closure without the tendency of the ordinary suture to overlap.

The *subcuticular suture* is a demanding stitch, but it has many rewards. It avoids the 'railroad-track' scars which follow most other closures, eliminates often arduous suture removal (especially in children), and provides precise approximation of epidermal tissues. This stitch can be done as a pullout suture with 3/0 monofilament nylon (Ethilon) or polypropylene (Prolene) or with a buried absorbable suture, such as 4/0 polyglactin 901 (Vicryl).

18–22

The *buried subcuticular suture* is begun with a stitch near the far edge of the wound; the needle is then brought out precisely at the corner to begin the suture line. The needle picks up about 1 mm of dermis just below the level of the epidermis, in progressive stepwise fashion along the length of the wound. The stitch can be ended by bringing it out at right angles to the wound or by tying a small slipknot in the end of the suture. The suture line is then painted with a skin adhesive, such as tincture of benzoin, and stabilized with a half-inch strip (Steri-strip) or a piece of paper tape. Tension is maintained on the suture until the paper strip has been placed; it can then be cut off flush with the skin.

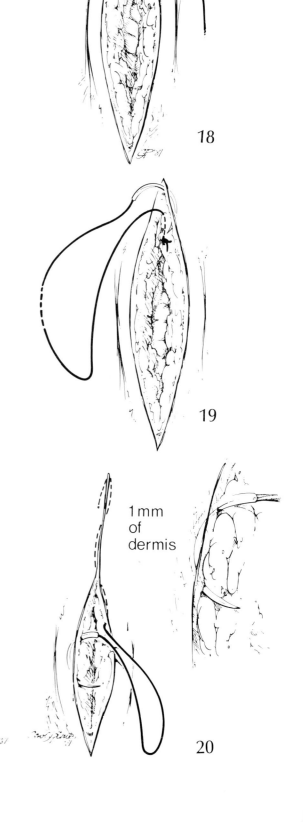

18

19

22

21

1 mm
of
dermis

20

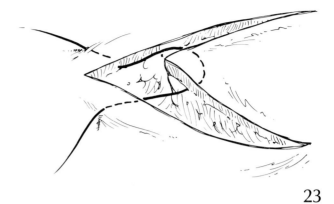

23

23, 24 & 25

The *corner stitch* is useful for the repair of jagged lacerations, for Z-plasties, and for the approximation of T incisions. The suture picks up the corner just below the epidermis, guides it precisely into the adjoining tissues and avoids the problem of necrosis of tissue in the angle that is sometimes caused by strangulating interrupted sutures.

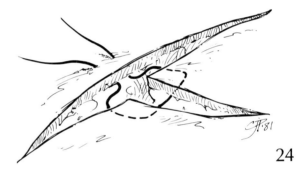

24

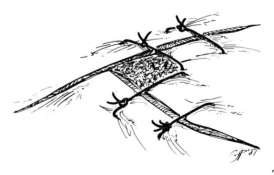

25

NEW SKIN CLOSURES

Tradition dies hard and at the time of writing most wounds are still closed with sutures. Many descriptions will be found throughout this book and its companion volumes. However, new techniques, some based on old ideas, are now taking hold.

26a–e

Clips and staplers

The old Michel clip (a) has the merits of simplicity and cheapness, but it is sometimes difficult to avoid the edges turning in. Newer devices are disposable and have a magazine of many staples (b). For the insertion of both clips and staples the wound edges must be held up beyond the point of application (a and b) though with the automatic device and sufficient hands, a slight eversion may be practised (c). Clips and staples are easily removed, usually with purpose-designed forceps (d and e).

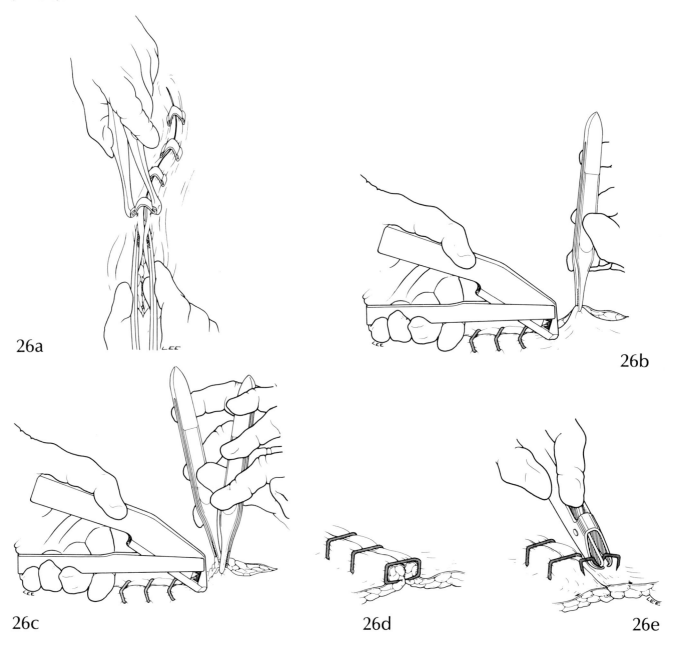

26a

26b

26c

26d

26e

27–30

Tape

Microporous adhesive tape (Steri-strip; Ethistrip) or, more recently, microporous film (Op-Site) may be laid across the wound. The cosmetic result is excellent. For this purpose it is essential that the wound edges are quite dry. A light spray of quick drying but sticky material (e.g. tincture of benzoin or collodion) may be used with advantage to aid adhesion.

In all these techniques of coaptation a sub- or intradermal stitch should be used to reduce distractive forces at the line of incision.

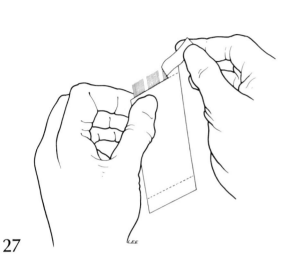

27

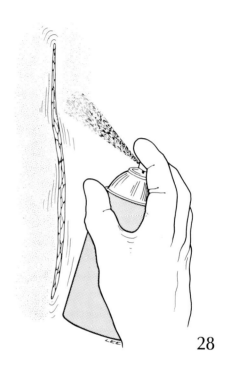

28

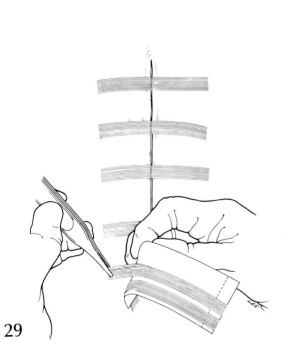

29

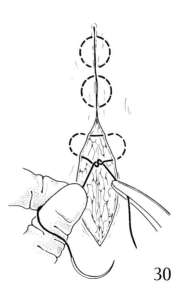

30

Further reading

Aston, S. J. The choice of suture material for skin closure. Journal of Dermatological Surgery 1976; 2: 57–61

Conn, J., Oyasu, R., Welsh, M., Beal, J. M. Vicryl (polyglactin 910) synthetic absorbable sutures. American Journal of Surgery 1974; 128(1): 19–23

Deveney, C. W., Dunphy, J. E., Heppenstall, R. B., et al. Wound management in selected tissues. In: Hunt, T. K., Dunphy, J. E., eds. Fundamentals of wound management in surgery, p. 456. New York: Appleton-Century-Crofts, 1979

Edlich, R. F., Rodeheaver, G. T., Thacker, J. G., Edgerton, M. Technical factors in wound management. In: Hunt, T. K., Dunphy, J. E., eds. Fundamentals of wound management in surgery, p. 364. New York: Appleton-Century-Crofts, 1979

Horton, C. E., Adamson, J. E., Mladick, R. A., Carraway, J. H. Vicryl synthetic absorbable sutures. American Surgeon 1974; 40: 729–731

Laufman, H., Rubel, T. Synthetic absorbable sutures. Surgery Gynecology and Obstetrics 1977; 145: 597–608

Martyn, J. W. Clinical experience with a synthetic absorbable surgical suture. Surgery Gynecology and Obstetrics 1975; 140: 747–748

Postlethwait, R. W., Smith, B. M. A new synthetic absorbable suture. Surgery Gynecology and Obstetrics 1975; 140: 377–380

Van Winkle, W., Hastings, J. C., Barker, E., Hines, D., Nichols, W. Effect of suture materials on healing skin wounds. Surgery Gynecology and Obstetrics 1975; 140: 7–12

Wounds: principles of management of different tissues

Charles G. Rob MD
Professor of Surgery, Department of Surgery, School of Medicine,
East Carolina University, Greenville, North Carolina

Introduction

A wound may be clean, it may be potentially infected or it may be infected. An example of a clean wound is one which is made and closed in the operating room. A potentially infected wound is a recent traumatic injury as is seen in a traffic or industrial accident or during a war. An infected wound is one of the above which is so grossly contaminated that infection is inevitable or one which has been neglected so that pus and inflammation are already present.

We will discuss the soft-tissue wound which is potentially infected because many lessons have been learnt from the care of this type of wound both in war and peace. The medical management of a wound should begin as soon as possible after injury. First steps include the control of haemorrhage by pressure or occasionally a tourniquet, the application of a sterile dressing, splintage if necessary, and smooth rapid transfer to the hospital. Today, intravenous solutions can be administered in the ambulance, if prescribed by a doctor. In hospital, tetanus toxoid will be administered, the patient examined and prophylactic antibiotics begun.

The clinical picture may be divided into the patient's general condition and the local condition around the wounds.

The general condition varies considerably but certain findings are common to battle casualties and many road or industrial injuries. The patients are dirty, tired, often cold, thirsty, and all battle casualties want an operation. It is a curious fact that a wounded soldier both expects and welcomes an operation; he feels that something is being done for him. The majority have no other general abnormalities, but a minority with severe wounds or gross blood loss are suffering from varying degrees of circulatory failure (shock). The worst patients have a blood pressure which cannot be recorded, a pulse which cannot be palpated at the wrist and a very sluggish peripheral circulation.

The local condition depends upon the wounding agent. A knife wound may appear to be clean. The modern high velocity bullet produces an explosive wound. Industrial and farm injuries may be extensively contaminated as may be pedestrian, bicycle and motorcycle injuries. Shell or bomb explosions cause multiple injuries. Certain special missiles, such as the phosphorus bomb, cause peculiar problems.

In warfare, the multiplicity of wounds is astonishing. In a series of abdominal wounds treated in World War II[1], in over half of the patients other injuries were present in addition to the abdominal wound; and in 20 per cent these other wounds were of a major character such as open fractures, traumatic amputations, thoracic or cerebral wounds.

Surgical intervention

Every wound that penetrates the skin should be treated by a surgeon. However, the type of treatment will vary widely depending upon the tissues which are injured, the degree of contamination and the time interval between injury and treatment.

MANAGEMENT OF A CONTAMINATED WOUND INVOLVING MUSCLE

These wounds should be excised if the operation can be performed within 12 h of wounding. After 12 h wound enlargement or cleansing, but not complete excision, should be practised. The correct, two-stage management of such wounds was established during World War II, when it was used for gunshot wounds. At the first operation the wound was excised and at the second operation the wound was closed by delayed primary or secondary suture. An exception was a low velocity through-and-through bullet wound, when even in early cases, excision of the whole wound track was not practised.

Wound excision

After the induction of anaesthesia, the wounded areas are washed and shaved. They are then painted with Betadine or an antiseptic of the surgeon's choice. In patients with multiple wounds the decision has to be made as to which wounds are to be treated first. Wounds that interfere with the airway, cause cardiac tamponade, require the urgent control of haemorrhage or an immediate amputation or that have much damaged muscles are top priority. It has been estimated that if the amount of damaged muscle equals or exceeds the size of two clenched fists then early excision is necessary to avoid renal shutdown.

Wounds of the back which necessitate rolling and turning the patient for their excision present a special problem. For example, a patient with a buttock wound in association with an abdominal wound should in many instances have the buttock excised first, because usually he will withstand the necessary movement much better before rather than after the laparotomy.

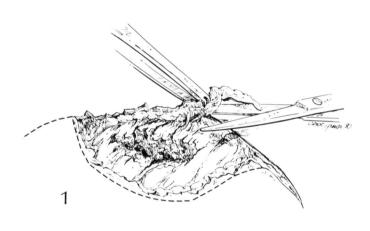

1

Excision of the skin and superficial layers

The first step is to enlarge the wound in such a way that delayed primary suture can be performed with minimum difficulty. This means the conservation of skin at all costs and enlarging incisions which follow the skin folds and creases if possible. It is unfortunate that the skin is the easiest tissue to excise; skin must be conserved and only removed if devitalized. Damaged and contaminated subcutaneous tissue and fat are excised and the deep fascia incised to the same extent as the skin. If necessary incisions may be made in the fascia at right angles to the skin incision, so that the damaged muscle is widely exposed.

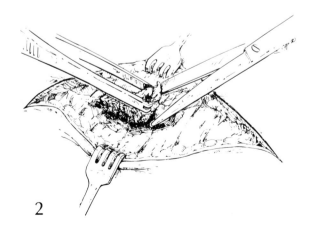

2

Excision of damaged muscle

All damaged and devitalized muscle should be removed and all pockets laid open so that the wound presents a saucerized appearance in which exudate will not accumulate. A metallic foreign body, if it comes to hand, is removed, but an extensive search is unnecessary. The importance, however, of removing non-metallic foreign bodies, such as clothing or earth, cannot be overestimated. After haemostasis has been achieved, the wound is copiously irrigated with saline.

3

The wound dressing

Experience during all the wars of this century has shown that the primary closure of wounds in warfare is a mistake. For many civilian wounds the same is true. No sutures of any kind are placed in either the deep fascia or skin. The saucerized wound is not packed but is dressed by placing a flat dressing over the wound. Drains are not required, because the wound is shaped by the surgeon so that these are not necessary. Large wounds are best immobilized in plaster of Paris. The antibiotics, which were begun before surgery, are continued for the first 3–5 days after the operation.

Wound closure

This will usually be by the operation of delayed primary or secondary suture. During the interval between wound excision and wound closure, the wound should not be inspected or dressed. If inspection is required, then it should be carried out in an operating room with full aseptic precautions. The importance of this was demonstrated by Edwards in 1945[2]. Of 869 consecutive wounds, 163 had been dressed on the ward before closure and 48 per cent of these were infected with pathogenic bacteria; 706 were not dressed until closure in the operating room and 33 per cent of these wounds were infected with pathogenic bacteria.

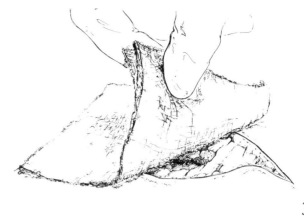

3

4

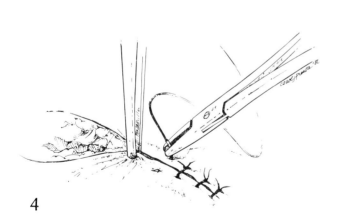

4

Delayed primary suture

This should be performed in the operating room. The dressing is removed, preferably 4 or 5 days after wound excision. The decision is then made for or against delayed primary suture. Contraindications to delayed primary suture include: acute inflammation (the presence of bacteria or pus is not a contraindication), the presence of gas in the tissues, incomplete wound excision and excessive skin loss. Most wounds that have been properly excised are suitable for delayed primary suture.

The operation consists of undermining the skin edges by blunt dissection, trimming off any redundant tags of skin or fascia, irrigation of the wound with saline and accurate closure of the skin with interrupted sutures; a fair degree of tension is permissible. In many wounds a dead space remains after closure. It is better to drain this rather than attempt to close it with deep sutures. Amputations are particularly suited to delayed primary suture, but here drainage with a suction drain should be employed for 3 days.

The presence of open fractures is not a contraindication to delayed primary closure. However, in open fractures of the tibia, it may be mechanically impossible; and in open fractures of the femur, it is often wise to leave the posterior wound open, because exudate may collect in this region.

5, 6, & 7

Secondary suture

Delayed primary suture is possible during the 4–10 day period after wound excision. After this, the closure procedure of the wound changes to secondary suture, which can be performed at any time after the tenth day.

The operation consists of excising the granulation tissue, removing a very thin strip of the skin edge and undercutting the skin for a sufficient distance to make suture possible. The skin is then closed with interrupted sutures. Wound drainage should usually be undertaken for 48 h with a Penrose drain.

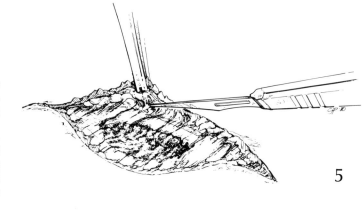

5

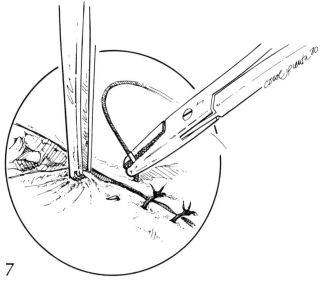

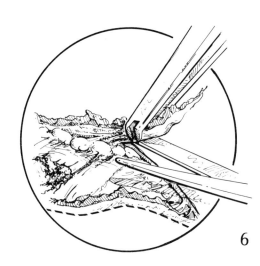

6

7

Skin grafting

This should be reserved for those patients on whom secondary or delayed primary suture has failed or was impossible.

Split-skin grafting with patches is the usual method employed, though sheets can also be used. The cosmetic result is not always satisfactory and so this method should not be used in exposed areas where the aesthetic outcome is important. If necessary these patients should be referred to a plastic surgeon.

8

Splintage

A good principle is to splint a wounded extremity if there is extensive muscle injury and of course if there is a fracture. When in doubt, splint. The cast must be padded and must be split along each side. In no circumstances should adhesive tape encircle the limb under a cast. Unless ischaemia is present the limb should be kept moderately elevated after the operation.

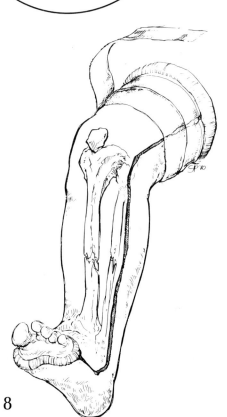

8

WOUNDS INVOLVING BONE

9

The presence of shattered bone in a wound introduces technical problems. The bone fragments are managed in the following way.

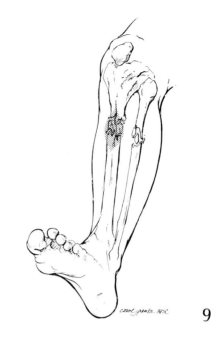

9

10

As much bone as possible is saved. All small, detached and therefore non-viable fragments of bone are removed. All bone fragments, regardless of their size, which retain muscular attachments are considered viable and are left *in situ*.

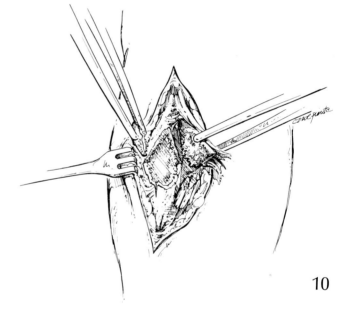

10

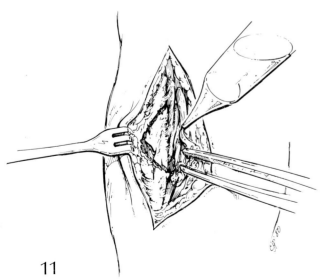

11

11

Soiled fragments are cleaned with a curette and a rongeur and are copiously irrigated with saline. Large detached bone fragments may be cleaned and then considered for use as a bone graft.

As a general rule internal fixation is not used if the wound is likely to become infected. Immobilization by a well padded and split or a bivalved plaster of Paris cast is satisfactory, but the plaster must be split throughout its entire length and down to the skin in order to accommodate swelling of the extremity, which invariably occurs immediately after the operation.

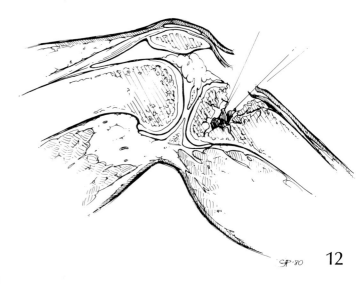

12

WOUNDS OF JOINTS

12 & 13

The arthotomy incision must be large enough to provide satisfactory exposure of the interior of the joint. It may be made by enlarging the traumatic wound. All blood clots, foreign bodies and loose bone or cartilage fragments are removed and the area thoroughly irrigated.

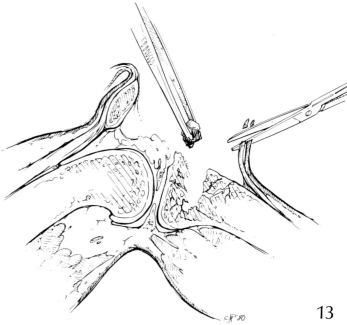

13

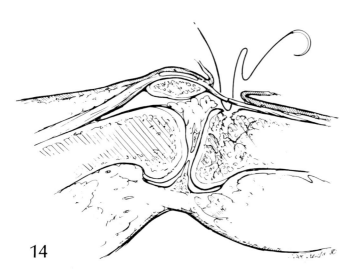

14

14

Closure of the joint is mandatory, either the capsule or the synovial membrane being closed, depending upon which is easier. The joint is then immobilized in a padded and split plaster cast.

UNHEALED WOUNDS

In spite of good treatment a small percentage of wounds remain unhealed. The common causes are bone infection, a retained foreign body, inadequate drainage of an abscess cavity and in the case of wounds of the trunk a faecal or urinary fistula or a chronic empyema. The first step is to find the cause. This will include X-rays and possibly a sinogram. Then, treatment may require removal of a retained foreign body, adequate drainage and full wound exploration.

15

WOUNDS OF ESSENTIAL BLOOD VESSELS

The first step is to control haemorrhage by the application of vascular clamps but not haemostats. Unimportant arteries, such as the internal mammary, are clamped with haemostats and ligated. Wounds of all essential arteries should be assessed for repair. During wound debridement, it is important to examine the artery with great care. In gunshot wounds more than one arterial laceration may be present and knowledge of such additional arterial wounds should be obtained before repair is started. Lateral repair should rarely be used. It is better to repair arterial injuries by end-to-end anastomosis, a blood vessel graft or a patch graft angioplasty. Autogenous veins are preferred over all other arterial graft materials except for the repair of wounds of the aorta and its major branches, when a Dacron prosthesis is preferred.

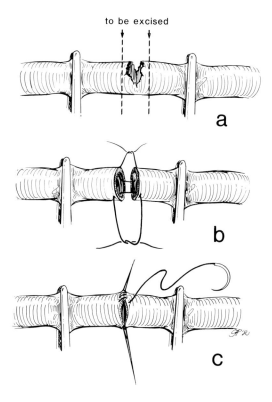

to be excised

a

b

c

15

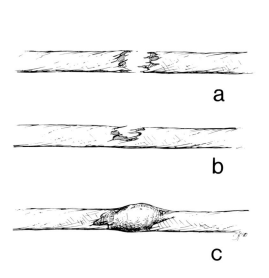

a

b

c

16

16

WOUNDS OF PERIPHERAL NERVES

Apart from procedures for the relief of pressure, surgical exploration of closed peripheral nerve injuries is never indicated at the time of initial injury. For patients with open wounds which require debridement, a search is not made for injured nerves. If the nerve is seen, its appearance should be recorded. The notes should state specifically whether the nerve trunk was anatomically intact or a gap in continuity was found. Intact nerves should be disturbed as little as possible. No attempt should be made to fix the nerve ends, and markers should not be placed at the site. Primary suture of a divided nerve should not be attempted at the time of initial wound surgery, unless it is a clean incised wound, which is to be closed primarily.

WOUNDS OF TENDONS

Soiled and frayed tendons must be resected. Tendon repair should only be attempted at the time of initial surgery if the wound is clean and primary suture is to be carried out. For all other tendon wounds, repair is delayed until the wound is healed and infection is no longer present.

Postoperative care

Some wounds heal more rapidly than others. This depends in part upon the blood supply. For example the sutures from a neck or facial wound may often be removed after 48 h whilst it may be wise to leave the sutures in a wound of the back for 14 days or more. If delayed infection occurs it will require drainage.

An important part of wound management is rehabilitation. Joints must not become stiff and muscle tone must be maintained. Splintage is often required but joints proximal and distal to the splinted region should be exercised actively. For example, when the forearm is injured the shoulder should be exercised and the fingers and toes should be exercised whenever possible. In many patients treatment in a rehabilitation unit is of great value.

References

1. Rob, C. G. The diagnosis of abdominal trauma in warfare. Surgery, Gynecology and Obstetrics 1947; 85: 147–154

2. Edwards, H. C. Revival of early wound closure. Two stage operation, as applied in Italy. Lancet 1945; 1: 583–585

Further reading

United States Department of Defense. Emergency war surgery, NATO handbook. Washington, DC: US Department of Defense, US Government Printing Office, 1958

Illustrations by Carol J. Pienta

Principles of small grafts and flaps

Edward G. Flickinger MD
Associate Professor of General Surgery, School of Medicine,
East Carolina University, Greenville, North Carolina

Introduction

A well healed wound, the hallmark of a successful surgical endeavour, combines restoration of structural integrity and unencumbered function with an acceptable appearance. The surgeon works toward this desirable goal by gentle handling of tissues, careful debridement, meticulous haemostasis and a layered wound closure that is free of tension. When deficiencies in function and appearance might result from primary wound closure, it should be avoided. Clinical judgement will direct the surgeon to alternative measures in such situations.

Additional skills required for management of the moderately complex wounds frequently encountered in general surgery include grafting of autologous skin and use of small local skin flaps. Skin grafts and flaps are useful adjuncts to basic wound care when the surgeon combines a thorough grasp of their underlying principles with a precise application of their technique. Both methods may be practised in the clinician's office, in the emergency department or in standard operating suites, without any expensive, sophisticated instruments. Type, size and location of the wound will determine the best place to operate and whether local or general anaesthesia is appropriate.

The patient can benefit in terms of reduced pain, shorter treatment time and less anxiety, if the surgeon uses skin grafts and small local flaps with foresight. This chapter will cover the techniques of those skin grafts and flaps which are a useful part of every surgeon's armamentarium.

Skin grafts

1

Free autologous skin grafts are classified according to thickness. A graft of epidermis and superficial dermis containing dermal appendages is a partial or split-thickness graft. The donor site for such a graft will heal spontaneously, by re-epithelialization, much as an abrasion heals. A graft including all layers of skin is a full-thickness graft, and the donor site for such a graft must undergo partial-thickness skin grafting or primary reapproximation when possible. Generally speaking, the thinner a free skin graft is, the more likely it is to take, possibly at the expense of wound contracture. Conversely, the thicker the graft, the less predictable is its take; but if a thick graft is successful, contracture will be minimal.

When a wound requires grafting, the surgeon must decide upon the appropriate thickness of the graft, both for immediate coverage and for long-term functional and cosmetic result.

Free skin grafts should be avoided in grossly contaminated or previously irradiated wounds. Similarly, grafting is contraindicated over areas of exposed tendon, cartilage or bone. The probability that the graft will take may be improved by careful surgical technique, maintenance of stability of the recipient bed and graft apposition, and control of infection, particularly streptococcal infection.

The techniques of partial-thickness and full-thickness skin grafts will be presented in detail.

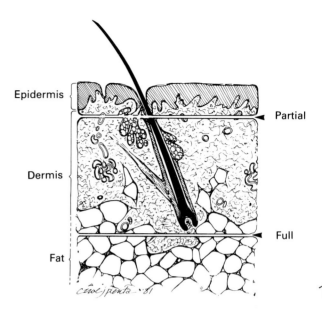

Epidermis
Dermis
Fat
Partial
Full

1

PARTIAL-THICKNESS SKIN GRAFTS

Partial-thickness skin grafts are appropriate for situations in which maximum take is the primary consideration. Thin partial-thickness grafts may take even though the recipient bed is less than ideal. Such grafts may also be useful when a minimum of donor skin is available, such as in a large surface area burn. Frequent recourse to the common donor site is possible when this approach is used. A case that seems likely to progress to wound contracture over a period of time would better be treated by some method other than a partial-thickness skin graft.

Instruments

2

Dermatomes are finely calibrated instruments used for obtaining skin grafts of varying partial thickness. The Braithwaite and Watson knives operate manually, whereas the Brown dermatome requires electrical or compressed-air power to provide the necessary reciprocating blade action. Simple dial adjustments alter graft thickness by 0.001 inch increments. Both techniques can be rapidly mastered. Preference for one instrument over the other is a personal choice, although the size of graft needed may be influential. The Brown dermatome easily harvests uniform long skin strips up to 7.5 cm (3 inches) in width, while the Braithwaite or the Watson knife may produce narrow, irregular pieces unless skilfully used. Naturally the blades of either instrument must be sharp for best results.

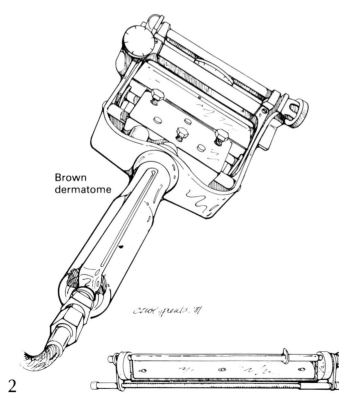

Brown dermatome

Braithwaite knife

2

Graft procurement

Careful selection of the donor site is imperative. A flat or minimally contoured surface, with skin colour and texture resembling that surrounding the wound is best. Care must be taken to match glabrous skin grafts to appropriate sites, hairy grafts to defects in hairy areas. A further consideration in choice of donor site may be the size of the wound to be covered. Finally, the defect remaining after harvesting of the graft should not further handicap the patient.

3

Common donor sites for partial-thickness skin grafts are the anterolateral aspects of thighs and flanks.

Once a site has been chosen, local hair should be clipped or shaven and the area thoroughly cleansed. It may be desirable to use cleansing agents that will not discolour the skin (PHisoHex, saline rather than povidone-iodine) during the graft harvest.

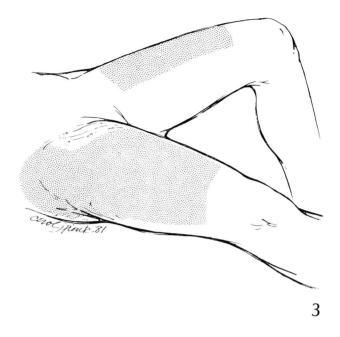

3

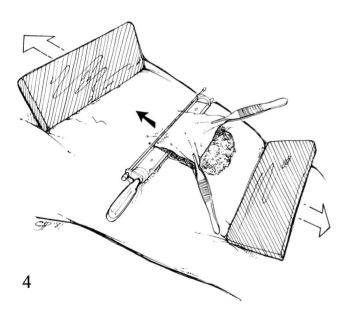

4

4

The entire donor site is painted with mineral oil to provide lubrication during the procedure. Wooden skin boards are then used to flatten the skin at the proposed donor site and adjusted as needed to facilitate graft harvest.

5

Braithwaite knife and Brown dermatome harvest skin grafts by controlled advance of the reciprocating blade. Both instruments are applied firmly to the skin during the procedure; it is impossible to cut too deeply into the dermis because of inherent safety features of the instruments. Irregularities in graft thickness will occur when the pressure is uneven. Once the desired graft has been obtained, it may either be applied directly to the wound or stored briefly in saline-soaked gauze. If surplus skin has been obtained, it should be reapplied to the donor site or stored in a skin bank, if such a facility exists. The donor site is then covered with either fine mesh gauze or Xeroform and a protective dressing.

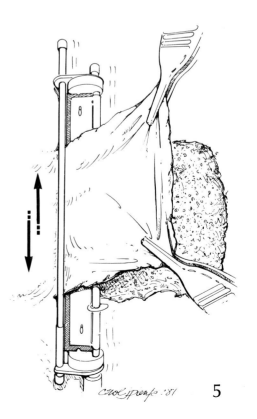

5

Graft application

6

Before direct application of the partial-thickness graft, the wound should be cleansed gently and debrided if necessary. Any areas of hypertrophic granulation tissue should be smoothed in order to obtain a uniform bed on which the graft will lie. If the graft is to be meshed, to cover a larger surface area, this is done immediately before application.

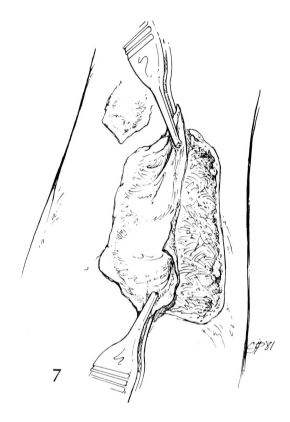

7

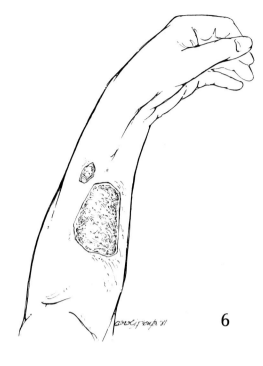

6

7

The graft is then positioned to cover the wound, with care to maintain direct graft–wound apposition.

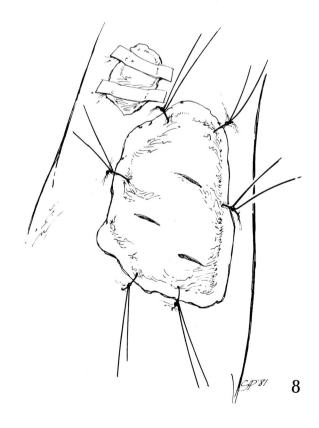

8

8

Small grafts can be held in position with adhesive strips, while larger ones are best secured by fine sutures. Several small cuts may be made into the graft to provide drainage for any accumulation of serum or blood.

Fine-mesh gauze or Xeroform is applied as a topical dressing. Then, depending upon the size and location of the wound, either a pressure dressing or a cotton stent may be used to maintain direct graft–wound contact. At times it may even be necessary to enclose a grafted extremity in a cast to prevent motion between the wound and the graft. The original dressing is maintained for 5–7 days, during which time the graft will take. When the dressing is removed, great care should be taken not to disrupt the healing process. Any problems will usually be apparent at the time of the first dressing change.

PINCH GRAFTS

9

Pinch grafts may occasionally be useful in sites where, over time, partial-thickness grafts are likely to break down because of predictable wear and tear. Certain wounds of the hands and feet and those over bony prominences are suitable for pinch grafting.

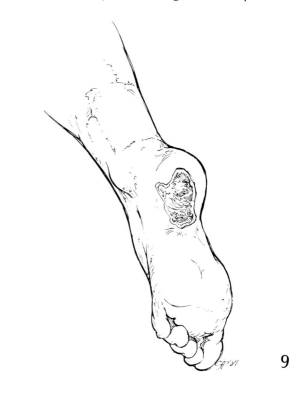

9

10

Pinch grafts are small discs of skin (approximately 1 cm in diameter) with both partial- and full-thickness elements. The thicker elements provide better protection against local trauma, while the partial-thickness elements provide a better chance of take and a margin for re-epithelialization. This form of grafting is no longer as popular as previously, but its principles and techniques may occasionally be useful.

The advantage of pinch grafting is that it can be performed under local anaesthesia by those with minimal experience in other forms of grafting. Its main disadvantage is the final pebbled appearance of both the donor and the grafted sites.

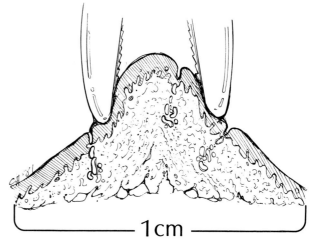

1cm

10

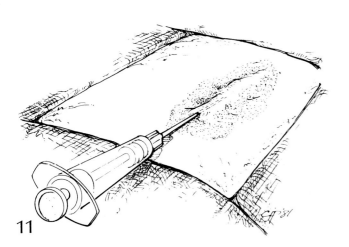

Graft procurement

11

The defect requiring grafting will dictate the surface area of skin to be prepared for harvest. The local hair should be trimmed away and the skin cleansed. A local anaesthetic agent is then administered subcutaneously by a fine-gauge needle in an area sufficient for providing the desired number of pinch grafts to be harvested.

12

After satisfactory anaesthesia has been obtained, a small mound of skin is elevated by the tip of a straight needle or fine forceps. A standard scalpel blade is then used to excise a disc of skin measuring approximately 1 cm in diameter. In this fashion, multiple grafts are obtained. The donor site is then dressed sterilely to allow for healing by granulation and re-epithelialization.

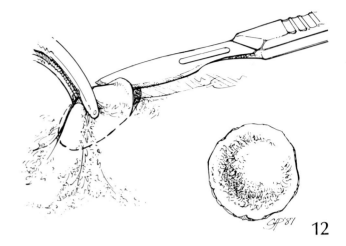

12

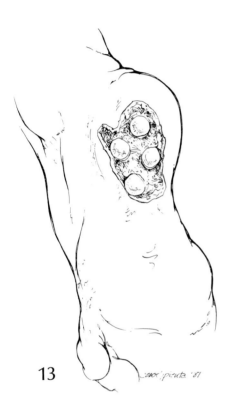

13

13

Graft application

The wound is prepared for receiving the graft by gentle cleansing and minor debridement when necessary. The pinch grafts are applied to the wound, allowing about 1 cm between graft margins. Fine-mesh gauze or Xero-form, together with a sterile dressing, protects the grafts during the healing phase. About 5 days are required for graft take.

FULL-THICKNESS SKIN GRAFTS

Full-thickness skin grafts are recommended for small wounds of the face and neck where cosmesis is a crucial consideration. Appropriate colour, texture, contour and durability can be achieved with minimal contraction in a well executed full-thickness graft.

Because its rate of take is less predictable, a full-thickness graft should be applied only when the wound exhibits either a fresh or a rich granulating surface conducive to healing.

14

The lesion is excised with an appropriate margin, with the long axis of the wound aligned with the wrinkle lines for the best cosmetic result.

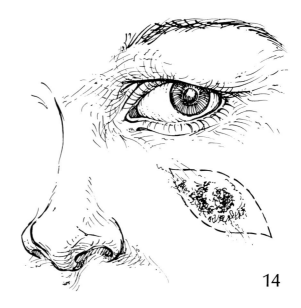

14

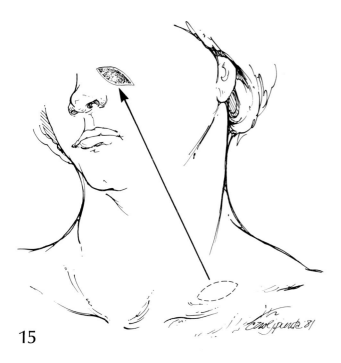

15

16

The graft is excised at the interface of dermis and subcutaneous fat, with special care being taken to protect the graft edges from unnecessary trauma.

Graft procurement

15

The final appearance of a grafted wound of the face or neck is critical; thus the donor skin should be similar in colour and texture to that of the face and neck. The groin and supraclavicular area of the neck are frequently chosen sites. Occasionally the anterior and lateral chest may serve.

After an appropriate site has been selected, the hair is clipped and the skin cleansed as in other grafting procedures. The surgeon should measure the wound carefully, transcribing its exact dimensions to the donor site. The proposed graft is then outlined by a marking pen.

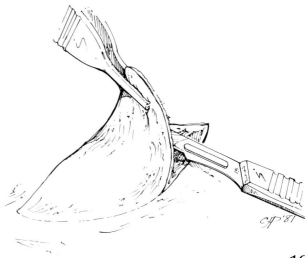

16

17

Before graft application, all residual fat adherent to the dermal surface should be meticulously scraped off with the edge of a scalpel blade to assure the best chance of graft take.

18

The donor site is closed by approximation of the edges.

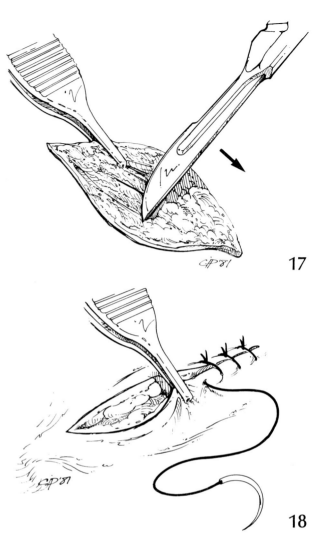

17

18

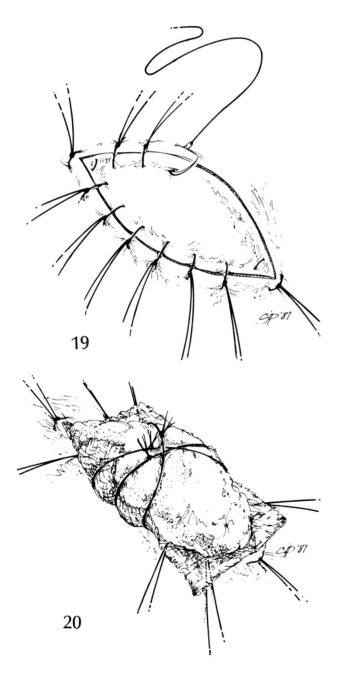

19

20

Graft application

19

The full-thickness graft is placed directly upon the clean wound and anchored in place with fine sutures.

20

It is usually desirable to tie these sutures over Xeroform and a cotton stent to provide continuous graft–wound apposition. Five to seven days will be required for the graft to take securely.

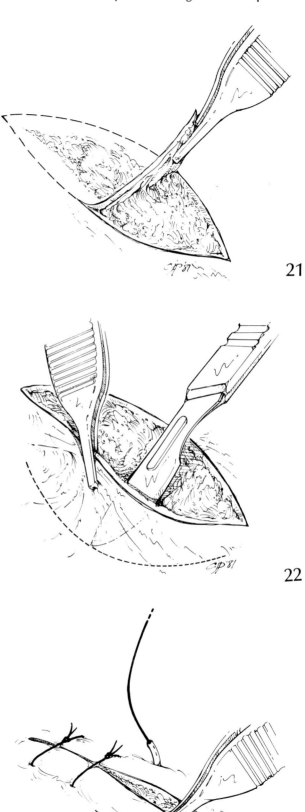

21

22

23

Local skin flaps

General surgeons frequently face wounds involving full-thickness loss of skin and exposed tendon, bone or cartilage. These may be managed best by reorienting nearby skin flaps of like colour and texture. Such wounds include avulsion injuries or excision sites, the edges of which cannot be approximated primarily without undue tension or an unsatisfactory final appearance. Other wounds requiring local flaps include lacerations through and perpendicular to natural skin folds or across joints. Primary closure of such defects could produce an undesirable cosmetic result or functional impairment. Proper management of these cases requires a working knowledge of advancement flaps, rotation flaps and Z-plasty.

A great deal of forethought in designing a skin flap, combined with meticulous technique, is essential for successful healing. Well vascularized and redundant skin adjacent to the wound is desirable if local flaps are to be used. When redundancy is lacking, a secondary donor defect is often the price paid for satisfactory coverage of the primary wound. Such a defect, when covered by a partial-thickness skin graft, should not be cosmetically undesirable or functionally limited.

ADVANCEMENT FLAPS

21, 22 & 23

Local undermining

The simplest form of advancement flap technique involves local undermining of skin edges to allow approximation without tension.

Utilization of adjacent skin

24

When simple undermining is insufficient for satisfactory closure, an advancement flap can be designed, utilizing adjacent lax and vascularized skin. The dimensions of the flap are ultimately limited by the blood supply derived from the base of the flap. While vascularity varies in different parts of the body, one should avoid flap length-to-width ratios exceeding 2:1.

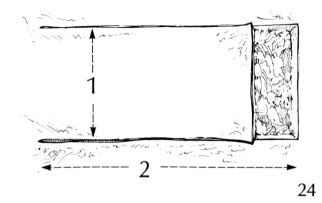

24

25

The lesion is excised, with a rectangular margin to accommodate the flap. The flap edges are incised and the skin undermined through fat.

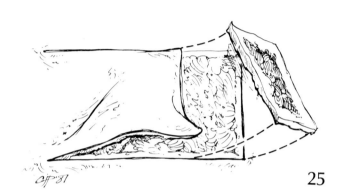

25

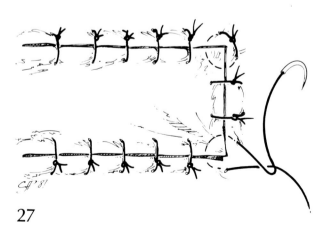

26

26

Gentle handling of the flap with fine skin hooks is essential for preventing necrosis along the margins.

27

The flap is advanced to cover the primary wound and sutured into place. This is what one generally hopes for but rarely achieves without excessive tension or an unsightly 'dog-ear'.

27

Excision of dog-ear

28 & 29

As suturing progresses toward the base of the flap, a dog-ear on one side or both may become apparent. In this event, an incision should be made at right angles to the flap; the triangle so formed is undermined and excised.

30

The flap may then be sutured securely into place. Even with this modification, the practical application of advancement flaps may be limited, because suture line tension cannot be totally avoided.

Second incision

Dog-ear

28

29

30

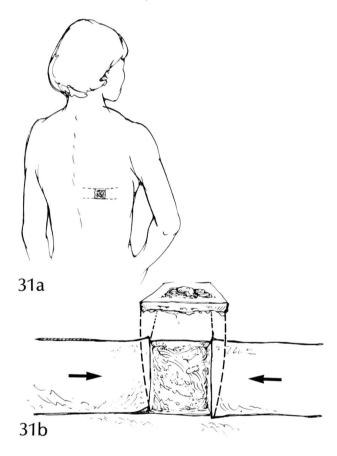

31a

31b

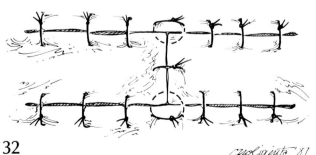

32

31 & 32

Wide excision

A modification of the advancement flap technique can be used in closing large defects of the back created by widely excising a lesion, such as a malignant melanoma. The so-called 'bra-strap closure' is completed by creating bilateral advancement flaps with medial approximation of one flap to the other.

ROTATION FLAP

33a & b

A rotation flap is applicable for covering triangular defects. The apex of the triangle defines the base of the proposed flap to be rotated over the defect. Before any incision is made, the proposed flap should be accurately measured and drawn out to ensure appropriate dimensions. The base of the triangular defect is continued radially to inscribe the flap margins. The defect itself is a segment of the inscribed arc.

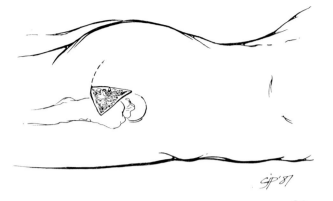

33a

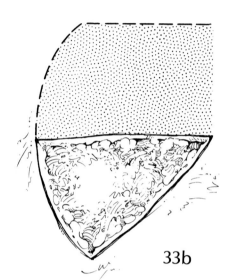

33b

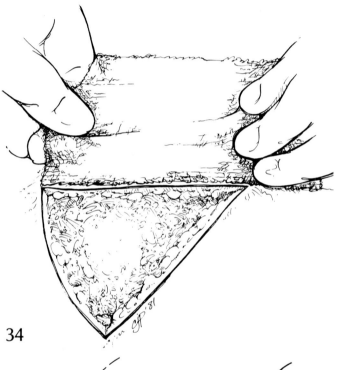

34

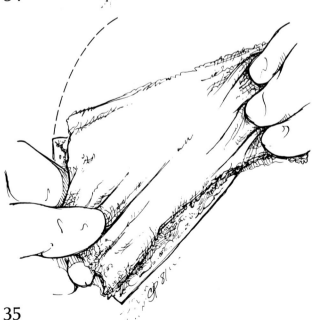

35

34 & 35

The flap's adequacy may be confirmed by using a mock-up of a strip of cloth with dimensions the same as those of the proposed flap, rotated over the defect as a trial. The flap's base must be sufficiently wide to provide adequate vascularity once the flap is developed.

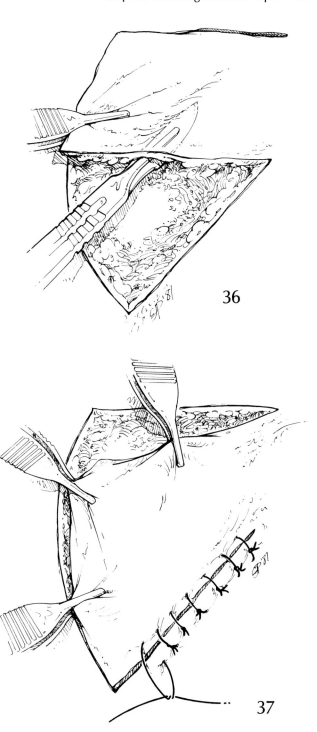

36 & 37

The flap is finally rotated over the primary defect and sutured into place by redistributing the tension. If excessive tension develops at the suture line, grafting may be necessary to close the secondary defect.

Proper planning and meticulous surgical technique can spell the difference between failure and success. Sound principles must never be bypassed for the sake of merely closing the wound. A flap with marginal vascularity under tension is doomed from the start.

Z-PLASTY

38

A Z-plasty involves transposition of two triangular skin flaps which functionally lengthen a wound while redistributing tension across it. Although a Z-plasty is usually employed as a secondary procedure to revise an unsightly scar or release a contracture across a natural skin crease, it may be used in the primary closure of certain wounds. By using a Z-plasty as a primary mode of wound care, a laceration is broken up into several components, many of which can be neatly camouflaged in natural skin creases. This technique is particularly useful in dealing with certain lacerations of the face or ones which traverse joint creases. Forethought in designing an appropriate Z-plasty can frequently ensure a pleasing cosmetic result while maintaining function.

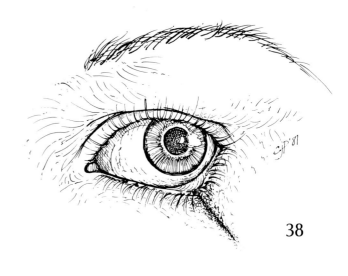

38

39

A Z-plasty is performed only after it has been carefully mapped out. The central aspect of the Z represents the primary laceration or the scar to be revised. The two limbs of the Z are parallel lines that intersect the central portion at a 60° angle. In constructing the Z, all segments should be of equal length to provide maximum wound lengthening.

39

40

After the procedure has been clearly thought out, the appropriate incisions are made and flaps developed.

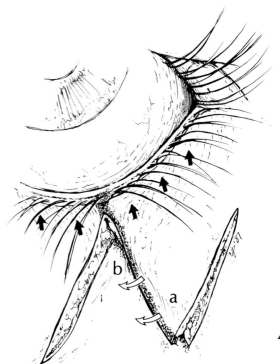

40

41 & 42

The two newly constructed triangular skin flaps are then transposed and sutured in place.

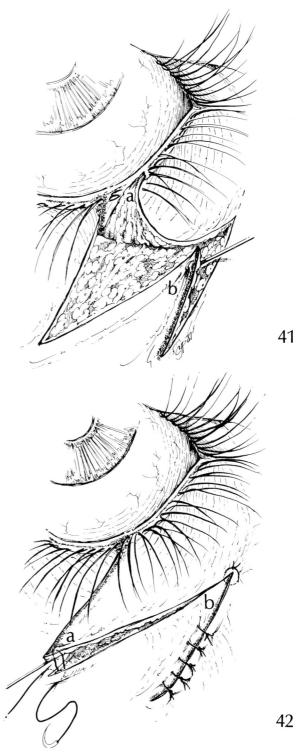

41

42

43

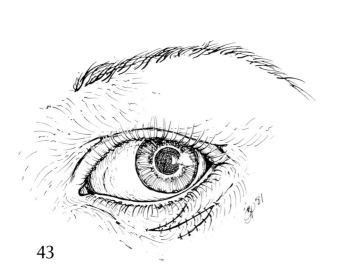

43

This series of manoeuvres creates a new Z, the central portion of which lies perpendicular to the original defect. Ischaemia and necrosis of wound margins, particularly of the tips of the skin flaps, represent potential complications, best avoided by meticulous surgical technique throughout.

Illustrations by Gillian Lee

Wound drainage

A. M. van Rij FRACS
Senior Lecturer in Surgery,
University of Otago, New Zealand

Introduction

The use of drains has been recorded since the time of Hippocrates, who used drainage tubes in the treatment of empyema. Despite this long history controversy continues about their use, including the indications, the materials used and their configuration as well as methods of placement. The description of new drains continues, suggesting that current drains are not always ideal. The successful use of drains is dependent on a clear recognition of those circumstances in which they are appropriate and of their limitations as well as their potential hazards.

Purposes

Drains may be used for several different purposes.

1. The encouragement of the discharge of pus as in the drainage of a localized abscess without the premature closure of the overlying wound.
2. The removal of transudate from a wound to facilitate healing and to reduce complications. This is most appropriate in those sites which are prone to collection of fluid, such as underneath skin flaps following simple mastectomy.
3. The provision of an early warning of a complication such as bleeding or bile leak following biliary surgery.
4. The approximation of tissues or indirect splinting of a wound by the use of negative pressure applied through the drain as used under the skin flaps of a radical neck dissection.
5. The provision of a means of irrigation, particularly in infected and heavily contaminated tissues and in the serous lined cavities as well as joint spaces.

Complications

Drains should be used with caution as they may themselves complicate the surgery in several ways.

1. Perforation of adjacent structures, particularly when rigid materials are used or too vigorous suction applied.
2. Infection may be introduced from the external environment along the track or through the lumen of a drain. This occurs more often in drainage systems that are directly open to the atmosphere and in sump drains that entrain contaminated air. This hazard increases the longer a drain remains in place.
3. Inhibition of the healing process may result from the increased inflammatory reaction induced by the drain material and from direct mechanical obstruction by the drain.
4. Failure of a drain to perform the intended role will lead to unsatisfactory results in the associated procedure. In these circumstances a false sense of security leads to delays in the management of the underlying problem. Failure of a drain to function is often the result of the drain and its perforations being of inadequate size; increased thrombogenicity of the material, predisposing to blockage by blood clots; as well as the collapse of a drain with excessive suction. Drains obviously fail in their function if they come out prematurely and this is often the result of inadequate methods of attachment.

Some of these problems are avoided by the use of smooth, soft, non-irritant materials. In addition, drains in clean wounds should be carefully protected from bacterial contamination, preferably by the use of closed drainage systems. When feasible a closed system is also desirable in infected wounds to reduce the handling and spread of organisms.

1a–e

Types of drains

(a) Soft latex rubber tubing (Penrose tubing in North America; Paul's tubing in the United Kingdom) is one of the most widely used drainage materials and has the advantages of being 'floppy' and adaptable to the wound form.

(b) Corrugated material—rubber or plastic—is similar to Penrose drain but not often used outside the United Kingdom.

(c) Fine multiply perforated tubing is most useful for closed vacuum suctioning. A compromise must be found between rigidity and flexibility so that on the one hand the holes remain patent and on the other the drains do not damage adjacent structures.

(d,e) There are two varieties of open suction drains. In one (d) air is drawn in down the narrower tube and air and liquid evacuated up the wider. The air effectively prevents the holes from being occluded by the suction. In the other (e) the outer tube acts as a sump and the liquid percolating into it is scavenged, along with air which passes down into it from the surface, up the narrow tube.

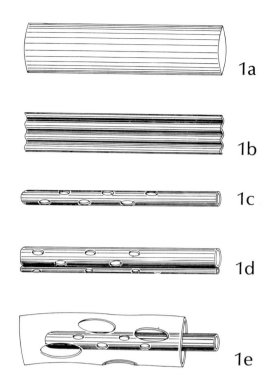

1a

1b

1c

1d

1e

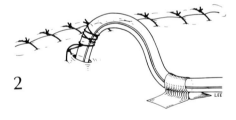

2

2

Fixation

The fixation of a drain should be carried out with particular care. A doubly safe approach by suturing the drain to the skin and taping so as to take the drag from the drain is preferable.

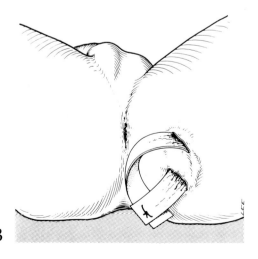

3

3

Abscess wound

In wounds through which abscesses are drained, soft Penrose tubing or corrugated drains are convenient and effective in maintaining an opening for drainage. These drains may be readily dislodged if not carefully secured.

The use of two stab openings into an abscess and inserting a single length of drain with the ends sutured together is an effective approach to this problem. As this type of drain may also disappear into the wound at least a safety pin should otherwise be attached outside the wound on these drains.

4a & b

Wound apposition

For splinting a wound or the removal of transudate in a wound a multiperforated drain with a negative pressure applied to it using one of a variety of portable suction devices is quite effective and now widely used. These systems have the advantage of being closed drains.

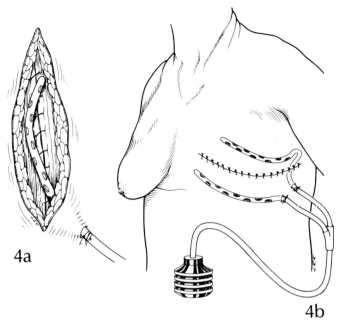

4a

4b

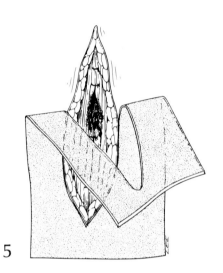

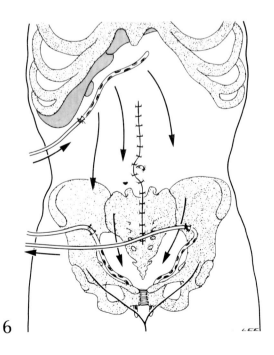

5

5

Open wounds

Although many open wounds are appropriately managed with absorbent material directly applied to the wound, an alternative approach is necessary when such wounds are associated with excessive loss of fluid, as for example from a fistula. Protection of the skin is achieved by the use of an adhesive skin barrier to which a collecting device may be attached. A suction catheter may in addition be passed through such a device to lie in the wound and aspirate the irritant fluid more directly.

6

Peritoneal drains

Drainage of the peritoneal cavity is generally ineffective with most of the systems devised because of the prompt apposition of adjacent intraperitoneal structures about the drain to close it off from the rest of the cavity. Sump drains which draw in air through a second channel do not necessarily overcome this difficulty. The most effective means of maintaining continuity between a drain and the peritoneal cavity is by the use of intermittent infusion of a lavage solution into the cavity which after a short period of 20–30 min is drained by a number of tubes in suitably placed dependent sites. This may be used in heavily soiled peritoneum; lavaging is carried out with a balanced dialysate solution containing gentamicin sulphate 15mg/l. A similar drainage system can be used in acute pancreatitis with one infusing drain placed in the lesser sac. Care should be taken to monitor and correct any electrolyte disturbances and protein losses which may occur. It is probably not advisable to use this technique in the presence of gastrointestinal anastomoses as wound healing may be impaired.

Wound dressings and techniques

Diane Meelheim RN, FNP
Department of Surgery, School of Medicine,
East Carolina University, Greenville, North Carolina

Introduction

Indications for dressing a wound are the following.

Protection of the wound, surrounding skin and underlying structures
Containment of wound drainage
Debridement of necrotic tissue; removal of wound exudate
Application of medications
Immobilization and/or support
Aesthetics

The appropriate dressing will aid in wound healing, reduce contamination, promote early ambulation and help patients to feel better by comfortably and securely covering aesthetically unpleasant wounds. Redressing should take place as often as is required to deal with the purposes listed above.

Wound and skin protection

This is most often provided by gauze bandages held in place by tape, gauze wrap, elastic wrap or rigid dressings. Gauze pads are commercially available in many different weaves, thicknesses and sizes. Cost and use dictate the choice. The quality of commercially available bandages has continually improved and the majority of those marketed today are lint free. Gauze wraps have also been consistently improved so that they no longer have loose strands that find their way into healing tissues. It is now feasible to use these products alone for wound coverage. Care should be taken in applying these wraps as they can have a tourniquet action if applied too tightly. They should be rolled on or applied in a figure-of-eight pattern and secured with tape or elastic nylon tubing.

Absorbent pads that do not adhere to wounds are sometimes useful. This is a particularly important consideration for thermal or abrasion burns or for other wounds with much exudate. Another type of non-adherent dressing is fine-mesh gauze impregnated with various petroleum-based medications. Some companies offer dressings impregnated with antibacterials. With all of these, one medicated layer of the dressing is laid directly onto the wound and covered with additional layers of dry dressing materials.

Protection of the wound and surrounding skin can also be accomplished by use of a semipermeable transparent membrane which adheres to dry skin but allows for evaporation of moisture and the accumulation of exudate, thereby not interfering with healing in some wounds. The technique of application is easy to master. These films are unlikely to induce an allergic reaction and because the dressing is transparent, the wound can be assessed without removing the dressing; thus the patient is spared the discomfort formerly associated with dressing changes. This dressing is particularly useful for wounds with little exudate and for wounds in areas that may be difficult to dress. The film is quite flexible and so is far more comfortable than more rigid dressings. Whilst it is generally agreed that dressings should be kept dry in order to reduce the risk of cross-infection, it may be necessary to protect the structures underlying the wound (e.g. tendon, joint capsule, gut) with moist dressings. An outer plastic covering will maintain such a moist environment, or it may be achieved by continuous saturation dressings (see *below*).

161

Containment of wound drainage

Thick absorbent dressings or collection bags can be used to contain wound drainage.

Absorbent dressings

The thick absorbent dressing may be constructed of numerous layers of gauze or non-woven pads with a covering (to prevent fluff from entering the wound). The dressing may be applied wet to keep it from becoming hardened by serous drainage; saline or similar irrigants are generally used for this purpose.

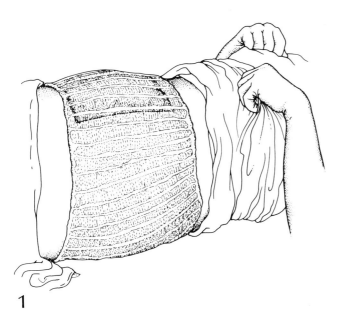

1

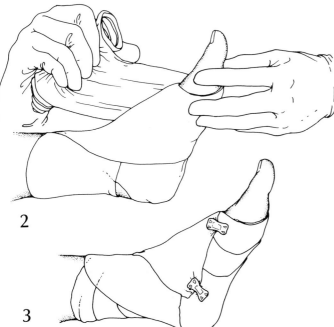

2

3

Methods of anchoring dressings

Dressings of all types must be held in place. The most common way of doing this is with tape, available in many widths and types. Nowadays most tapes are hypoallergenic, such as paper tape, silk tape or plastic tape. Paper tape is made of non-woven material and therefore is to some degree stretchable; it will generally conform to areas with many creases and can be used as the only dressing on dry, clean wounds. Adhesive or cloth tape does not stretch and will cause blisters if it is pulled too tightly during application. Many patients have suffered allergic reactions to the adhesive used in such tape; the resulting burns or reactions must be treated as open wounds. Stretchable adhesive wraps are useful for pressure dressings, but tape burns are a frequent complication of their use.

Another type of commercially available dressing combines the gauze pad and tape into one. Many varieties, shapes and sizes are available with non-adherent or gauze pads, and with plastic or adhesive tape.

1

A comfortable way of anchoring dressings is with knitted elastic tube, available in sizes to fit arms, head, legs and trunk. It can be cut to the proper length, handled with ease and washed and reused many times.

2 & 3

Elastic bandages are occasionally used to anchor dressings but they are difficult to apply properly, slip easily and must be frequently adjusted or reapplied. They should be applied in a figure-of-eight pattern to eliminate tourniquet action; this may require several attempts until the desired arrangement has been achieved. The elastic wrap is secured by small separate clips or by fasteners sewn to one end of the wrap.

Collection bags

Collection bags, the alternative to absorbent dressings, may be applied directly to the skin or to a skin seal. Many brands of such bags are commercially available. Appliances that may be cut to fit a particular wound are of most use postoperatively. These collection bags may be left in place for many days and irrigations and inspections can be carried out through the bottom opening without removing the bag.

Debridement or cleansing of wounds

This may be aided by dressings with one layer of fine-mesh gauze resting directly on the wound surface. Any exudate or necrotic tissue will adhere to this gauze, provided it is not of the non-adherent type and the gauze can then be removed daily or as frequently as seems desirable. Debridement and cleansing of wounds may require the use of active agents topically. Gauze dressings soaked in desloughing agents may be applied directly to necrotic areas.

4, 5 & 6

A continuous saturation dressing is useful in the debridement of wounds where viable skin edges are not immediately apparent, as in the necrotic diabetic foot wound, or necrosis caused by extravasation of drugs. A constantly moist, absorbent dressing, it brings about maceration and debridement of dead tissue while allowing healthy tissue to begin healing. One layer of fine-mesh gauze is first placed directly on the wound followed by a thick layer of gauze sponges. The end of a catheter is positioned directly over the covered wound and gauze layers and catheter are secured in place by wrapping with bulky gauze roll. To ensure that all layers are kept in contact, with no air spaces, an elastic bandage is rolled on as the outer layer. An intravenous set with normal saline or other chosen solution is then attached to the catheter and all layers of the dressing are thoroughly moistened with the solution. The intravenous flow is adjusted to maintain a slow, continuous drip onto the dressing. The continuous saturation dressing should be changed daily. Wounds may be irrigated with active agents, desloughing or bactericidal agents at the time of redressing. Active agents may be applied directly to the wound or an impregnated dressing laid over the wound.

Proprietary products are also available in the form of 'soft cast' which may be poured into the wound, forming a solid but flexible plug specific to that wound. Such products may contain active ingredients or may be of an absorbent nature allowing the wound to drain.

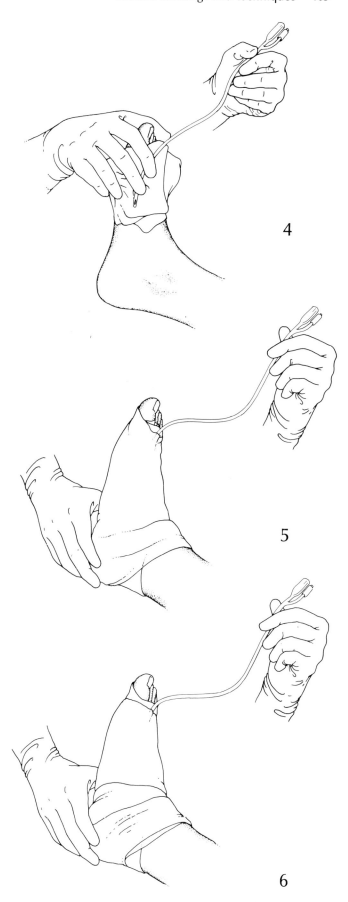

4

5

6

Application of medications

A gauze wrap impregnated with zinc oxide, glycerine and gelatine – Unna's paste – is most frequently used on the lower extremities, applied directly to the wound. It is useful for stasis ulcers, strains, sprains or, occasionally, stumps. Because it does not stretch, it limits oedema. Additionally, it is very absorbent and even though it may not look attractive externally, inside it will be quite clean at the wound site, actually serving to debride the wound in some instances. An Unna's paste dressing need not be changed often and may remain in place safely for up to 2 weeks, though most patients will request that it be changed sooner because of soiling and odour. Care should be taken in application of this bandage to use even, slight tension in rolling it on in a figure-of-eight or spiral pattern to prevent tourniquet action. Removal is best accomplished with large bandage scissors while the extremity is elevated.

Immobilization and/or support

Rigid dressings

Well padded rigid dressings (plaster casts) are frequently applied, with the limb in the position of function, to below-knee or above-knee amputations as the operating room dressing. This approach is very effective in preventing oedema or contamination by urine or faeces. The cast may look very soiled on the outside but remain quite clean inside. Such a dressing is particularly helpful as protection for the suture line when a patient is confused or disoriented. Rigid dressings may be applied over closed-vacuum drains. Removal of the dressing should not be necessary when the drains are discontinued. The whole dressing should be light enough for the patient to lift and must be quite smooth on the outside to protect the other extremity from scrapes. Should the patient complain of pain in the extremity or develop an unexplained fever, the rigid dressing must be removed to allow examination of the limb. For this purpose a cast may be bivalved to allow examination of the wound; it may then be retaped or secured with an elastic bandage. Dry dressings soaked with blood from a wound may act as rigid dressings, thus offering another means of support or immobilization.

Articles of clothing

Adequate wound support may be provided in some cases by articles of clothing. A brassiere can be most helpful postoperatively for the breast biopsy or reconstruction patient; a small dry dressing next to the wound can be held in place by the brassiere, obviating the need for tape.

Supportive garments

These are manufactured by several companies. To be effective they must be properly fitted. The garments – usually stockings or corsets – are expensive and the cost may be a considerable factor in deciding whether to use them or some other means of support. Some patients may

lack the manual dexterity required for applying the garment and in some instances could possibly obtain the same benefit from a more flexible and less tailor-made appliance.

Aesthetics

The external appearance of the wound is important from the point of view of both the patient and those who must care for him. Wounds that are unpleasant to look at should be covered. Dressings should permit maximum function, appear clean and be as unobtrusive as possible. There should be no unpleasant odour. Redressing of wounds should enhance a patient's feeling of well-being and analgesia should be administered as necessary before this procedure. For major dressings of raw or discharging surfaces this means intravenous opiate supplemented by chlorpromazine or diazepam. It is important that wound drainage tubes are secured to permit their correct function and to allow the patient maximum mobility (see p. 159).

Important factors in prescribing dressings are the cost and skill necessary for application of the dressings, as well as the time required for proper care. A detailed description of the prescribed dressing should be given to those who will be caring for it. This description should list the necessary supplies and should give step-by-step instructions on the proper method.

There are times when no dressing is required. The patient may like the idea that something is being done for him in that a dressing is being fashioned and applied, but if the dressing is not actually needed for the reasons enumerated on p. 161 then no dressing should be used and the benefit of fresh air circulating around the body part should be welcomed.

Table 1. Summary of types of wound dressings

	USA	UK
Gauze wraps	Kling, Kerlix	Crinx
Absorbent pads non-adherent	Telfa	Melolin Perfron
Non-woven pads	ABD Combipads	Mesoft Softnet
Non-adherent dressings	Vaseline gauze Xeroform gauze Xeroflo gauze Scarlet Red gauze	Paraffin gauze Paranet Welnet Release, 'N–A'
Transparent film	Op-Site	Op-Site
Tapes – non-stretch self-adhesive	Transpore Coban	Transpore Coban
Stretch	Elastoplast	Elastoplast Murofoam
Elastic bandages	Ace	Elastocrepe Lestreflex
Skin seals	Stomahesive Karaya Hollihesive	Stomahesive Karaya

Local care of burns in the early surgery of the burned patient

Anne B. Sutherland MD, MB ChB, FRCS(Ed.)
Consultant Plastic Surgeon, Regional Plastic and Maxillofacial Surgery Unit,
Bangour General Hospital, Broxburn, West Lothian, Scotland

Preoperative assessment

Assessment of burn depth

This assessment is all important in selecting the local care of any individual patient. Surgery is not required for the *superficial burn* (first degree) which, given good local care by any currently accepted method (exposure or dressing), should heal within 3 weeks. The *deep dermal burn* (second degree) may heal with delay and a poor scar. The *deep burn* (third degree) will eventually slough and granulate.

There is still no completely accurate bedside test of burn depth. The appreciation of pin-prick with a hypodermic needle will usually indicate the more superficial injury and its absence one of greater depth. Additional help is obtained by considering the thickness of skin in the part involved, the age of the patient, the heat and duration of contact of the agent and the appearance of the burned surface (*see* colour plate section facing p. 172).

Assessment of extent of burn

When the area of deep dermal or deep burn is small, for example under 10 per cent of the body surface area, surgery can and should be performed within 48–72 h of injury. In the more extensive burn involving 20 per cent or more of the body surface area, adequate resuscitation will usually demand a delay of some days, the involved areas being treated temporarily by simple dressing or exposure before excision. However, 5–7 days' delay is considered maximal if infection is not to supervene.

Site involved

Position may influence the procedure adopted. A small circumscribed deep burn on the trunk or limb may be suitable for excision while one of similar size and depth on the face may not. A severe destructive deep burn of a limb may be best treated by amputation.

Age of patient

The elderly patient and the infant may be considered to be at greater risk, but age alone should not preclude surgical intervention. Young children especially stand major surgery well, providing adequate fluid replacement is given during and following the procedure.

Additional injury

The burn may be complicated by other injuries which have priority in care or because of which aggressive treatment of the burn wound is contraindicated. Many injuries are complicated by the effects of inhalation of smoke or other noxious fumes. This can cause respiratory damage severe enough to endanger life and in many instances contraindicate general anaesthesia.

Bacteriology of the burn wound

It is vital to establish what organisms are present before any surgical intervention. The presence of a β-haemolytic streptococcus is an absolute contraindication to surgery and should be treated with penicillin for 48 h. Other infections can be treated with the appropriate antibiotic, begun just before surgery.

Extensive injury

A plan should be worked out beforehand for extensive burns. While the aim of surgery is still the closure of the wound at the earliest possible moment, the lack of sufficient unburnt area to provide autograft skin poses the major problem. Little is achieved if excision leaves a wound which cannot be closed. The areas selected for excision in such patients should be those where autografts will have a good chance of taking completely, for example one surface of the trunk or limb. Careful preoperative planning can do much to avoid technical difficulties imposed by a position on the operating table which does not take into account the accessibility of the excision and donor areas.

Circumferential injury

The dangers of circumferential burning of the limbs or trunk must be appreciated. These by their tourniquet effect may prejudice the distal circulation or impair local blood supply at the site of the burn and thus increase tissue destruction. On the trunk such burns can interfere with adequate respiratory excursion. Release incisions may be required within hours of injury and often must precede the formal surgery of the burn wound itself.

Operative procedures

Scalpel excision

Scalpel excision is usually taken to the level of the deep fascia, although in some instances where the burn is less deep it can be through the subcutaneous fat. The resultant raw area is closed by a split-skin graft or by a skin flap, the latter being necessary if bone, tendon, joint, major vessel or vital structure (such as brain) lie in the base of the excision wound. The graft can be applied at the time of excision or delayed 48–72 h. Such delay is advisable when adequate haemostasis is difficult to secure.

Tangential excision

In this technique successive slices of the necrotic tissue are removed until punctate bleeding is obtained. Split-skin grafts are then applied to close the defect. When this form of excision is used grafting should be immediate, otherwise further necrosis may ensue. In burns where the depth has been in doubt this technique may also be diagnostic.

In smaller injuries excision by either the scalpel or tangential method followed by complete closure is usually possible. In extensive injuries the excision may have to be staged, but either method can be used. Autograft sites will, of course, be limited and available donor sites will be unlikely to provide sufficient skin grafts to obtain complete cover. In such instances there are three choices.

1. Excise only what can be covered with available autografts.
2. Excise and cover with a combination of autograft, allograft, xenograft* or synthetic skin**.
3. Excision and mesh grafting.

Use of a skin graft mesher allows expansion of the graft and thus a larger area of cover than would be possible by autografts in strips. The usual mesher expands the graft 3:1. If the grafts are to be meshed it is preferable to use the electric dermatome as the width of the graft is controlled and will be no greater than the width of the mesher. Narrower grafts can, of course, be meshed. If meshed grafts are used following tangential excision they should be covered with xenograft to prevent necrosis of the excised areas between the interstices of the mesh. Mesh grafting leaves an uneven surface which may be cosmetically objectionable and require later replacement.

Preoperative preparation

Minor excision

The general condition of the patient must be assessed, particularly regarding fitness for possible general anaesthesia. In those unfit, excision and grafting can be carried out under local anaesthesia or regional block. The bacteriological state of the surface should be known.

Major excision

The general state of the patient must be assessed in terms of adequate volume replacement given over the period of the initial fluid loss and also fitness to withstand major surgery and anaesthesia lasting 1½ h. Immediate preoperative estimation of blood urea, creatinine, electrolyte concentration and haemoglobin or haematocrit level must be available. Sufficient cross-matched whole blood to make good the estimated loss from the excision areas and the skin graft donor sites is vital.

The bacteriology of the burn surface, the nose, the throat and the rectum should be available to exclude especially β-haemolytic streptococcus and *Pseudomonas pyocyaneus*.

Antibiotics should not be given routinely, but where large raw areas are being created a 5 day course of a broad spectrum antibiotic, started 24 h preoperatively, is wise. The choice will be influenced by any pathogens isolated in the routine cultures. Not only should there be an overall plan but also each procedure should be worked out in advance, including the availability of accessible veins for intravenous infusion. Where more than one area is being excised, two teams will help to keep the operating time to an acceptable length.

Measures must be taken to prevent heat loss through the large raw area created at the time of surgery and either a hot water blanket should be available or arrangements made to keep the theatre temperature to around 25–30°C (80–85°F)

Special equipment

1. Skin grafting knives, preferably with disposable blades – for example, Watson and Humby
2. Skin graft boards
3. Electric dermatome
4. Skin graft mesher
5. Water blanket for the operating table

*Armour Porcine Skin (Ethicon Corethium)
**Epigard (Parke Davis)

The operations

SCALPEL EXCISION AND AUTOGRAFT

1

Removal of necrotic tissue

The whole of the involved area is excised at a sufficient depth to obtain a viable base. Usually this will be at the level of deep fascia, but can be at the level of sub-cutaneous fat.

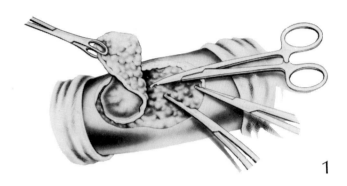

1

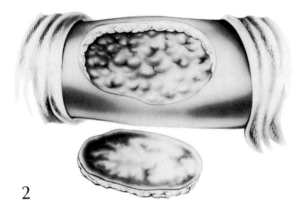

2

2

Control of bleeding

Larger vessels are tied, and smaller ones coagulated. Hot packs are applied.

3

Grafting the defect

Thin to medium split-skin grafts are cut and, following removal of the packs, are applied to the excision area and sutured in position. Haematomas are evacuated. If large sheets of skin are being used, small random perforations may be made to assist in evacuation. The grafts are then dressed with a simple tulle gras padded dressing or left exposed. The graft can be secured with sutures or Steri-strips.

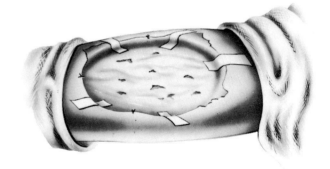

3

TANGENTIAL EXCISION AND AUTOGRAFT

4

Removal of necrotic tissue

The grafting knife is set as if to cut a medium thickness split-skin graft. The area of the burn and the surrounding skin is put on the stretch, if necessary using a skin grafting board. Successive slices are removed until punctate bleeding is seen, one or two usually being sufficient.

Completing the excision

The whole of the involved area is so treated. No further slices should be taken once punctate bleeding is seen. Haemostasis is secured with saline packs while the skin grafts are being cut. These should be of thin to medium thickness.

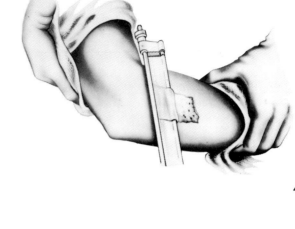

4

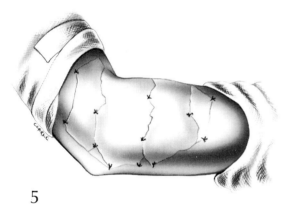

5

5

Grafting the excised area

The packs are removed gently and the grafts laid on the raw surface. The grafts must be applied edge to edge to avoid drying out and necrosis of the uncovered areas. They can be secured with a few fine sutures – 3/0 silk, nylon or synthetic absorbable – held with Steri-strips, or simply laid on without fixation.

Any small haematomas are evacuated and the grafts dressed with a simple tulle gras padded dressing, or left exposed.

PARTIAL EXCISION OF EXTENSIVE BURN

6

Excision of the selected area

The area of burn to be excised is removed by scalpel excision, tangential excision, or by a combination of the two methods. Haemostasis is secured.

Cover of the excised area

Available split-skin grafts are taken and used in one of the following ways.

7

1. Part of the excised area is covered with autograft, while allograft, xenograft or synthetic skin is used on the remainder. (Stippled area represents allograft/xenograft/synthetic skin.)

8

2. Alternating strips of autograft with allograft, xenograft or synthetic skin are applied. (Stippled area represents allograft/xenograft/synthetic skin.)

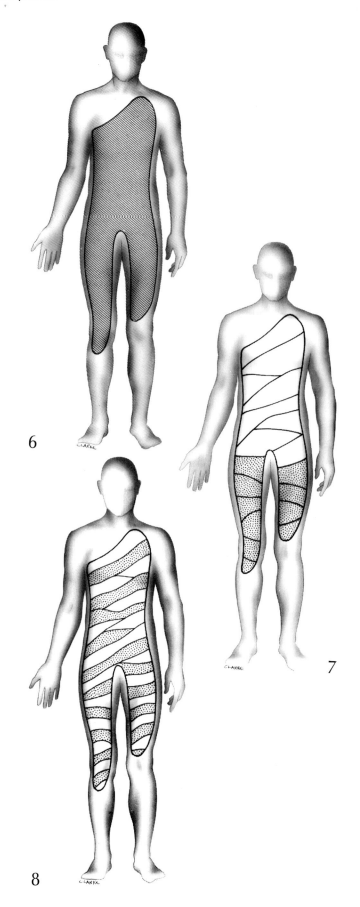

6

7

8

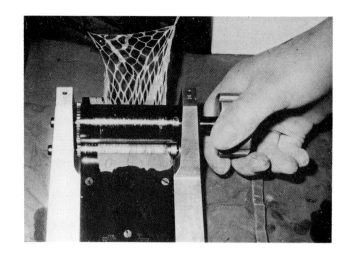

9a & b

3. The autograft can be meshed.
   (a) The grafts are taken with a skin grafting knife or electric dermatome and passed through the skin graft mesher.
   (b) The graft is expanded and laid on the excised surface. It can be combined with sheet grafting if sufficient skin is available.

If doubt exists about the possibility of the autograft taking or if the patient's general condition makes the additional trauma of taking autograft skin inadvisable, the whole excised area can be covered with allograft, xenograft or synthetic skin. The grafting procedure is delayed for 3–4 days.

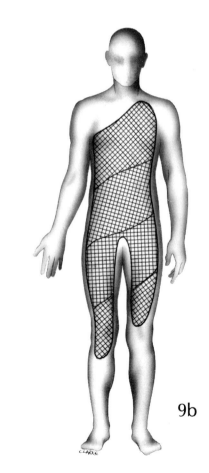

9b

RELEASE INCISION

10

Incision in limbs

A zig-zag incision is made down to deep fascia. In some instances the deep fascia may also need to be incised. The incision should gape widely. Careful haemostasis is important.

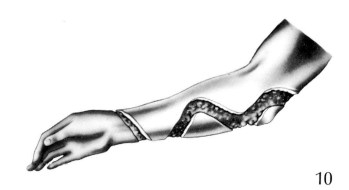

10

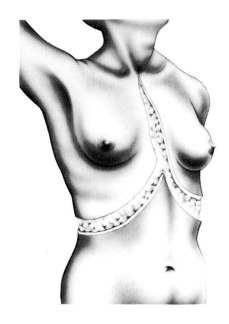

11

11

Incision on trunk

Incisions are made over the areas of maximal tension, the incision being taken to deep fascia.

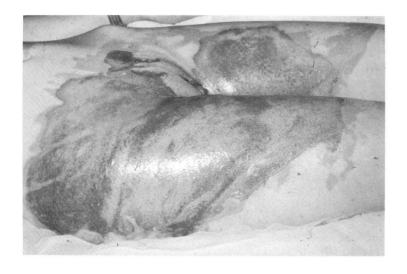

Superficial burn
Note pink moist-looking surface

Deep dermal burn
Note the whitish appearance typical of deep dermal involvement and the more superficial areas around the periphery

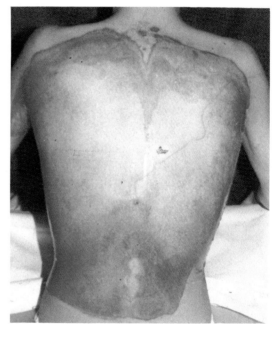

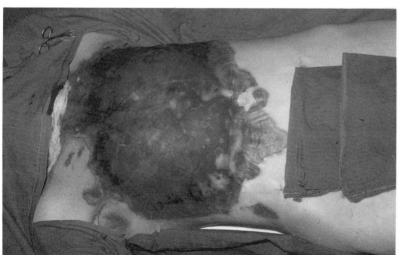

Deep burn
Note dry dark brown colour with thrombosed vessels evident in the eschar

Postoperative care

Blood loss

Following excision, there will be continuing blood loss both from the excised area and from the donor site. Adequate replacement must be ensured.

Pain

Postoperative pain from areas of excision and skin graft donor areas can be severe. Opiate analgesia should be prescribed in adequate dosage. This will also help to avoid unnecessary movement in recently grafted areas.

Care of grafts and dressings

The grafts themselves may be exposed or dressed depending on the associated nursing problems. Where possible, grafts on the chest wall are better left exposed, to avoid the shearing forces between graft and dressing which occur with respiratory excursion.

If dressed, the time of dressing change will depend on the state of the surface at the time of grafting. For example, if haemostasis has been difficult to achieve, inspection at 3–4 days may be indicated. Otherwise, there is no reason to redress in under a week. In the dressed grafts, there must be free circulating air around the dressing to allow evaporation and to avoid maceration. The same is true of the donor sites. In either, any soakage to the outside of the dressing is an indication for dressing change.

In the US antibacterial ointments such as Sulfamylon and silver sulfadiazene are widely used to control surface infection. Silver nitrate is also effective but can cause serious electrolyte disturbances and is a nuisance because it permanently spots linen and clothing.

In the major excision, dressings should be changed every 3–4 days, the old allograft/xenograft removed and fresh dressings applied. The process should be repeated until the donor areas have healed and can be reused (about 3 weeks). Then the allograft/xenograft can be replaced with autograft. Several crops of grafts may have to be taken from the same areas before skin cover of an extensive burn is achieved. A similar technique can be used where the burn slough has been allowed to separate spontaneously, for example in a patient where other factors have precluded early excision. The granulating areas are protected by frequent changes of allograft/xenograft until autograft cover is possible.

Further general anaesthesia, or good analgesia, will be required for these dressing changes, but the increased protein and energy needs of these patients must be maintained.

Later care

Once the grafts have consolidated and the donor areas are soundly healed, they should be treated with a simple hydrous ointment, for example Unguentum Aquosum, to avoid excessive dryness. Where the lower limbs have been involved, ambulation must be preceded by carefully graded exercises, first in the bed and then with increasing dependency before free movement is allowed. Support to the limbs is provided by Tubigrip and crêpe bandage, which should be worn continuously for 2–3 months to avoid late blister formation and breakdown.

Further reading

Artz, C. P., Thompson, N. J. Early excision of large areas in burns. Surgery 1968; 63: 868–870

Artz, C. P., Moncrief, J. A., Pruitt, B. A. Burns: a team approach. Philadelphia, London: W. B. Saunders, 1979

Cason, J. S. Treatment of burns. London: Chapman & Hall, 1981

Jackson, D. M. Tangential excision and grafting of burns. The method and a report of 50 consecutive cases. British Journal of Plastic Surgery 1972; 25: 416–426

Janžekovič, Z. A new concept in the early excision and immediate grafting of burns. Journal of Trauma 1970; 10: 1103–1108

Pruitt, B. A., Curreri, P. W. The burn wound and its care. Archives of Surgery 1971; 103: 461–468

Illustrations by Gillian Lee

Principles and practice of drainage of abscesses

R. G. Lightwood FRCS
Senior Surgical Registrar, St Mary's Hospital, London

Introduction

The treatment of an acute pyogenic abscess involves the evacuation of the contents, by either open or closed drainage. Open drainage is performed by incision of the abscess wall, after which the cavity may be closed primarily or left open to drain and heal by secondary intention. Closed drainage by the aspiration of pus is an alternative method, which is appropriate to specific sites, particularly pleural and hepatic abscesses.

Preoperative

Indications for drainage

Drainage is indicated as soon as there is evidence of localized pus. Fluctuation is the most reliable sign in a superficial abscess though it may not be demonstrable if the abscess is very tense. Fluctuance is a late sign in tissues which have a strong network of fibrous tissue, such as those of the neck, breast and ischiorectal space. In these areas, considerable pus formation may be present before the classic tightness of the skin and ballottement of fluid develops. In suspicious cases, aspiration of the inflamed area is strongly advised. Early drainage can prevent the considerable danger of a destroyed breast or an uncontrollable pararectal infection. It is important not to incise an aneurysm by mistake! Preliminary needle aspiration should be used when there is doubt.

The decision to drain a deep abscess is based on systemic signs together with imaging investigations which show the cavity, the displacement of surrounding structures, or abnormal distribution of radionucleide-labelled white cells.

Preparation

Once indicated, drainage should not be delayed. Routine preparation is made for anaesthesia and hair removed from the operation site. It is preferable to have a separate theatre reserved for septic cases; otherwise decontamination must take place before the next clean operation.

Anaesthesia

A small superficial abscess can be incised after freezing the skin with an ethyl chloride spray. General anaesthesia or a regional nerve block is used for any larger abscess. Local anaesthesia by infiltration is avoided because the procedure is painful and may result in the spread of infection.

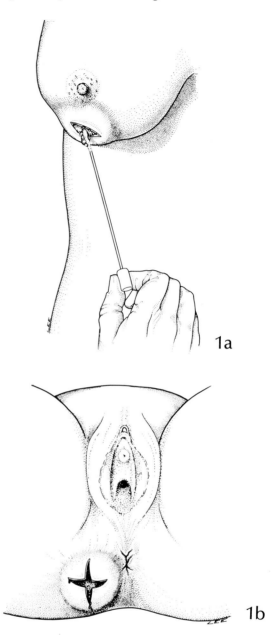

1a

1b

The operation

1a & b

The incision

(a) A small superficial abscess is incised over the centre of fluctuation in Langer's lines (in fact, the skin wrinkle lines), avoiding damage to any important local structures. The moment pus flows a specimen is taken for bacteriological examination. If necessary the incision can be enlarged by making a cruciate incision (b). For an extensive abscess a counter-incision may be added to provide drainage in more than one direction.

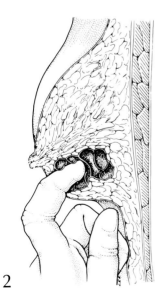

2

2

The cavity is entered with a blunt instrument, such as a sinus forceps, and a finger is used to explore the abscess and to break down any loculi.

The pus is evacuated. The wound can either be closed at once with antibiotic cover, or left open to drain and heal by granulation. Primary closure reduces the need for dressings, allows rapid healing and is suitable for the small superficial abscess when the spectrum of antibiotic sensitivity can be anticipated. The larger abscess cavity is best left open, as is also the case when the nature of the organism and thus its antibiotic sensitivity remain in doubt. Experience dictates the choice of method.

3

Primary closure

Before primary closure the abscess wall is removed by thorough curettage, to allow the penetration of systemic antibiotics; a single dose of these is effective, given 1h before operation[1]. The wound is then closed with interrupted non-absorbable monofilament skin sutures, placed deep enough to obliterate the cavity, so as to avoid the formation of an infected haematoma. If later there are signs that pus has reaccumulated, then the wound must be reopened.

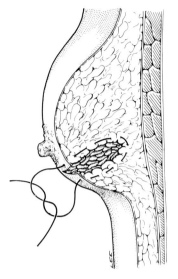

3

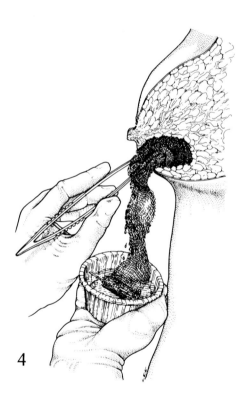

4

Packing

4

The evacuated abscess cavity is *filled* with sterile ribbon gauze soaked in antiseptic solution, such as Eusol, mixed with liquid paraffin to enable the pack to be removed with the least discomfort to the patient. The pack must be changed frequently until the discharge stops.

An alternative method is to fill the cavity with silicone elastic foam which sets after a few minutes to provide an absorbent non-adherent pack which is easy to remove and clean when redressing (*see also* chapter on 'Wound dressings and techniques', pp. 161–164). This may be done by the patient using the same pack until a smaller one is needed as the cavity closes[2].

An ordinary dry dressing is substituted when the cavity has almost healed.

DRAINAGE

5

Following the initial incision, continued drainage is needed for large or deeply situated abscess cavities. Drains must be of adequate size, placed in the cavity, preferably in a dependent position, and fixed securely to the patient. The best method of fixation is to place a strong suture through both the drain and the adjacent skin on each side. There must be no hesitation is using more than one drain.

A drain should not be removed until a track has been formed – usually at least 5–6 days – or before the cavity has closed. Soluble X-ray contrast medium injected down a tube drain will demonstrate this. When a drain is removed, there is no advantage to be gained from progressive shortening.

Types of drain

Many different sorts of drain are available, derived from the basic patterns of the open corrugated drain and the closed tube drain. All drains should have radiopaque markers.

6

Corrugated drains

These are suitable for relatively superficial abscesses and both ends can be used to provide drainage in two directions. Drainage is directly into the dressings, which may need frequent changing. Variations in design are the Yates and Ragnell drains, neither of which has any specific advantage.

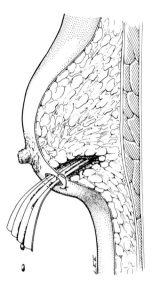

5

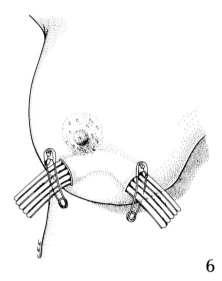

6

7

Tube drains

For deep cavities a tube drain with side holes at the distal end is more suitable. It is attached to a drainage bag which provides a closed system and reduces the need for redressing.

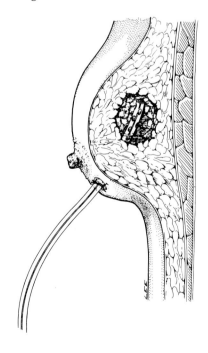

7

8

Sump drains

These double-lumen tube drains enable suction to be applied to the cavity without blockage of the drain. They are most useful in the management of abscesses associated with gastrointestinal fistulae.

Closed drainage

The closed method of drainage is used most often for abscess cavities in the liver and the pleura.

9

Needle aspiration

The skin is infiltrated with local anaesthetic and a wide-bore aspirating needle is introduced into the abscess. Pus is aspirated until the cavity is dry, and a specimen is sent for bacteriological examination. The appropriate antibiotic is injected before withdrawing the needle. The procedure is repeated at intervals until the cavity closes.

10

Closed tube drainage

Under local or general anaesthesia, a drainage tube is placed in the abscess cavity using an introducer, guided by ultrasound or computerized tomography. The use of a Foley balloon catheter enables the drain to be self retaining and the cavity may be irrigated through the additional channel of a three-way catheter[3].

References

1. Blick, P. W. H., Flowers, M. W., Marsden, A. K., Wilson, D. H., Ghoneim, A. T. M. Antibiotics in surgical treatment of acute abscesses. British Medical Journal 1980; 281: 111–112

2. Wood, R. A. B., Williams, R. H. P., Hughes, L. E. Foam elastomer dressing in the management of open granulating wounds: experience with 250 patients. British Journal of Surgery 1977; 64: 554–557

3. Kraulis, J. E., Bird, B. L., Colapinto, N. D. Percutaneous catheter drainage of liver abscess: an alternative to open drainage? British Journal of Surgery 1980; 67: 400–402

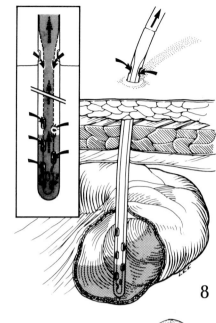

8

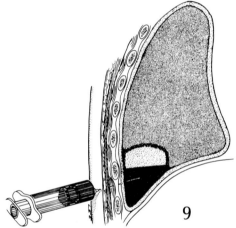

9

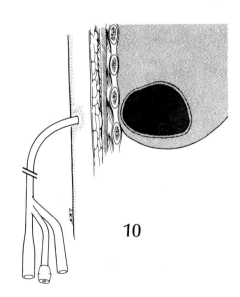

10

Illustrations by Patrick Elliott

Hand sepsis

D. J. Williams FRCS
Consultant Orthopaedic and Trauma Surgeon, Queen Elizabeth II Hospital,
Welwyn Garden City, Hertfordshire and Hertford County Hospitals

Introduction

The treatment of hand infections will not be successful unless it has been preceded by correct diagnosis. The emphasis of this chapter will be towards diagnosis.

Since antibiotics became widely available, complete restoration of function should be possible in practically every infected hand. There are three reasons for bad results.

1. Delay by the patient before seeking treatment.
2. Delay by the physician in referring the patient to hospital.
3. Bad hospital treatment, which is most often the consequence of mistakes in diagnosis and the wrong timing of operations.

A full and detailed history is the best safeguard against mistakes in diagnosis and management. Hand sepsis conforms to a definite time pattern from onset to localization. Antibiotics can achieve resolution of hand infections if correctly given within 48 h of the onset of infection. If given later, antibiotics do not usually influence the time of localization.

The history of an injury is remembered by 60 per cent of patients and gives a valuable clue to the anatomical diagnosis. Infections that begin on the dorsum of the hand are usually boils or carbuncles. The palm must be examined to exclude palmar infection as the cause of dorsal swelling.

A 1–2 day history of throbbing pain, with swelling and one sleepless night caused by the pain, accompanies an acute cellulitis or a tendon sheath infection. The infecting organism is often *Streptococcus pyogenes.*

A 4–5 day history of pain, swelling and one sleepless night on account of throbbing indicates that pus is present. The infecting organism is usually *Staphylococcus pyogenes.*

This information is summarized in the flow chart (p. 180)

The patient's occupation should also be taken into account when making the diagnosis.

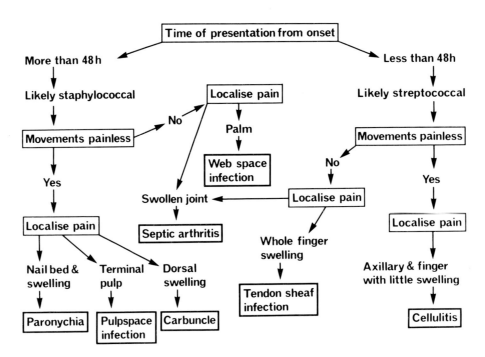

Treatment principles

Rest and chemotherapy when infection is diffuse

The infected hand should rest in a sling in an elevated position relative to the heart. Chemotherapy must begin as soon as the diagnosis is made. Patients who are pyrexial should be admitted for bed rest, as should patients with lymphangitis. Systemic antibiotics should be given to these patients.

The choice of antibiotic

Over 85 per cent of infections are caused by staphylococci, 10 per cent by streptococci. All will be sensitive to flucloxacillin and this is the antibiotic of choice. Tetracycline should be given to the patient with a history of hypersensitivity.

Five per cent will be the result of a mixed infection and co-trimoxazole (Septrin) is the antibiotic of choice.

The sling

The sling should support the hand to prevent a secondary painful dependency-swelling which will occur if the sling is not appropriately placed.

Relief of pain: preventing deformity

A dorsal plaster of Paris splint which immobilizes the wrist in dorsiflexion, with the metacarpal phalangeal joints in 90° flexion and the interphalangeal joints slightly flexed in the position of function, is essential for relief of severe pain, especially in tendon sheath infections and septic arthritis. Adequate analgesia should be prescribed in addition, but elevation and rest with splintage often brings more significant pain relief than analgesia alone.

Topical application

The local application of highly osmotic wet solutions must be avoided because the skin will become macerated and there is no evidence that resolution is helped.

Regular review

Outpatients must be seen daily. Continued throbbing pain after evacuating pus means incomplete evacuation. Most pulp space infections and acute paronychia need to be drained at the first attendance.

Techniques for localized infections

Instruments

A few small fine instruments are necessary.

Sharp pointed 12 cm scissors.
Dissecting forceps.
Fine probe.
Small curette.
Sinus forceps.

Preoperative preparation

The patient should wash and dry both hands. The area of maximum tenderness and the size and direction of the proposed incision should be marked out with a skin pencil. The incision should be small and along the direction of normal skin tension lines. Midline incision should be avoided in infections of the proximal and middle pulp spaces so as to protect the tendon sheaths. A bloodless field is essential and can be achieved by elevation of the arm for 2 min, followed by the application of a tourniquet.

Anaesthesia

General anaesthesia

This is necessary for any infection proximal to the middle phalanx of the finger. A general anaesthetic is also indicated for:

very nervous patients;
children under the age of 14 years;
operations when bone infection is suspected;
patients with deficient circulation of the fingers;
patients with cellulitis where pus needs to be drained.

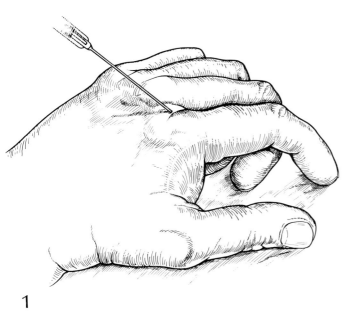

1

Local anaesthesia

Where possible, local web space ringblock anaesthesia with 1 per cent lignocaine hydrochloride without adrenaline should be used and gives excellent results; 2.5 ml are injected around each digital nerve. If the needle is inserted subcutaneously into the loose tissue of the web and then directed forwards, it is not painful. Complete anaesthesia takes 5 min to reach the tip of the finger where most lesions occur.

1

Specific infections

PARONYCHIA

This is an infection around the base of the nail which is often caused by rough manicuring or by picking a hang-nail.

Acute infection

Treatment

If less than 48 h from onset, the hand should be rested and chemotherapy given.

2

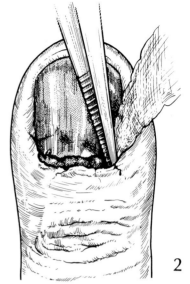

2

If longer, the pus should be drained. Incision is made only where the pus lies. Adequate drainage is provided by deroofing the abscess with scissors and exploring the cavity with a blunt probe, but leaving the nail intact if there is no pus under the nail fold.

3 & 4

Late treatment

In patients who present late there is often a subungual abscess. Transillumination of the finger tip will show the pus as an opaque area. The proximal half of the nail should be excised to drain the abscess by cutting the loose nail across with a pair of scissors. The wound should be dressed daily with moist dressings.

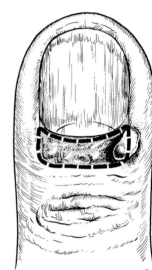

3   4

Chronic infection

5

This affects many nails simultaneously. The nail fold is hypertrophic and the nail grows in thickened ridges. Fungal infection is often the cause. Occasionally, tuberculosis may be the underlying lesion and must be especially considered in a susceptible population.

Treatment

The hands should be kept dry, clean and protected from immersion by wearing rubber gloves with cotton liners. The nail should not be removed. Appropriate antibiotics should be continued for at least 24 months, if indicated. Castellani paint may be applied twice daily to the affected nail fold.

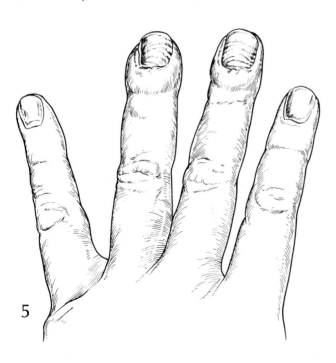

5

TERMINAL PULP SPACE INFECTIONS

6

These may present as a subcuticular abscess which will be of collar stud type, the deeper pulp infection having decompressed into the subcuticular space. The more sinister infection is the red, swollen, throbbing fingertip of 5 days' duration – deep pus under pressure will be present and requires drainage. Failure to recognize this may lead to the pressure rising above the closing pressure of the blood vessels, causing necrosis of the distal four-fifths of the terminal phalanx with an osteomyelitic sequestrum.

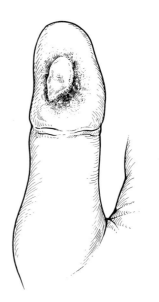

6

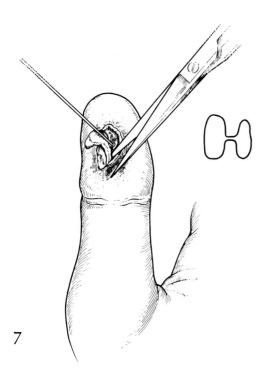

7

Treatment

This is urgent. Local anaesthetic is effective.

7

Collar stud abscess

The superficial cavity is deroofed with scissors. The size of the communicating deeper cavity is defined by a blunt probe. Adequate drainage is effected with sinus forceps; granulations are curetted out. The wound is dressed daily but drain or wicks are not inserted.

Deep pus under pressure

The correct site for incision is directly over the site of maximal tenderness which should be determined with a fine blunt probe. The pus is drained after defining the cavity with the probe and enlarging the small linear incision into a diamond shape with fine scissors.

Complications

Inadequate drainage of pus will not relieve the patient's symptoms. Osteomyelitis of the phalanx may be established or occur. Necrosis of the phalanx may follow.

APICAL PULP SPACE INFECTIONS

This infection will either be localized or will have spread subungually. The cause is always local trauma and nail biters are most vulnerable.

8

Localized abscess is deroofed and the wedge of nail excised opposite the point of maximal tenderness at the apex.

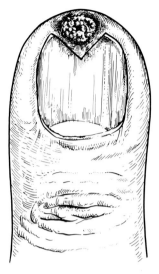

8

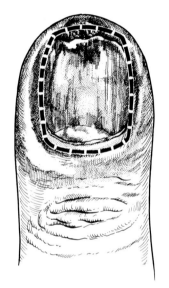

9

9

If subungual spread has occurred the nail should be removed and the abscess cavity deroofed.

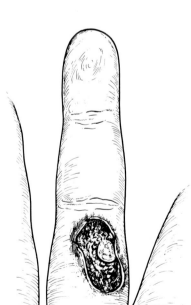

10

10

OTHER PULP SPACE INFECTIONS

These are almost always of the collar stud variety and should be treated in the same way as terminal pulp infections. Iatrogenic injury of the flexor sheath or neurovascular bundles is very unusual as the pus pushes these vital structures out of the way. The neurovascular bundles will be protected by the surgeon's constant awareness of their anatomical position (see Illustration 17) and by probing deeper structures with sinus forceps or blunt probes.

NEGLECTED TERMINAL PULP INFECTIONS COMPLICATED BY OSTEOMYELITIS

This is extremely rare but will occur if the pulp infection has not been adequately drained within 7 days of onset. The bone sequestrum will prevent healing until it has been removed. The dead bone which is loose should be removed and curetting of the cavity carried out until bleeding from the bone is obvious.

PALMAR INFECTIONS

Web space infections

11 & 12

These may follow infected blisters on the palm of the hand. Adduction of the affected finger is painful. Early cellulitis and dorsal oedema develop.

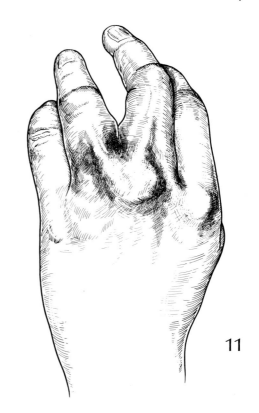

11

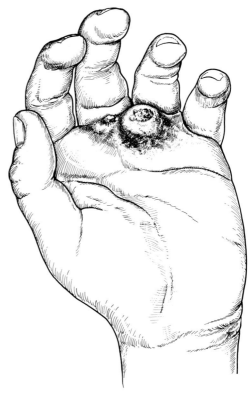

12

13

Treatment

The blister is deroofed and probed for a deeper extension. Gentle pressure will show pus welling up from these cavities. Sinus forceps should be passed to effect drainage. If there is no blister and pus is present, a transverse incision is made in the palmar skin 2 cm proximal to the skin on the edge of the affected web but the sinus forceps are used to explore the deeper layers.

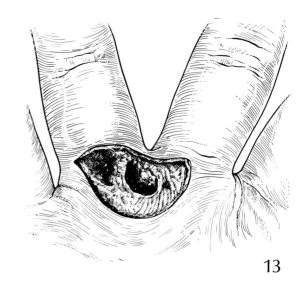

13

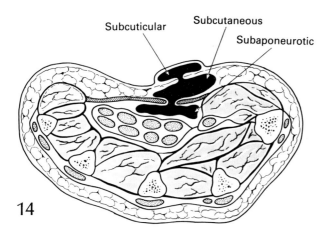

Subcuticular   Subcutaneous

Subaponeurotic

14

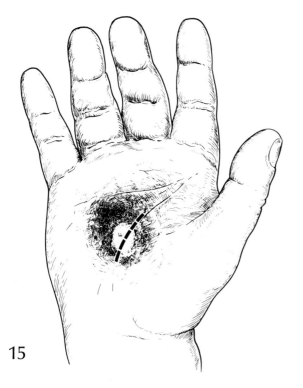

15

14 & 15

Palmar abscess

This is a collar stud type of abscess and should be managed in a similar manner to that in the pulp space.

TENDON SHEATH INFECTIONS

16 & 17

These may occur without any history of injury though the onset of severe symptoms within hours of a midline injury to the volar aspect of the finger or palm will suggest the diagnosis. The infecting organism is usually a streptococcus. The finger is uniformly red, hot, swollen and held slightly flexed. There is acute tenderness directly overlying the surface markings of the sheath. Any attempt, active or passive, to extend the finger is severely painful.

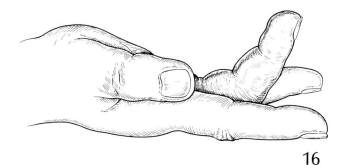

16

Treatment

The infection may resolve if diagnosed early, i.e. within 48 h, and flucloxacillin administered parenterally for 5 days. The hand *must* be immobilized in a plaster cast which is applied on the dorsum with the hand in the position of function. The arm must be elevated in a sling so that the hand is higher than the heart. Tetracycline is not used for patients with a history of sensitivity to penicillin because of a high resistance rate. Erythromycin is a preferable alternative.

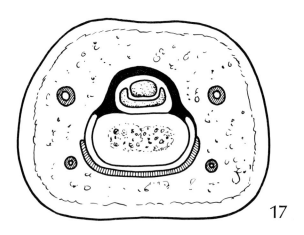

17

Late diagnosis

In such patients the site of the original injury should first be explored by a transverse incision over the sheath. In severe infections, in addition, both ends of the sheath may have to be opened. In less severe cases only the proximal end of the sheath will need to be opened as well. The sheath should be washed through using normal saline. Rest, splintage and elevation should be continued for a further 48 h, then gentle mobilization of the fingers should begin.

Acknowledgements

I should like to thank Joan Sneddon, MD, MRCPsych, Lecturer in Psychiatry, Sheffield University, for allowing me to base this work on her chapter published in the 3rd edition. I should also like to thank her and the artist Patrick Elliott for agreeing to let me make use of the illustrations, which have been prepared for Dr Sneddon's chapter 'Infections' in *The Hand* volume, 4th edition.

Further reading

Bolton, H., Fowler, P. J., Jepson, R. P. Natural history and treatment of pulp space infection and osteomyelitis of terminal phalanx. Journal of Bone and Joint Surgery 1949; 31:B499-504

Lowden, T. G. Prevention and treatment of hand infections. Postgraduate Medicine 1964; 40:247-252

Petrie, P. W. R., Lamb, D. W. Severe hand problems in drug addicts following self administrated infections. Hand 1973; 5:130-134

Sneddon, J. The care of hand infections. London: Edward Arnold, 1970

Illustrations by Robert Lane

Procedures for pilonidal disease

Douglas Millar FRCS, FRCS(Ed.)
Surgeon and Surgical Tutor, Essex County Hospital, Colchester

Introduction

Numerous surgical treatments for postanal pilonidal sinus have been employed; they have varied in their effectiveness and carried significant failure rates. The choice of the procedure has been influenced by changing opinions as to the cause, significance of recurrence, the presence of infection and secondary sinuses. The expense and lack of availability of operating theatre facilities and of inpatient hospital care has also stimulated the use of the more simple and purely outpatient procedures. The wider excisional procedures were introduced on the basis that the sinus originated in a congenital cyst which had to be completely extirpated. The use of more simple procedures is based on the sinus being a granulating cavity analogous to a septic foreign body reaction to hair and other buried material. The simple procedures require a more accurate outpatient follow-up procedure which might not be available in a widespread community. Multiple and extensive tracks from the main sinus can influence the choice of procedure in that these may require more extensive curettage and longer inpatient hospitalization, but it seems that this situation is unusual.

SIMPLE NON-OPERATIVE MEASURES

In small central sinuses with no tracking the simple measure of removal of hairs from the sinus with forceps without anaesthesia, followed by meticulous local hygiene and shaving of the surrounding skin can give comparable results to surgery. A small foreign-body granulomatous sinus will heal provided the foreign material is removed and sound healing is obtained. Local shaving is helpful to keep the hairs short until the scar is sound but the dose of irradiation required for effective epilation is unjustifiable.

SIMPLE OPERATIVE METHODS

Principles

Simple midline sinuses can be dealt with under local anaesthesia but more extensive cavities and the presence of lateral tracks extending more than 5 cm usually require general anaesthesia. The essential technique is to excise the midline sinus pits to allow free drainage of a cavity after careful cleansing. Lateral tracks are cleaned out with the excision of the external orifice or alternatively laid open throughout the whole length. The raw areas are allowed to heal from the base by granulation but supervision is required to ensure that the patient maintains good hygiene and that the skin edges do not bridge over the cavity.

Position of patient

The patient lies on the left side turned slightly face downwards. The right buttock is retracted by an assistant or by adhesive plaster to open up the natal cleft. Alternatively a prone position can be used but this complicates the general anaesthetic procedure.

Anaesthesia

Local anaesthesia can be given in the form of an injection of 1 per cent lignocaine and 1:200 000 adrenaline around the midline pits and around the openings of any lateral tracks. General anaesthesia is indicated particularly in the presence of an abscess or local fibrosis caused by previous operative procedures, and in cases where tracks extend 5 cm or more from the midline epithelial pits or extend into both buttocks.

The operation

1

Preparation of site

The area immediately around the midline pits and the lateral sinuses is meticulously shaved for a distance of 5 cm. Any residual hair that was long enough to enter the operation wound might interfere with healing. After careful shaving, midline epithelial pits which were not previously visible may sometimes show up.

The elliptical lines indicate the lines of surgical excision. They closely surround the midline pits and the lateral sinus openings.

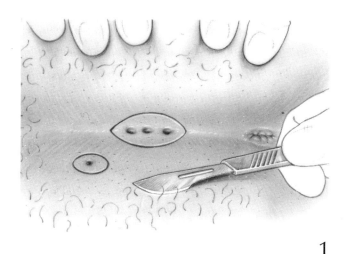

1

2

Excision of midline pits

The midline epithelial pits are excised in an elliptical fashion, removing not more than 0.5 cm of skin on either side. This excision is carried down into the underlying granulomatous cavity from which any hair is carefully removed and debris is cleaned out. No attempt is made to excise the cavity completely.

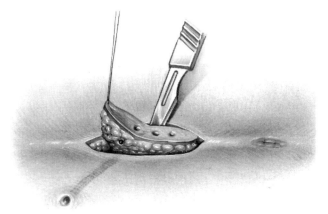

2

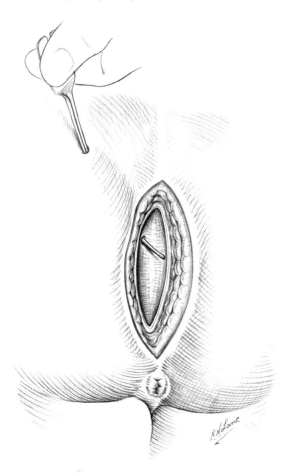

3

Demonstration of lateral sinus track

The lateral sinus track is probed to demonstrate its connection with the main central cavity. The track can then be enlarged with sinus forceps.

3

4

Excision of lateral sinus opening

The opening of the lateral sinus is excised with a circular incision to gain good access to the connecting track. If there is a lateral abscess this must be unroofed by a similiar circular incision to obtain full drainage.

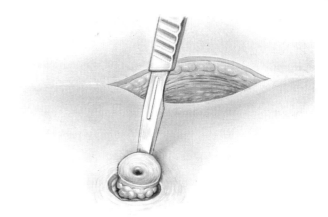

4

5

Debridement of cavity and sinus tracks

All hair and foreign material must be removed by thorough cleaning of the midline cavity and of the lateral sinus tracks. Hair is removed with forceps and the cavity curetted. Hair in the lateral sinus and foreign material can be removed by inserting successively small bottle brushes and a spoon curette. These are rotated and moved backwards and forwards to clean out the track.

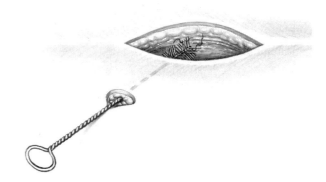

MODIFIED SIMPLE PROCEDURE

5

As an alternative the lateral track can be incised throughout its full length into the main cavity. The granulomatous track and its contents and hairs are then curetted out and cleaned.

MARSUPIALIZATION (ADDITIONAL PROCEDURE)

In very obese patients or cases in which the exposed sinus cavity appears to be overlapped by the skin edges with a danger of bridging-over, marsupialization may be employed.

Interrupted chromic catgut sutures are placed between the raw skin edge and the margin of the opened-up sinus. The object is to turn in the skin edge to prevent a skin bridge healing over the site.

Postoperative care

Care of the wound

After the simple procedures all that is required is a dry gauze pad for a dressing. On the first postoperative day a bath is taken and the dressing removed. After careful drying of the area the gauze pad is replaced. This procedure is repeated daily and can be carried out at home by the patient. Leisure and work activities may be resumed immediately and only restricted by any local discomfort.

Subsequent care

It is essential that the patient attends an Outpatient Clinic at at least 2-weekly intervals until complete firm healing in the area has been achieved. At this time any bridging of the skin across the deeper cavity can be broken down so that the healing takes place from the base towards the surface. Any accumulated debris is cleaned out and the hair is shaved on the surrounding skin for a margin of 5 cm. Following complete healing the patient is advised on careful personal hygiene and the use of a simple astringent lotion, allowing the scars to become pale and firm. This type of follow-up procedure is essential to ensure the minimal hospitalization, earliest return to work and minimal recurrence rate.

Alternative major surgical procedures

Introduction

Total excision of the whole granulomatous area and tracks has no advantage over the simple measures. Split-skin grafting of these areas may accelerate the produced delayed healing but only leads to prolonged hospitalization. Other methods of excision and direct suture with rotation flaps or Z-plasty require longer hospitalization, but although suitable for extensive tracking are contraindicated in anything but a quiescent condition. Badly infected or extensively tracking sinuses carry a higher recurrence rate with these methods.

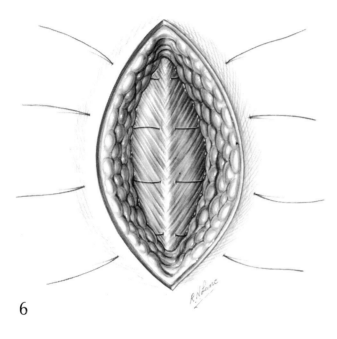

6

EXCISION AND SUTURE

This method is suitable for a local sinus without tracking where the hospitalization time is not important and the follow-up attendance for the patient is difficult to achieve.

6 & 7

Following wide excision of the sinus, wound closure can be maintained by direct sutures through the sacral fascia.

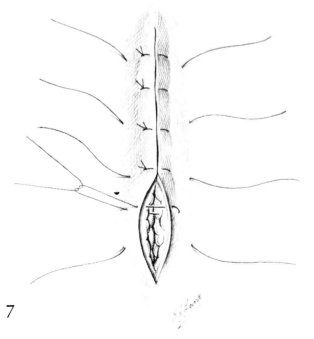

7

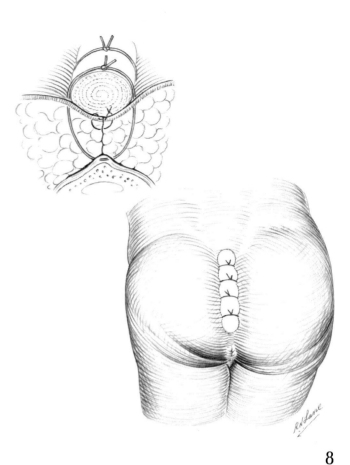

8

The sutures are tied externally in order to hold a gauze pressure dressing in place.

8

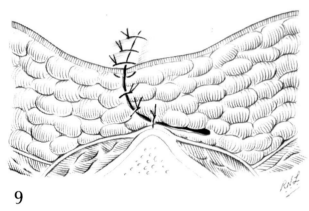

9

9

Undermining of the lateral flap can reduce tension, thus producing an increased incidence of primary healing.

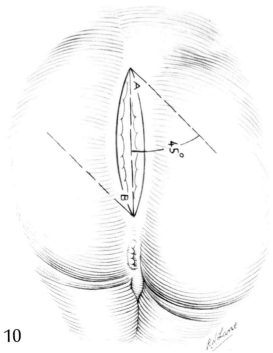

10

10

For extensive lateral tracking a Z-plasty flap can be fashioned but requires extensive mobilization of the buttock tissues.

These methods produce a cure rate comparable to other methods but are not superior. They have the disadvantage of longer hospitalization but probably require less meticulous follow-up.

Acute pilonidal abscess

A simple incision over the pointing abscess results in a very high recurrence rate and should be regarded therefore as a temporary expedient before definitive surgery. If, however, sinus pits are excised and the whole cavity laid open and thoroughly cleansed into the lateral tracks a high percentage of cures result, requiring no further surgery.

Recurrent pilonidal sinus

A simple excision of sinus pits and laying open of the underlying cavity with cleansing, with or without marsupialization, is as effective as any other treatment and simpler. It is generally inadvisable to attempt to re-excise totally a recurrent pilonidal sinus.

Further reading

Simple treatment techniques

Edwards, M. H. Pilonidal sinus: A five year appraisal of the Millar-Lord treatment. British Journal of Surgery 1977; 64: 867–868

Goodall, P. Management of pilonidal sinus. Proceedings of the Royal Society of Medicine 1975; 68: 675

Notaras, M. J. A review of three popular methods of treatment of postanal (pilonidal) sinus disease. British Journal of Surgery 1970; 57: 886–890

Ortiy, H. H., Marti, J., Sites, A. Pilonidal sinus: A claim for simple track incision. Diseases of the Colon and Rectum 1977; 20: 325–328

Primary suture techniques

Bentivegna, S. S., Procario, P. Primary closure of pilonidal cystectomy. American Surgery 1977; 43: 214–216

Goligher, J. C. Surgery of the anus, rectum and colon, 3rd Ed. London: Baillière Tindall, 1975

Flap–suture techniques

Fishbeir, R. H., Handelsman, J. C. A method for primary reconstruction following radical excision of sacrococcygeal pilonidal disease. Annals of Surgery 1979; 190: 231–235

Middleton, M. D. Treatment of pilonidal sinus by Z-Plasty. British Journal of Surgery 1968; 55: 516–518

Karydakis, G. E. New approach to the problem of pilonidal sinus. Lancet 1973; 2: 1414

Surgery of hidradenitis suppurativa

L. E. Hughes DS, FRCS, FRACS
Professor of Surgery, Welsh National School of Medicine, Cardiff

W. P. Morgan BSc, FRCS
Senior Registrar in Surgery, University Hospital of Wales, Cardiff

Introduction

Hidradenitis suppurativa results when apocrine sweat glands, obstructed by keratinous plugging of the hair follicles, become secondarily infected. Recent work has suggested that anaerobic organisms are the principal pathogens. Because the glands are frequently destroyed by the inflammatory process, the diagnosis of hidradenitis is essentially a clinical one based on the known distribution of the glands and the characteristic behaviour and macroscopic appearance. Since apocrine glands lie deep to the dermis, the lesions typically occur as indolent deep abscesses, which may temporarily regress and take weeks or months to discharge; and as deep burrowing sinuses and retracted scars resulting from the infection. Radical measures should only be undertaken where the diagnosis is considered certain.

Preoperative

Diagnosis

1

Apocrine glands are normally found in relation to the hair of the axillae and puboinguinoperineal region. Hidradenitis is thus most commonly seen in the axillae, and almost as commonly in the inguinal region, especially the inguinoscrotal or inguinovulval groove. Although apocrine glands are present in the scrotal skin, the disease rarely extends onto the scrotum in Caucasians, although there may be racial differences in site distribution of the disease. Differential diagnosis is from staphylococcal abscesses, which are recognized by their rapid course, bacterial culture and healing without deep, retracted scars.

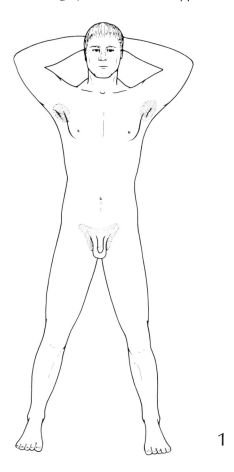

1

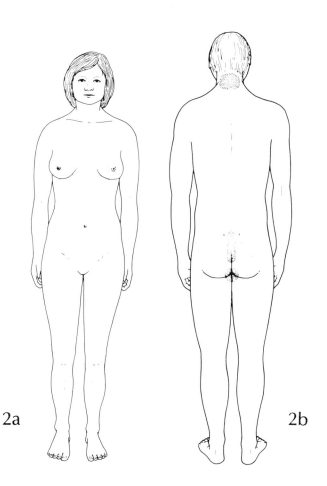

2a   2b

2a & b

Less common, 'ectopic' sites are on the anterior chest wall, periareolar and periumbilical regions, and around the anus and natal cleft. Of the anterior sites, only the presternal area in the male and the submammary and intermammary regions in the female have been affected in our experience. Differential diagnosis from cystic acne is an extremely difficult problem. In very severe cases, a surgical approach can be used without precise differentiation of the two conditions. The same is true of the back of the neck. Natal cleft disease may be confused with pilonidal sinus, and the two conditions frequently coexist, raising the possibility of a common factor. Perianal hidradenitis may be confused with Crohn's disease, mucoid carcinoma and simple perianal fistulae. Unlike the other areas described, the authors have little personal experience of management of perianal disease, which has been uncommon in their series. A useful reference to this site is that of Ching and Stahlgren[1].

Indications for surgery

Although conservative measures have little effect on the course of this disease, surgical excision should be reserved for chronic cases when the extent, protraction and severity of the disease seriously impair the patient's quality of life. This is obviously a matter of clinical judgement, which must balance the severity of the disease against the facts that its course is unpredictable, that a cure cannot be guaranteed and that only radical excisions can be relied on to give a reasonable chance of control.

The severity of the disease must be assessed in part by the patient, since the external appearance, especially between attacks, may be misleading. The process of subcutaneous nodules developing into abscesses which finally burst is very painful, particularly because of movement and the sensitivity of the axillary and groin areas. Mild cases may be intermittent or even regress completely, but once the patient has frequent attacks with short periods of quiescence, and persisting deep sinuses, it is unlikely that the disease will settle spontaneously – at least until late middle age.

Cure cannot be guaranteed with this condition, and the patient should be aware of this fact. In particular, the following should be noted.

1. Local excisions clearing overt lesions by 1 cm or less, to allow direct or rotation flap closure, are frequently followed by recurrence. The radical excision of apocrine-gland-bearing areas described here is very rarely followed by local recurrence in the axilla. This is not always true in the inguinoperineal regions, where even radical excisions may be followed by recurrence at the edge or towards the anus.
2. After eradication of the condition from involved areas the disease shows a distinct and unfortunate tendency to appear at previously uninvolved sites, and patients should be warned that successful surgery may be followed by the development of new disease at another site. At present there is no way of predicting which patient will go on to develop the disease at another site.
3. At 'ectopic' sites, such as the back of the neck and anterior chest wall, apocrine glands tend to be widely distributed and peripheral recurrence is common after surgery.

Preoperative preparation

Determining the extent of excision

In clinical practice the extent of excision is usually delineated according to the known distribution of apocrine glands, particularly in relation to the hair-bearing area. Apocrine glands open into hair follicles and are most numerous and obvious in relation to overt axillary and pubic hair. Occasional, randomly scattered glands can be shown to extend centrifugally from the main areas. These can usually be ignored, but tend to be most numerous in patients with very severe disease, in whom ectopic sites are often affected. In these patients such peripheral glands may lead to recurrent clinical disease.

The distribution of apocrine glands has been clarified by the use of the atropine/oxytocin test[2]. While tedious and unnecessary as a routine measure this test is useful when excising hidradenitis of less common sites or recurrent disease. In brief, eccrine sweat glands are blocked with atropine, and intravenous oxytocin is then used to empty the apocrine glands. The apocrine sweat droplets are mapped out by a paste of alcoholic iodine solution and starch applied to the skin.

Bacteriological study

Where skin grafting is to be used, bacterial swabs should be taken for culture and sensitivity. Skin graft failure caused by infection is common, even with delayed application, and intensive prior use of antibiotics normally given as part of conservative management may result in the presence of resistant organisms. Appropriate antibiotic cover should be considered during the grafting period. Bacteriological assessment is not necessary where healing is to be by open granulation, unless such healing is inexplicably delayed.

The operations

AXILLARY DISEASE

The extent of excision

3

Axillary apocrine glands can usually be removed by clearing the axillary hair by a 1 cm margin, with an extension upwards and forwards along the anterior axillary fold. Less radical excisions related only to overt disease are followed by a high incidence of recurrent disease.

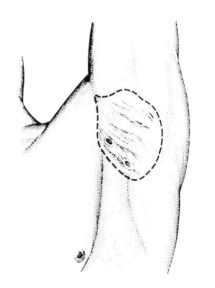

3

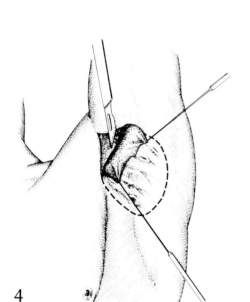

4

The excision

4

The area to be excised is mapped out and excised to a depth of 0.5 cm of subcutaneous fat. This is adequate to excise the apocrine glands, and deeper excisions risk damaging the lymphatics. Sinuses which burrow deeply into subcutaneous fat should be laid open in preference to deeper radical excision. Haemostasis is obtained and the wound suitably dressed – a gauze roll soaked in acriflavine/paraffin emulsion is very satisfactory.

5

If a skin graft is to be used it is taken at this stage, usually from high on the inner aspect of the thigh, and stored for delayed application[3]. Thin split-skin grafts are best because they take more readily, and the greater tendency to late contraction is of no significance at this site.

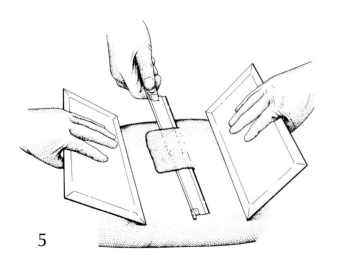

5

Repair

The wound may be managed by delayed skin grafting or allowed to heal by secondary granulation. Both are satisfactory for axillary wounds and each has advantages and disadvantages.

Skin grafts

Skin grafts give a very satisfactory result with rapid convalescence and good function when they are accepted wholly or in large part. However, grafts frequently fail because of the unsatisfactory bed of infected adipose tissue. Further disadvantages are those of the donor site and the necessary 10 days of immobilization – tiresome on one side but virtually unacceptable for simultaneous bilateral excisions.

6

On the second or third day, the packing is gently removed under adequate sedation and analgesia, and the skin graft applied by the delayed open method. The arm is immobilized on an aeroplane splint until the graft is firmly attached. Because of the unsatisfactory recipient base this usually takes 10 days or more. Where the skin graft fails in part or whole, the management reverts to Silastic foam dressing. Rapidity of healing is such that a second grafting procedure is not worthwhile.

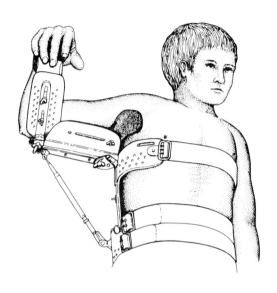

6

Granulation

Healing by granulation using a Silastic foam dressing gives certain though more protracted healing, greater comfort during the healing phase and a better cosmetic result because of the smaller scar. Average healing is 6–8 weeks, of which two are spent in hospital. The functional result is usually as good as with grafting, especially in women where the breast provides greater mobility of skin up into the axilla. In a controlled study of bilateral excision in patients where one axilla was grafted and the other allowed to granulate, the overall results favoured healing by granulation. The authors' current practice is to allow female patients to heal by granulation. With male patients skin grafting is attempted in unilateral cases, or on one side·in bilateral cases. Primary repair by local flaps or direct suture depends on conservative sacrifice of skin and consequently leads to a high recurrence rate. The authors have abandoned their use.

The technique of Silastic foam dressing of granulating wounds does not differ from that described for inguino-perineal wounds below.

PUBOINGUINOPERINEAL DISEASE

The extent of excision

7a

Inguinal hidradenitis in the female occurs mainly in the medial halves of the groin and outer aspects of the labia majora, but a wider surgical excision is required to provide a low incidence of recurrence. This removes the pubic hair, extends laterally along the inguinal ligaments and the groin skin with a 2 cm clearance lateral to the groin crease, and medially removes the outer aspect (only) of the labia majora. The skin excision broadens lateral to the posterior commissure of the perineum to clear any overt disease by 2 cm. In the midline, a narrow strip of skin is preserved between the anus and vagina. Although the perianal skin contains apocrine glands it is not practicable to carry out wide excision of perianal skin at one sitting in continuity with the radical puboperineal excision described. Fortunately, perianal hidradenitis is· relatively uncommon and the authors therefore reserve formal excision for cases with clear clinical involvement, excising this area as the secondary procedure when the anterior wound is fully healed.

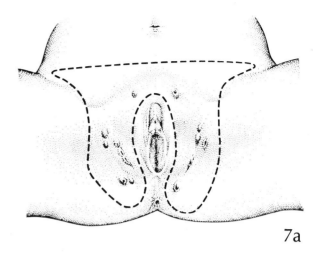

7a

7b

The amount of skin removed appears somewhat frightening, but should cause no concern providing care is taken to preserve a rim of skin at the base of the mons pubis around the clitoris, the inner aspect of the labia majora and the skin of the perineal raphe. The wound will heal predictably and with an excellent cosmetic result.

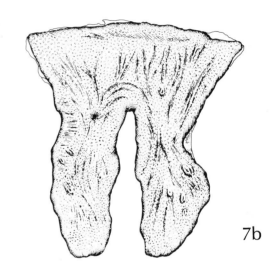

7b

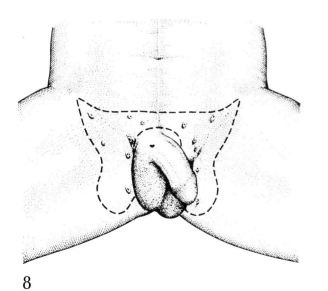

8

8

In the male the area of excision is similar, although most of the scrotal skin is preserved. Only a 1 cm wide strip of scrotal skin is excised from its lateral margin, in order to clear overt areas in the adjacent groin. It is paradoxical that the scrotal skin appears physiologically to be rich in apocrine glands as demonstrated by the oxytocin test, yet we have only seen two cases affected by hidradenitis suppurativa in this area.

The excision

9

With the patient supine, the legs and abdomen are prepared and the legs towelled with sterile tubular bandage
(Tubigrip), so that they can be manipulated during the
posterior perineal part of the operation. The area is
excised to a depth of 0.5 cm to avoid interference with
lymphatics. Special care is taken to avoid deep excision in
the region of the root of the penis and mons pubis,
otherwise postoperative preputial or labial oedema, normally moderate and transitory, may be gross and slow to
resolve. Deep excision of the labia majora is unnecessary
and will lead to troublesome bleeding.

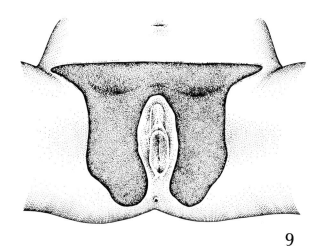

9

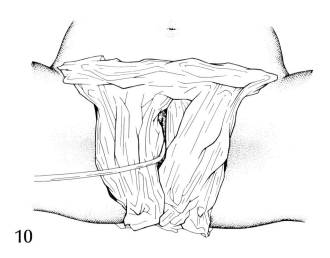

10

10

Haemostasis is obtained, a urinary catheter inserted, and
the wound packed with gauze generously soaked with
acriflavine/paraffin emulsion. On the second or third
postoperative day the dressing is removed in theatre
under general anaesthetic, as removal is extremely painful. It is immediately replaced by a Silastic dressing.

Repair

With wounds following radical excision in this region,
healing by granulation using a Silastic foam dressing is
comfortable, predictable and without complication, and
gives excellent cosmetic and functional results. Healing is
complete in about 12 weeks, of which 3 are spent in
hospital. The authors do not believe that split-skin grafting
has any role to play in this situation.

11

The Silastic foam dressing is made from two components,
a base – Silastic Foam Dressing Q79100 (Dow Corning)—
and a catalyst.

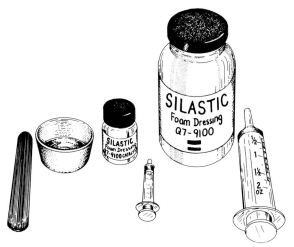

11

12

The two are mixed in a proportion of 100 parts of base to 6 of catalyst. For an axillary wound, 10 ml base and 0.6 ml of catalyst will be sufficient, but a large inguinal wound may require two pourings of 20 ml base and 1.2 ml of catalyst. The base and catalyst are drawn up in separate syringes, mixed in a plastic container and poured over the wound.

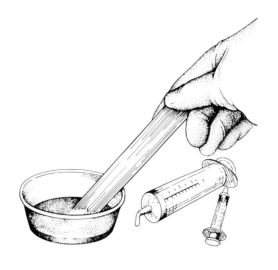

12

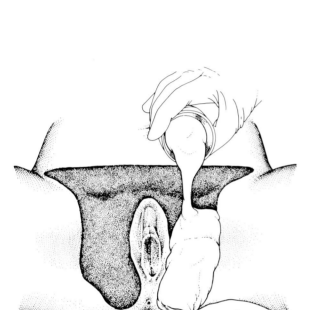

13

13

The dressing is usually poured from below upwards. It sets in 3 min, expanding to about four times its original volume as it does so. The final dressing will be about 1 cm thick.

14

The two sides usually require a separate pouring, but the material bonds together satisfactorily. When set, it may be removed and replaced with ease and minimal discomfort. The first dressing is poured with the legs slightly abducted to give a comfortable position for lying in bed. A second dressing is usually poured a few days later, and the legs adducted as the material sets to give a satisfactory shape for walking. The catheter is removed as soon as the patient is mobile.

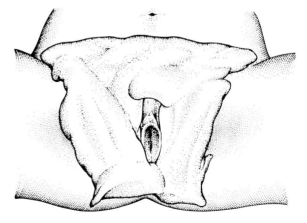

14

15

The dressing is held in place with Micropore tape and tight underclothes or Elastonet body stocking. The patients take a salt bath twice a day, wash the dressing in an antibacterial solution and replace it[4]. They are usually able to manage the dressing themselves at home after 2–3 weeks, returning each week for a new dressing.

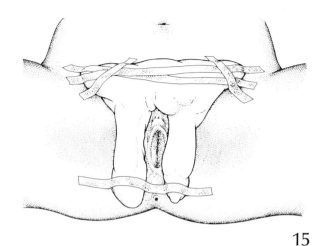

15

16

Healthy granulations rapidly develop and by 4–6 weeks the surface area of the wound has diminished by half. Secondary grafting could be considered at this stage, but complete healing can be expected in a further 6 weeks. Meantime the patients can remain at home and many resume their normal occupation during this period. Hence patients do not normally accept secondary grafting.

16

ECTOPIC DISEASE

Hidradenitis of other areas, particularly the presternal area and submammary folds, the nape of the neck and the gluteal and perianal regions, is less satisfactorily treated by surgery. It tends to occur in patients with apocrine glands scattered widely over much of the trunk and on the upper half of the body. The disease is not readily differentiated from cystic acne – indeed the two may overlap. It is impracticable to excise all apocrine glands and surgery is best confined to relatively conservative excisions, reserved for the most severely involved areas in severely affected patients.

Results

Our own series of 53 patients treated surgically have now been followed for up to 8 years. Axillary excision as described here has given excellent results in 27 patients. There has only been one recurrence – in a patient with extensive ectopic glands, and he was cured by a further minor local excision.

Radical excision gives excellent results in most cases in the perineal region as well. However, some recurrence will occur at the edge of the scar in about 30 per cent of patients. This is usually localized and gives little trouble, and if necessary can be dealt with by a conservative

excision under local anaesthetic. A smaller group, those with extensive areas of ectopic glands, will have major recurrence in the posterior perineal, perianal and intergluteal regions. We are not yet in a position to assess with confidence the results of excision of these more posterior areas of disease.

References

1. Ching, C. C., Stahlgren, L. H. Clinical review of hidradenitis suppurativa: management of cases with severe perianal involvement. Diseases of the Colon and Rectum 1965; 8: 349–352

2. Morgan, W. P., Hughes, L. E. The distribution, size and density of the apocrine glands in hidradenitis suppurativa. British Journal of Surgery 1979; 66: 853–856

3. Rees, B. I., Hughes, L. E. Delayed exposed skin grafting in surgery for breast cancer and melanoma. Clinical Oncology 1975; 1: 131–139

4. Wood, R. A. B., Williams, R. H. P., Hughes, L. E. Foam elastomer dressing in the management of open granulating wounds: experience with 250 patients. British Journal of Surgery 1977; 64: 554–557

Illustrations by Barbara Hyams from originals by Jean Loos

The gangrenes

J. Wesley Alexander   MD, ScD
Director, Transplantation Division,
University of Cincinnati Medical Center, Cincinnati, Ohio;
Director of Research, Shriners' Burn Institute, Cincinnati Unit

James A. Majeski   PhD, MD
Assistant Professor of Surgery,
Medical University of South Carolina, Charleston, South Carolina

Introduction

The gangrenes, for the purpose of this chapter, will be taken to mean the infectious gangrenes. Gangrene occurring as a result of vascular disease or other causes will not be discussed.

Fortunately, infectious gangrenes are relatively rare, but the mortality associated with this group of diseases remains high, partly because their uncommon occurrence leads to delay in recognition and institution of appropriate therapy. The infectious gangrenes develop most frequently in diabetic patients, debilitated malnourished patients, those patients with severe vascular disease, and the elderly. These infections are quite diverse both in aetiology and in clinical presentation. All are characterized, however, by progressive tissue necrosis and failure of a granulation tissue boundary (pyogenic membrane) to develop. Without treatment, virtually all afflicted patients will die.

There are possibly eight distinct clinical entities that may be classified among the infectious gangrenes:

1. Acute clostridial myositis
2. Acute clostridial cellulitis
3. Acute streptococcal myositis
4. Acute haemolytic streptococcal gangrene
5. Necrotizing fasciitis
6. Synergistic cutaneous gangrene (Meleney's gangrene)
7. Deep fungal infections (predominantly mucormycosis)
8. Necrotizing cellulitis

Preoperative

Making the diagnosis

Some of the infectious gangrenes clearly follow trauma, whereas for others the injury may be operative or even inapparent. In patients who are not receiving antibiotics, both acute clostridial infections and acute streptococcal infections are typically associated with high fevers and toxicity which may be profound, especially with the clostridial infections. Such infections should be suspected in anyone who develops these symptoms within the first 24 h after any operation, especially those for gastrointestinal or biliary surgery. Synergistic infections caused by other organisms may produce extensive involvement and necrosis with surprisingly minor symptoms and few physical signs. The initial diagnosis is especially elusive in the elderly, the diabetic and patients receiving antibiotics. Swelling of an extremity with cutaneous oedema may be the only physical indication of an extensive necrotizing fasciitis in such patients. The presence of subcutaneous air found by palpation or X-ray is an important and almost pathognomonic diagnostic clue. A high index of suspicion should lead to aspiration of potentially affected areas because obtaining small samples of fluid for microscopic examination is central to establishment of a tentative diagnosis in many instances. A Gram's stain of aspirated or excised material is mandatory to guide initial surgical and antibiotic therapy. *Table 1* can be used as a guide for the diagnosis of the infectious gangrenes.

Preoperative preparation

Patients should be prepared for operation as soon as possible once a diagnosis has been established. These patients usually have a moderate to severe volume deficit and acidosis. It would not be unusual for such a patient to be given 600 ml of fresh frozen plasma (as a source of opsonins), 1 litre of Ringer's lactate, and 20 mmol of sodium bicarbonate in the hour before operation. Preoperative antibiotics should be selected based upon the Gram's stain (*Table 2*). Steroids should be avoided.

Table 1 Guide to the diagnosis of infectious gangrenes

Primary site of necrotizing infection	Gram's stain	Working diagnosis
Subcutaneous tissue	Gram-negative rods	Necrotizing cellulitis
	Gram-negative rods	Clostridial cellulitis
	Streptococci alone	Acute streptococcal gangrene
	Staphylococci alone	Look deeper for fasciitis
	Mixed	Look deeper for fasciitis
	Fungi	Mycosis
Fascia	Streptococci	Necrotizing fasciitis
	Staphylococci	Necrotizing fasciitis
	Mixed or Gram-negative rods	Necrotizing fasciitis
Muscle	Gram-positive rods	Clostridial myositis
	Streptococci	Streptococcal myositis
	Mixed	Probable secondary infection
	Fungi	Mycosis

Table 2 Selection of preoperative antibiotics

Infection	Antibiotic
Presumed clostridia	Penicillin G plus a tetracycline
Streptococcus	Penicillin G
Staphylococcus	Nafcillin
Mixed infections	Penicillin plus an aminoglycoside or clindamycin plus an aminoglycoside
Fungi	Amphotericin B

The operations

Operations for these diseases may vary considerably, depending upon the site and extent of the involvement. Two principles must be strictly followed: (1) excision of all necrotic tissue; (2) establishment of wide surgical drainage. For clostridial myositis, it is necessary to excise all of the involved muscle. For deep fungal infections, excision or amputation must be complete as guided by intraoperative biopsies with frozen sections. For streptococcal and mixed infections, the excision may be less radical, and tissues of questionable viability are sometimes left. In all cases, the operative sites must be checked frequently during the first few days, and the patient should be returned to the operating room promptly for excision of any newly necrotic tissues.

During the operations it has been our policy to use electrocautery to control minor bleeding. When sutures or ligatures are required, we strongly prefer monofilament polypropylene or nylon.

Illustrations 1–11 show examples of operative procedures often necessary for treatment of necrotizing infections.

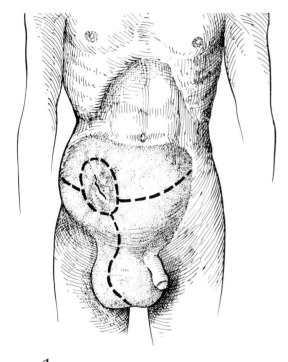

1

Necrotizing fasciitis following appendectomy

1

Wide debridement is essential to treat necrotizing fasciitis of the abdominal wall. There may be external discoloration only around the incision. However, the extent and seriousness of the infection should be suspected by extensive oedema of the lower abdomen and sentum. Extensive incisions are made across the inflamed areas. These incisions must extend into normal tissues to be certain that all infected material is easily visible and should be planned to conserve skin flaps for later reconstruction.

2

All of the frankly gangrenous fascia should be excised, exposing muscle whenever necessary. Fascia of questionable viability may be preserved at the initial procedure but should be removed once non-viability is established. It may be necessary to excise the entire investing fascia of the scrotum, sometimes with the skin, but the testicle is usually viable and should be preserved when possible. Implantation in a subcutaneous pocket in the thigh may be necessary. In this illustration the upper flap has been removed for clarity but only the gangrenous skin surrounding the appendectomy incision should be excised.

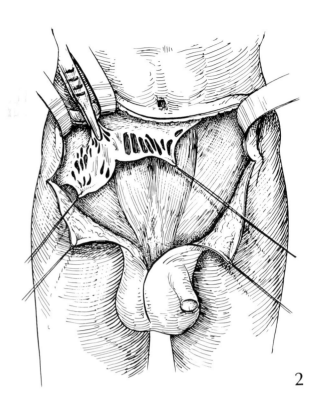

2

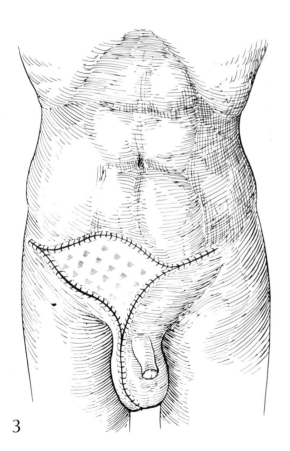

3

3

Reconstruction must be delayed until the infection is resolved. It is usually possible to cover the major portion of the wound by approximation of the preserved skin flaps, and the residual area can be treated with a meshed skin graft (artist's conception).

Clostridial myositis

4

A compound fracture of the tibia and fibula provi~~sier~~.
portal of entry. Because of the administration of anti
tics, the signs and symptoms of gas gangrene ma,
delayed in onset and/or masked.

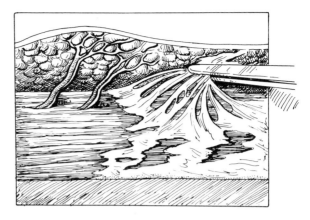

10

5

Gas formation in the muscle or subcutaneous tissue
X-ray is pathognomic.

11

A double-barrelled colostomy is used to divert the faecal
stream.

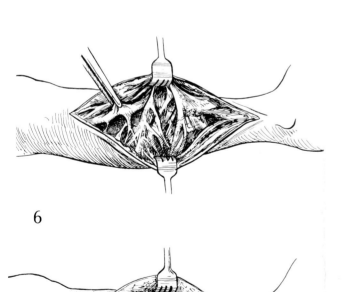

6

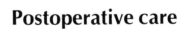

7

12

Extensive abdominal wall defects

Most defects over the trunk and extremities can be
covered with split-thickness grafts but abdominal wall
defects, as pictured here, usually need reinforcement with
a mesh made of Marlex or polyethylene. The mesh,
treated with Iodoform dressing, will be covered with
granulations and be ready for grafting in 7–14 days.

Postoperative care

Most patients with necrotizing infections either have or
will rapidly develop malnutrition. Therefore, we prefer to
be aggressive with nutritional support in an effort to
provide 1.5–2.0 times the patient's basal requirement for
energy intake with high-protein dietary supplements.
Serum transferrin levels are a good reflection of protein
nutritional status.

Extensive soft tissue defects may be a residual of serious
necrotizing infections, but reconstruction must be considered as secondary in importance when treating the intital
infection.

Antibiotic therapy may be altered according to sensitivity reports, and adequate antibiotic levels should be
evaluated by obtaining frequent peak and trough values.

Illustrations by Shian Hartshorn

Excision of surface lesions

R. C. G. Russell MS, FRCS
Consultant Surgeon, St John's Hospital for Diseases of the Skin
and The Middlesex Hospital, London

Introduction

The majority of skin swellings can be removed under a local anaesthetic as an outpatient. By their nature, these swellings present because the patient is aware of a blemish, and wishes to be rid of the lesion. Because excision of these lesions can be performed without upset to the body, skin surgery is frequently termed minor surgery, and is thus relegated to a secondary role. However, well performed skin surgery is a satisfying art which should be done with especial care to avoid complication, which is inconvenient for the patient and irritating to the surgeon.

The pathology of these skin swellings falls into two categories: benign and malignant.

Benign lesions

The management of most of these lesions is by surgical excision. Lesions that are of questionable origin require excision for histological examination. Excision biopsy is always preferable to an incisional biopsy, unless the lesion is large and the resulting excision would result in cosmetic deformity. Excision is indicated for skin lesions that itch, change in character or bleed; lesions that give rise to anxiety; or those whose location or appearance makes them cosmetically unacceptable.

Cysts

The entire wall of sebaceous and inclusion cysts should be removed in order to avoid recurrence. In the scalp, a simple incision can be made into the cyst's centre and the sebaceous material expressed. The cyst wall is then removed by twisting it out with a small haemostat. Unless the whole wall is removed, recurrence is inevitable and this technique should only be used when the operator can be sure of removing the whole cyst wall.

Foreign body tumour

These lesions should be excised using a simple ellipse.

Keratoses

Senile or actinic keratoses can be treated most satisfactorily by liquid nitrogen or 5-fluorouracil ointment. Seborrhoeic keratoses can be shaved off with good cosmetic result.

Warts

Treatment begins with caustic agents, such as trichloracetic acid; if this fails, cautery and curettage, liquid nitrogen or podophyllin may be used. In general, excision should be reserved for the intractable wart only.

Fibromas and histiocytomas

Surgical excision by a simple ellipse is the procedure of choice. However, the keloid should be approached with caution, and due attention given to adjunctive procedures (steroids, radiotherapy and compression bandages) necessary to prevent recurrence.

Naevi

These pigmented blemishes present in varied forms. In general, unsightly pigmented naevi around the face should be excised. Otherwise, removal is only indicated for a naevus which changes in colour, grows, becomes friable or bleeds easily.

Haemangiomas and lymphangiomas

Haemangiomas are the most common benign tumour of infancy. The two basic types are the capillary strawberry naevus (cavernous variety) and the port wine naevus.

The cavernous haemangioma is a compressible tumour that is nodular, lobulated and polypoid. Rarely, it can be flat. The strawberry haemangioma is composed of capillary loops with embryonic endothelium. It usually regresses in the first 5 years of life. Regression, shown by grayish discoloration, is a local ischaemic process which leads to self-destruction of the haemangioma.

The port wine haemangioma is a vascular tumour that consists of capillaries with adult vascular endothelium. It does not change during the patient's lifetime.

Lymphangiomas are developmental defects that are composed of excessive lymphatic tissue.

Surgical treatment is indicated for the lesions if they bleed, ulcerate, increase in size or threaten to occlude an orifice. The port wine stain is occasionally so large that excision cannot be undertaken and then reliance must be placed on cosmetics. Treatment of these lesions with the argon laser has yet to be evaluated.

Tumours of nerve fat and muscle

Surgical excision for histological examination is the preferred management for all these lesions. Most present as a lump, which is excised for diagnostic purposes.

Epithelial tumours

Diagnosis of the epithelial tumours, such as cylindromas, adenoma sebaceum, and sweat gland tumours is usually made after surgical excision of the skin lump. Occasionally, these tumours are malignant, in which case a wider excision is indicated.

Malignant lesions

Basal cell carcinoma

Basal cell carcinoma has many manifestations: it is a local malignancy which grows slowly, but in certain sites, such as the eye and nose, it may become aggressive and invade the underlying cartilage or bone. Regional metastases are most unusual. Treatment for these lesions can be by surgery, radiotherapy, cryotherapy, laser coagulation or chemotherapy. No extensive resection for a basal cell carcinoma should be undertaken without consultation with a radiotherapist specializing in skin cancer. Many large lesions, which would cause a cosmetic defect following extensive surgery, can be appropriately managed by radiotherapy with an acceptable cosmetic result. When excising these lesions, the minimum margin is 5 mm.

Squamous cell carcinoma

This is usually a more aggressive lesion than the basal cell carcinoma, and does metastasize to regional lymph nodes. Important in the management of these lesions are the predisposing causes, such as excessive sunlight and radiation dermatoses, which must be taken into account when planning treatment. Surgical treatment is preferable, but radiotherapy and chemotherapy are an integral part of the management of extensive lesions. Complete ablation is the cardinal rule. The minimum margin is 15 mm around the tumour.

Malignant melanoma

This is an unpredictable skin malignancy. Diagnosis and histological characteristics of the tumour should be established before the treatment is planned. Thus an excision biopsy is a necessary preliminary in the management of this tumour.

Preoperative

1

Preoperative preparation

The skin is cleaned with hibitane, care being taken to avoid 'drips' of fluid passing onto the rest of the skin or onto a mucosal surface. The area is then towelled with either conventional linen drapes or a single disposable laminated towel in which a hole has been shaped to the required size. The laminated towel has the advantage that on the face it does not obstruct breathing and shields the eyes from the intense light of the theatre lamp.

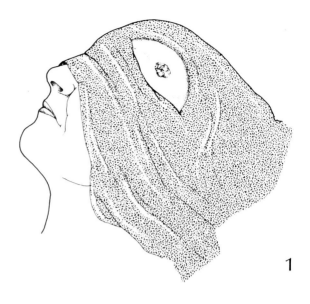
1

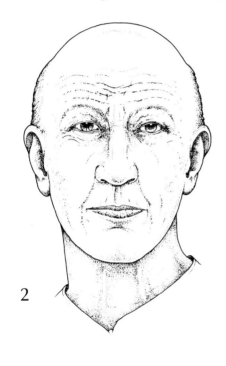
2

2

Planning the incision

The most favourable lines for scars follow the skin wrinkles, which form at right angles to the general direction of the contracture of the underlying muscles. By moving the skin, these lines soon become apparent, and the planned elliptical incision is drawn on the patient with a suitable marker. The length of the ellipse should be at least three times the diameter of the tumour to avoid 'dog-ears' on closing.

3

Local anaesthesia

Lignocaine 1 per cent with 1:200 000 adrenaline is suitable for most purposes. Adrenaline should not be added for anaesthesia of the extremities, especially if the circulation is compromised. Hyaluronidase 1500 u greatly aids the insertion of the anaesthetic in areas where the skin is tight, such as the scalp or the back. The local anaesthetic is inserted into the subdermal layer around the lesion over an area twice the size of the proposed excision. The surgeon then waits for 2 min with gentle pressure on the wound before starting.

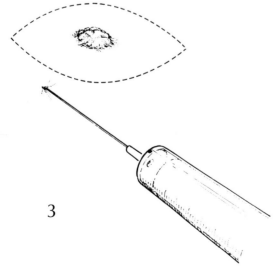
3

The operation

4 & 5

The incision

The first cut with the knife incises down to the mid dermis so that the skin maintains its shape until the whole ellipse has been made. The ellipse of skin containing the tumour is removed. The vast majority of skin tumours can be excised using a simple ellipse, which is well placed in a suitable skin crease and of sufficient length. Rotation flaps and other plastic surgical techniques can in the hands of a novice give worse scars than a well executed ellipse.

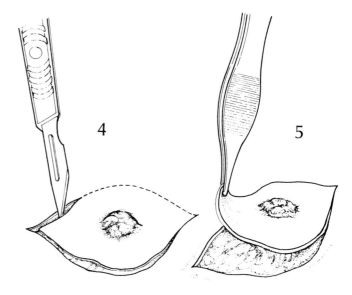

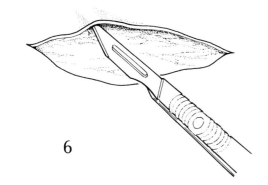

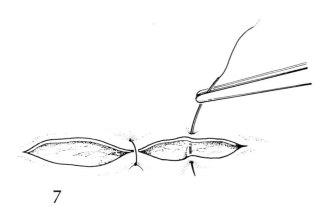

6

Preparation of the wound

The edges of the wound are undermined, in order to allow the skin to slide over the defect on suturing, without tension on the suture line.

Suture of the wound

The subcutaneous tissue should be stitched with fine interrupted suture, either polyglycolic acid or polypropylene, with the knots placed on the deep aspect of the wound. This should stop all bleeding and leave the dermis nicely apposed, without tension, for the final cutaneous suture. The cutaneous suture can be either an interrupted or a subcuticular stitch.

7

For the interrupted suture a fine (5/0) stitch of polypropylene should be used in a manner which neatly coapts the edges without tension. Sufficient sutures to appose the surface perfectly are required. However, too many sutures can be as harmful as too few. To assess the correct number of sutures, it is useful to halve each segment to be sutured until perfect apposition is gained.

8

The subcuticular stitch is ideally suited for this type of surgery, providing good apposition and ease of removal with the absence of suture marks. A fine polypropylene suture (5/0 or 6/0) on a small cutting needle (15mm or 19mm) is ideal. An initial suture is started away from the skin edge and brought out at the apex of the ellipse. The needle is then inserted at the dermal-epidermal junction, taking a bite of 2 or 3mm before emerging at the dermal-epidermal junction. The size of the bite is related to the thickness of the dermis, but should not be larger than twice the skin thickness. For the next suture, the needle is inserted at the apex of the wound on the opposite side, and the third needle insertion enters the dermal-epidermal junction at the site of exit of the first suture. Inserting the next suture at the site of the exit of the previous stitch on that side, prevents rucking of the wound on tightening the stitch. With this technique, it is advisable to insert four or five sutures before pulling the edges together. This means the contracting force is applied over a wider area and the suture will be less likely to 'cut out'. When the end of the wound is reached, the needle is inserted at the apex of the ellipse and brought out at least 1cm away from the wound.

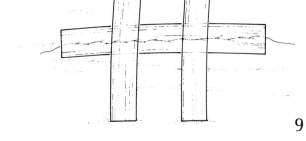

8

9

Dressing of wounds

In order to immobilize the wound and relieve tension on the suture line, paper strips should be placed along the length of the wound to include the ends of the suture, which were brought out some distance from the wound. To relieve the distracting force, strips are placed transversely to the wound. In wounds of the extremities, especially the lower leg, a compression bandage should be placed over the wound.

9

Postoperative care

The local anaesthetic will wear off in 2–4 h. As soon as the patient feels discomfort in the wound, a minor analgesic should be taken, and thereafter 2–4 hourly to relieve pain. The patient should be advised to take an analgesic before retiring to bed to prevent sleep disturbance. The sutures should be removed on the third day if the ellipse is on the face, the 10th day if the wound is on the body and the 14th day if the wound is on the leg. Problems arise with early removal of sutures, and, if interrupted sutures have been used, it is advisable to remove the sutures as early as possible and support the wound with paper strips in order to minimize these suture marks. On the other hand, if a subcuticular closure is used, it is advisable to leave the sutures in longer in order to prevent distraction of the wound during healing. With the subcuticular technique, there is no danger of stitch marks and the advantage of this technique is that the sutures can be removed at the patient's convenience.

Illustrations by Oxford Illustrators from originals by Paul Darton

Biopsy of specific tissues

R. C. G. Russell   MS, FRCS
Consultant Surgeon, St John's Hospital for Diseases of the Skin
and The Middlesex Hospital, London

Introduction

Biopsy of specific tissues is usually undertaken by the surgeon because a lump, whose nature is unknown, is present, or because a tissue diagnosis is required in a patient who is ill from a known or unknown cause. A biopsy cannot be performed without thoughts about a differential diagnosis because the tissue being removed for examination may not give the information sought, or the tissue being removed may not be the appropriate material for the group of conditions under consideration. In addition, it is important to be clear what examinations are required on the specimen to be removed and to have arranged these beforehand with due attention to the needs of the pathologist.

Many patients upon whom biopsies are required are unwell; careful consideration must therefore be given to the choice of anaesthesia – local, regional block or general anaesthesia. Because of the poor condition of many of these patients, it is useful to decide if further biopsies might be necessary to establish the diagnosis, and to carry these out, especially if they are uncomfortable (e.g. a bone marrow biopsy), under the same anaesthetic. It cannot be too strongly emphasized that these patients require a full assessment before the biopsy.

215

Lymph node biopsy (see also chapter on
'Managing the surgical operative specimen,' pp.
70–76)

This procedure is performed to elucidate the cause of enlarged nodes, the extent of a disease process or to determine the nature of a general illness in which there may or may not be lymphadenopathy. The biopsy must not impede future surgical procedures, nor compromise the clearance of a cancer. Other methods of achieving the diagnosis should have been excluded, e.g. laryngoscopy for a laryngeal carcinoma with cervical node metastases. On occasion, the surgeon is presented with a patient who has multiple nodes: in this case, the biopsy should be taken away from the site of any infection, the axilla or neck being preferable to the groin, and a site where discrete

nodes can be removed is chosen rather than a biopsy of a matted mass of lymphoid tissue. When the lymph nodes are only just enlarged, lymph nodes from several sites may have to be removed before a satisfactory diagnosis can be made; a firm node is usually a better prospect than a rubbery or diffuse node. At all times glands draining areas affected by an eczematous skin eruption should be avoided as these present particular histological difficulties. Whenever possible several nodes should be removed from the one site, and all nodes should be removed without damage to the capsule as this aids histological examination.

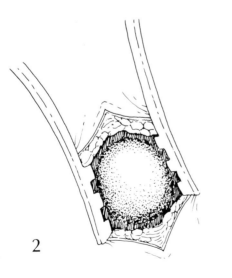

1

The incision

The line of incision should be planned to follow a suitable skin crease, which is usually apparent at sites where lymph nodes are commonly situated. To decrease bleeding, it is useful to inject adrenaline 1:200000 beneath the line of the planned incision and around the nodes which are about to be removed. The incision should be twice the length of the node which is to be excised or longer if it is deep in the axilla.

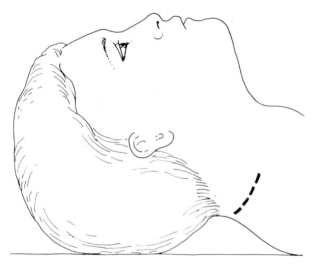

2

Exposure of node

The skin, fat and superficial fascia or platysma in the neck are divided to reveal a potential space in which the superficial nodes lie. A self-retaining retractor is inserted to hold back the deep fascia, so exposing the node or nodes.

3

Dissection of node

By blunt dissection the node can be exposed, leaving the vascular attachments intact. These vessels are now grasped with dissecting forceps and cauterized. By holding the vessel and surrounding fascia the lymph node can be enucleated without damage to the capsule. Haemostasis should proceed as the node is mobilized because haemorrhage obscures dissection and can be difficult to control once the node has been removed.

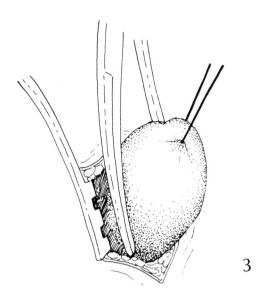

3

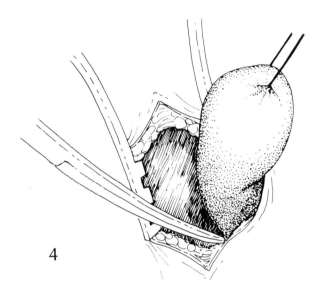

4

4

Exploration for further nodes

Once the main node has been removed the wound is explored for further nodes. Usually two or three adjacent lymph nodes can be enucleated through the same incision.

5

Closure of wound

The fascia is closed with interrupted sutures and the skin by a subcuticular polypropylene suture. The wound is supported by skin tapes. Drainage is unnecessary unless a large mass has been removed.

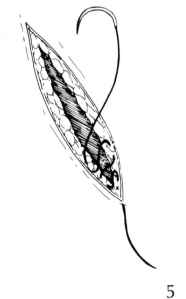

5

Biopsy of an artery

The commonest artery for biopsy is the temporal artery in order to confirm or refute the diagnosis of temporal arteritis. By definition the artery is prominent and easily palpable so that identification is not a problem. Local anaesthesia is quite adequate for this procedure.

6

The incision

After preparation of the skin and before injection of local anaesthetic the line of the vessel is marked. If the affected vessel runs close to the hairline, then the incision can be hidden in the hairline, otherwise the skin crease nearest the line of the vessel is chosen.

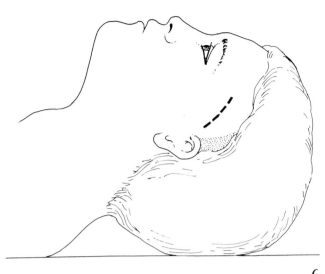

6

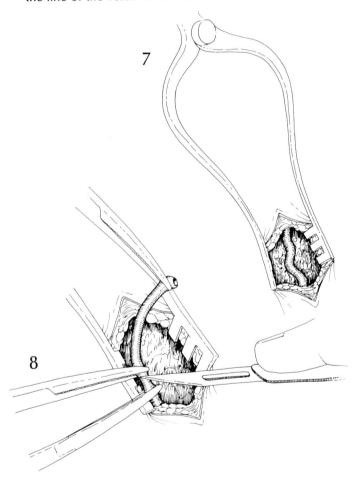

7 & 8

Dissection of artery

The incision is extended down to the temporal muscle on which the artery lies. A small self-retaining retractor is inserted. The vessel should be dissected out, starting proximally and avoiding handling the vessel. When the proximal end has been mobilized, two mosquito forceps are applied to the artery, which is divided. The proximal end is tied, while the distal end is mobilized for 2 cm before clamping and tying the distal end. Cautery should be avoided until the vessel is removed.

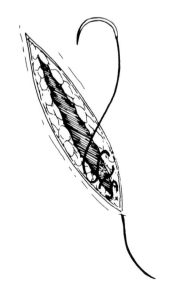

9

9

Closure

Two or three sutures are inserted in the fascia, and the skin is closed with a subcuticular polypropylene stitch, which is supported by skin tapes.

Muscle biopsy

The usual reason for a muscle biopsy is to confirm or refute the presence of dermatomyositis. A muscle affected early and commonly in this condition is the deltoid muscle. This muscle is suitable for biopsy under a local anaesthetic. The skin can be affected in dermatomyositis, and thus a skin biopsy should be performed at the same time.

10

The incision

After the injection of local anaesthetic beneath the skin and around the surface of the deltoid, a vertical elliptical incision is made and an ellipse of skin excised.

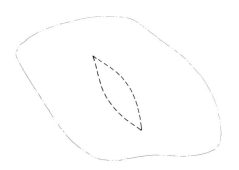

10

11 & 12

Procedure

The incision is deepened down to the muscle and a self-retaining retractor inserted. The fat is dissected off the muscle so that an area of muscle 2 × 1 cm is exposed. After ensuring that the muscle is anaesthetized, a segment of muscle 0.5 × 2 × 0.5 cm is excised. Sufficient muscle must be taken for conventional histology, electron microscopy and immunofluorescence as well as other special stains requested by the referring physician.

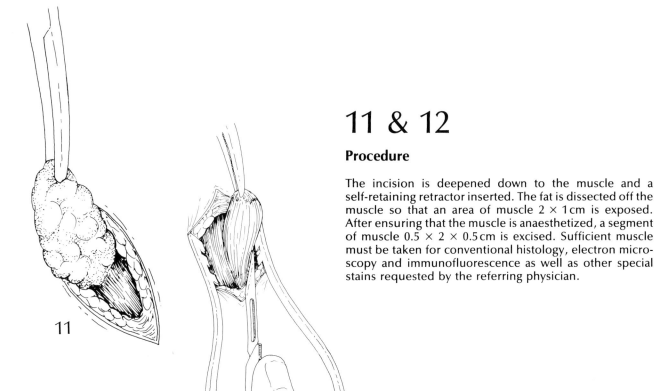

11

12

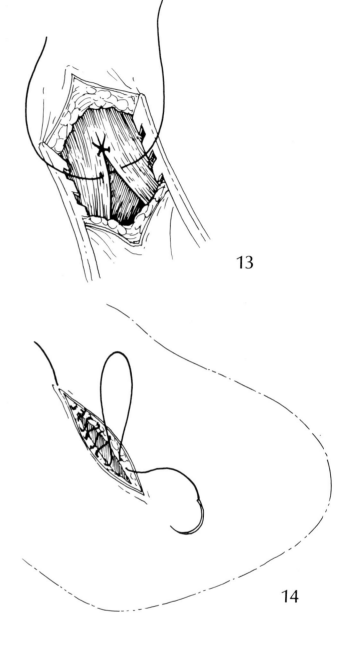

13 & 14

Closure

The muscle is closed with an interrupted suture, as is the fat. The skin is closed with a subcuticular polypropylene stitch and the wound is supported by skin tapes.

Nerve biopsy

A nerve biopsy is a rare request. Before undertaking such a biopsy the surgeon must be cognisant of the exact requirements of the physician, the type of nerve required and the techniques to be used for examination of the specimen. Once these criteria have been determined the selected nerve segment can usually be removed quite satisfactorily under a local anaesthetic. Care must be taken during the dissection not to handle the nerve, and cautery near the nerve should be avoided.

Postoperative care

No special care is required following these procedures. The main complication to be encountered is infection. The sutures should not be removed early as many patients requiring biopsies are ill, and the wounds may heal less well than usual.

Illustrations by Donald G. Powell

Operative management of cutaneous melanoma

Hilliard F. Seigler MD
Professor of Surgery and Associate Professor of Immunology,
Duke University Medical Center, Durham, North Carolina

Introduction

Primary cutaneous melanoma presents in three clinical forms and, before the surgeon can adequately plan for operative control of the primary, he must be aware of these different lesions.

Lentigo maligna occurs, for the most part, on the exposed surfaces of the body with the majority being found on the head and neck. The lesion is usually non-palpable until vertical growth has begun. In its earlier phases the lesion is mainly confined to the intraepithelial position. It is late to invade and metastasize.

Superficial spreading melanoma also has an initial radial growth phase which may reach 25–35 mm in width before vertical growth takes place. The latter is quite rapid and may be either black or pink and ulceration also occurs.

Nodular melanomas develop by direct tumour progression and do not have a clinical phase of radial growth. The nodule is easily palpable and is sharply delineated from the normal surrounding tissue.

Both the prognosis and the presence or absence of regional lymph node metastases can be correlated with the level of invasion of the primary tumour as well as its thickness[1]. Before primary surgery can be planned, an accurate diagnosis is vital. The pathologist must be provided with an optimal surgical specimen on which to measure the tumour thickness and determine the level of tumour invasion. Any minor surgery, such as electro-coagulation, curettage and shave removal, should be discouraged for suspicious cutaneous lesions.

The operations

1a & b

Biopsy

The entire gross lesion should be excised if the wound can be closed primarily. If the lesions are quite large or placed in anatomical positions that would involve a disfiguring procedure, then incisional biopsy should be done. The surgeon should select the most nodular area and extend the incision into the subcutaneous fat so that the greatest accuracy of diagnosis of the depth of penetration can be determined.

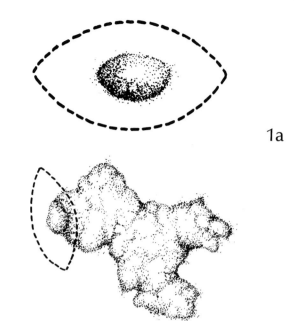

1a

1b

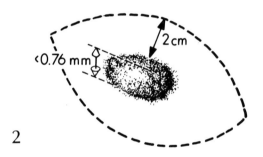

2

Operative control of the primary lesion

2

A margin of 2 cm from the gross lesion for melanomas that are less than 0.76 mm in thickness should be achieved.

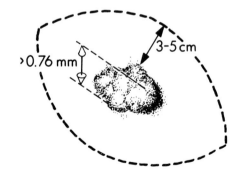

3

3

A 3–5 cm margin beyond all clinically visible tumour in those lesions greater than 0.76 mm in thickness is a reasonable guide line. The subcutaneous fat must be included if the proper depth of invasion is to be determined. On the limbs the surgeon can easily include the deep fascia as a guide line for depth of removal. This fascia thus becomes an easily recognized determinant for the area to be removed.

4

Subungal melanoma

Subungal melanoma should be managed by amputation without an attempt at local excision or coverage. For toe lesions the level of amputation should be at the metatarsal joint. For finger or thumb lesions, unless they are quite extensive proximally, the amputation should be carried out at the level of the distal interphalangeal joint. This procedure gives adequate functional results.

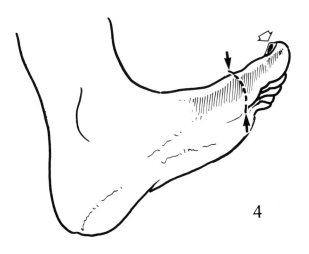

4

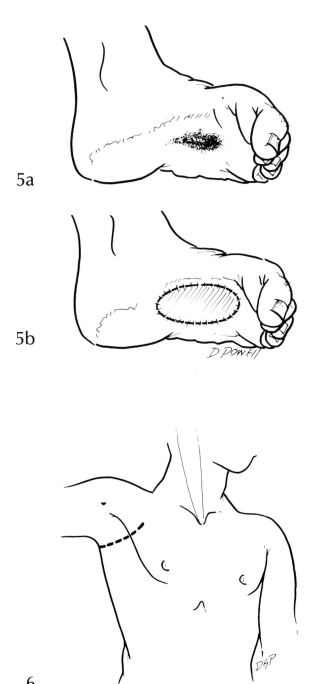

5a

5b

5a & b

Plantar or palmar melanoma

Melanomas that occur on the soles of the feet or the palms of the hands should be treated by wide local excision and full-thickness skin grafting.

The management of regional lymph nodes

When the surgeon is faced with centrifugal lymph node drainage to two regional areas such as the axilla and groin in certain cutaneous melanomas of the trunk, technetium-labelled antimony trisulphide injected around the primary lesion is a predictive and feasible diagnostic tool for documenting lymphatic drainage patterns. The three main lymph node chains involved are the cervical, axillary and ilioinguinal groups. Antecubital, popliteal and other superficial and deep lymph node groups are affected very rarely. If the lymph nodes are clinically involved the surgeon should complete nodal dissection.

Axillary lymph node

If an axillary lymph node is clinically evident then axillary node dissection with or without *en bloc* removal of the pectoralis minor muscle should be done.

6

The incision follows the skin lines so that a linear scar results and loss or range of motion in the upper extremity is obviated.

6

7

Using a cutting cautery, superior and inferior flaps should be developed to the anterior, posterior and superior borders of the dissection. Note that the pectoralis muscle is retracted medially and the lateral portion of the flap is dissected to expose the latissimus dorsi muscle.

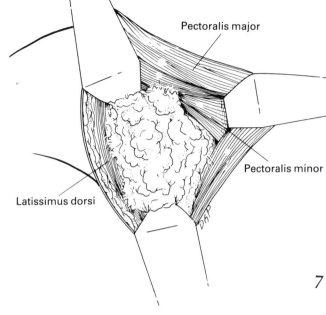

7

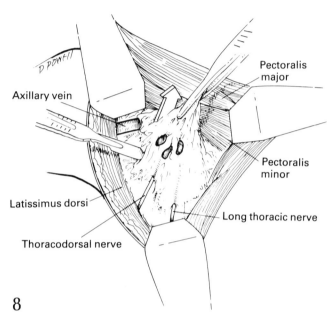

8

8

With blunt and sharp dissection the axillary vein is exposed and the dissection is carried along its sheath.

9

The major and minor pectoralis muscles are retracted superiorly and medially and the lymphatic chain is dissected away from the axillary vein at the level of the second rib. Staying in the avascular plane of the chest wall, the lymphatics are dissected laterally exposing the long thoracic nerve which is carefully left intact. At this point the neurovascular bundle is easily recognized; it is a useful landmark for identifying the thoracodorsal nerve. The neurovascular bundle is preserved and the specimen can be dissected away from the border of the latissimus dorsi muscle. The wound should be drained through a separate stab wound with a multiperforated drain and the incision closed in layers.

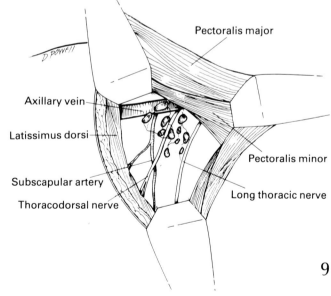

9

Inguinal lymph node

10

If an inguinal lymph node is palpable a superficial groin dissection should be undertaken using a transverse incision.

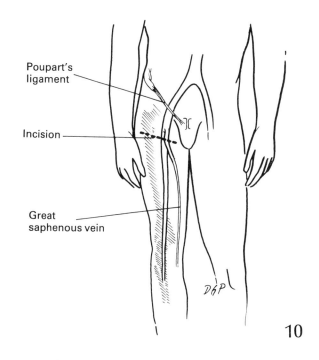

10

11

All the nodes around the confluence of long saphenous and femoral veins are removed down to the fascia of the quadriceps and adductor muscles. Superiorly, the dissection should be carried to the level of the inguinal ligament. The saphenous vein is divided at the bulb. The wound is drained through a separate stab wound, again utilizing a multiperforated closed drainage system.

The therapeutic benefit of a pelvic node dissection is doubtful; there is little question that if pelvic lymph nodes are involved the prognosis is quite poor. Very few patients with positive iliac nodes will survive longer than 3 years.

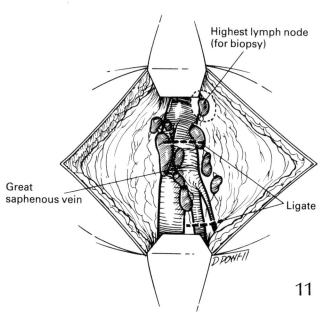

11

Clinical uninvolved regional lymph nodes

There is continuing controversy concerning the surgical management of patients with clinically uninvolved regional lymph nodes. A reasonable approach is that patients with primary cutaneous melanomas measuring less than 1 mm in thickness might be adequately managed without concurrent lymphadenectomy. Patients with primary lesions measuring 1–4 mm in thickness have a reasonable chance of micrometastasis to primary draining lymph nodes without distant disease and may indeed experience improved survival with simultaneous regional lymph node dissection. Patients with primary lesions measuring greater than 4 mm have a greater possibility of having distant disease and may not benefit from removal of first order lymph nodes[2].

Surgical management of cutaneous melanoma involving the head and neck

One-third of patients with a primary melanoma in these sites will have metastatic disease involving regional lymph nodes at the time of diagnosis. This group of patients has an extremely grave prognosis, but also two-thirds of patients with such primaries will have negative regional lymph nodes and should not undergo disfiguring radical surgery. Recent studies have suggested that for lesions involving the helix of the ear, excision in continuity with the posterior auricular, posterior cervical, infraparotid and superior and middle jugular nodes is adequate[3].

12

The incision is along a line projected upwards from the posterior border of the sternocleidomastoid muscle which is retracted anteriorly. The jugular vein can easily be preserved.

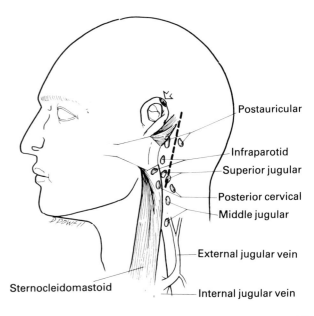

12

13

Primary lesions involving the parietal and occipital scalp should have simultaneous removal of the occipital, posterior auricular, infraparotid, superior jugular and posterior cervical lymph nodes. The internal jugular vein can again be preserved.

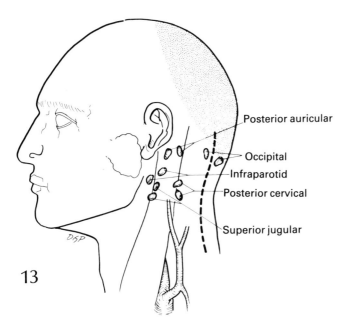

13

14

Primary lesions involving the forehead, preauricular region and anterior aspect of the ear require simultaneous superficial parotidectomy, thus removing the parotid lymph nodes; the operative field should also include the infraparotid nodes, the submandibular gland and its adjacent nodes, as well as the superior and middle jugular nodes.

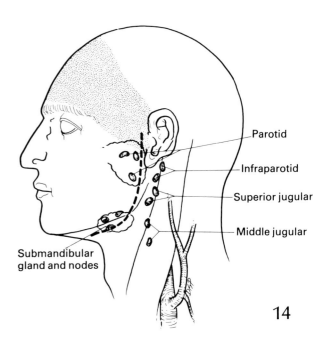

14

15

Facial melanomas that are below the zygomatic arch should have a simultaneous lymphadenectomy which includes the inferior pole of the parotid gland, the infraparotid, superior and middle jugular nodes and the submandibular gland with submandibular nodes as well as the submental nodes.

Primary lesions involving the neck should undergo lymphoscintography with removal of the lymph chains involved, as shown by the radionucleide study. This more selective approach to regional node dissection of melanomas involving the head and neck permits accurate pathological staging with minimal morbidity and cosmetic deformity.

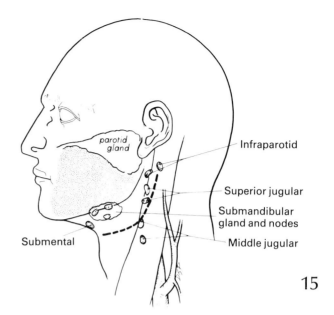

15

Recurrent local and distant disease

Local recurrent disease is generally defined as a lesion within 5 cm of the primary and not in lymph nodes. When melanoma recurs locally surgery continues to be the treatment of choice. The surgeon should accomplish wide excision with margins similar to those applied to the primary lesion and regional lymph node dissection.

Surgical removal may also be indicated in selective patients with symptomatic distant disease. Obstructing or bleeding resectable bowel lesions and excision of single, distant metastasis involving the lung or brain can result in long-term survival. Cytoreductive procedures may be indicated in patients with peripheral disease before beginning chemotherapeutic or immunotherapeutic regimens, even though the surgeon is aware that this will not be a curative operation. Hemipelvectomy and forequarter amputation for melanoma should be discouraged. Extremity amputation for bulky or diffuse local recurrent disease has been associated with a 20 per cent 5 year survival rate and this may provide an additional option for the surgeon managing this complicated problem[4].

References

1. Balch, C. M., Murad, T. M., Soong, S., Ingalls, A. L., Richards, P. C., Maddox, W. A. Tumor thickness as a guide to surgical management of clinical Stage I melanoma patients. Cancer 1979; 43: 883–888

2. Balch, C. M., Soong, S., Murad, T. M., Ingalls, A. L., Maddox, W. A. A multifactorial analysis of melanoma. III. Prognostic factors in melanoma patients with lymph node metastases (Stage II). Annals of Surgery 1981; 193: 377–388

3. Roses, D. F., Harris, M. N., Grunberger, I., Gumport, S. L. Selective surgical management of cutaneous melanoma of the head and neck. Annals of Surgery 1980; 192: 629–632

4. Fortner, J. G., MacLean, B., Mulcare, R. J. Treatment of recurrent malignant melanoma. In: McCarthy, W. H., ed. Melanoma and skin cancer, p. 453. Sydney: IUC and Australian Cancer Society, 1972

Isolated limb perfusion for chemotherapy of tumours

C. W. Jamieson MS, FRCS
Consultant Vascular Surgeon, Hammersmith Hospital, London;
Surgeon, St Thomas's Hospital, London

Introduction

This technique marries antitumour chemotherapy to a perfusion pump and oxygenator in a limb isolated from the systemic circulation by a tourniquet[1]. It permits perfusion of tumour in a limb with a high dose of a chemotherapeutic agent, but protects the patient from the systemic effects of this therapy. The limb is perfused and well oxygenated by circulation via its main artery and vein with warmed blood from a bubble oxygenator, and intermittent doses of the drug are added to the perfusion circuit.

The applications of the technique are strictly limited. It has apparently little value in the treatment of soft tissue sarcomas and its only established place is in the treatment of malignant melanoma[2,3]. The drug of choice remains phenylalanine mustard (Melphalan). More efficient agents now exist to combat melanoma, but multiple-drug regimens and other single agents which are slightly more efficacious unfortunately have unacceptably high inci-dences of arterial wall damage with the risk of catastrophic thrombosis. Melphalan itself is much more effective when used in an isolated limb perfusion circuit than it is when given systemically and response rates of up to 70 per cent have been reported, compared to the response rates of 15–20 per cent which accompany systemic intravenous administration. Several uncontrolled studies have now reported even better remission rates when the blood in the perfusion circuit is warmed to 40°C and to do this may be worthwhile[4]. However, this modification may add to the risk of damage to the limb[5]. This account is confined, therefore, to the treatment of melanoma of the limbs by normothermic isolated perfusion with Melphalan. Hyper-thermic perfusion with the addition of a heated blanket over the limb does not require any technical modifications of the procedure.

Indications

Overall improvement in the recurrence rates and survival figures of melanoma has been claimed when perfusion is added to conventional wide excision; large numbers of patients have been treated in this way in the United States. However, the survival figures in melanoma seem to vary internationally in an extraordinary manner, being, for example, better in Queensland[6] than in the United Kingdom[7], though the racial characteristics of the inhabitants are similar and the treatment virtually identical. Thus, it is a great pity that a large clinical trial of the efficacy of adjuvant isolated limb perfusion in melanoma has not been performed because it is very difficult to compare uncontrolled results of therapy from different centres. It is unlikely that such a study will be made, as the possible improvement in 5 year survival will not be more than 8–10 per cent, so a trial containing over 400 patients would be required to reveal a statistically significant difference. This number of patients with primary invasive melanoma without evidence of dissemination is not available at any centre within a reasonable time scale. Multicentre studies suffer from discrepancy in perfusion technique and the ethical criteria used by clinicians involved. However, the fact remains that extremely good response rates, 5 year survival figures and low morbidity have been published by those centres with the greatest experience of this technique, suggesting that it has some place in the management of melanoma.

Prophylactic perfusion is not generally recommended for superficial melanomas which carry a good prognosis. The slight risks of the procedure outweigh any marginal benefit, but we do recommend now that patients have a prophylactic perfusion after wide complete excision of a primary melanoma known to carry a *poor* prognosis, i.e. with involvement of fat and lymphatic channels. Less than 50 per cent of these patients survive following conventional surgical treatment[8] and it is probable that perfusion improves this figure without, in experienced units, an unacceptable morbidity[9, 10].

The greatest value of the technique is its effect on residual or recurrent tumour confined to one limb, a situation which is only too commonly encountered in this disease. There is at least a 50 per cent worthwhile remission rate after perfusion alone and also good evidence that it lessens the risk of further recurrence if it is combined with surgical removal of recurrent nodules. As a first line of attack, isolated limb perfusion is highly preferable to massive excision of skin and subcutaneous tissue or radical amputation. Occasionally, we recommend that fulminating limb metastases be controlled by perfusion, even in the presence of definite systemic spread of melanoma. The treatment in these circumstances has some palliative value and, in a tumour noted for its occasionally unpredictable behaviour and spontaneous regression, the odd miraculous long-term remission has been observed. Isolated limb perfusion, when not combined with an ablative operation or block dissection of glands, is not a particularly traumatic operation and causes little postoperative discomfort, so it does not add to the suffering of patients with a bad prognosis, and a good response is a great boost to morale.

Technique

The operation may be performed alone or combined with surgical excision of tumour. In these circumstances a skin graft is often necessary. The skin may be taken at the time of surgical excision; preferably, it is stored for 2–3 days in a refrigerator and then applied. Otherwise it may suffer from the high concentration of Melphalan in the subcutaneous tissues at the end of the perfusion. Block dissection of the groin is performed more rarely in melanoma without clinical or lymphographic evidence of nodal metastases in that its value as prophylactic therapy has yet to be clearly defined and it seems unlikely that it is beneficial. However, block dissection is still often necessary in the management of patients with obvious metastatic glands and may well be combined with perfusion.

The operation

1

General technique

The general diagram of the perfusion circuit and the operation is shown.

The operation consists of isolation of the main artery and vein of the limb, the dissection of these vessels, isolation of the limb's circulation by a tourniquet and cannulation of the vessels. The cannulae are connected to a bubble oxygenator and the limb perfused with oxygenated blood and Ringer's lactate for approximately 1 h. During that period divided doses of Melphalan are added to the perfusion circuit and at the end of perfusion the limb is washed out with fresh Ringer's lactate via the arterial perfusion line before the tourniquet is removed. It is of interest and some value to measure the leak from the perfused limb into the systemic circulation during the procedure. This can be indirectly calculated by adding a radioactive tracer such as 51 chromium tagged red blood cells to the perfusion circuit. Systemic blood from the patient is sampled every 15 min after the start of perfusion and the leak can be calculated from the concentration of the radioactive tagged agent in the systemic circulation. This, of course, presumes that the leak of Melphalan is comparable to that of the tagged agent; this may not in fact be the case as the drug tends to sequestrate in the limb, to be washed out after the tourniquet is removed. However, it does allow one to determine whether there is a gross inadequacy of the tourniquet causing an excessive leak, in which case it may be necessary to compromise in the dose schedule. At the end of the perfusion, the vessels are sutured and the wound closed.

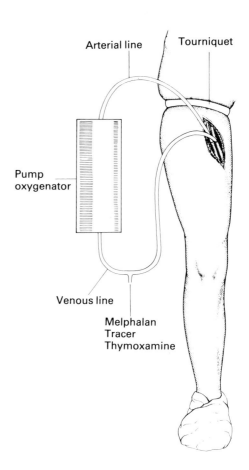

Arterial line

Tourniquet

Pump oxygenator

Venous line

Melphalan
Tracer
Thymoxamine

1

LOWER LIMB PERFUSION WITHOUT BLOCK DISSECTION

The patient is placed supine upon the operating table and the affected limb is prepared and draped to allow exposure of the whole limb and the groin. Tourniquets consisting of 1 cm diameter, thick wall rubber tubing are placed around the root of the limb and left loose. The perfusion apparatus is prepared; it consists of a disposable bubble oxygenator and pump with arterial and venous lines. Tapered arterial and venous polyethylene cannulae, with lines which may be passed by the surgeon to the perfusion team to be connected to the lines on the machine, are placed on the instrument tray. The perfusion circuit is primed with 500 ml of suitable cross-matched blood, Ringer's lactate 1 litre and 5000 u of heparin. Melphalan in three divided doses which total 1 mg/kg of the patient's weight is prepared. The radioactive tracer is supplied by a clinical isotope laboratory.

2

The incision

An incision approximately 12 cm long is made along a line which overlies the anterior border of the sartorius muscle, connecting the anterior superior iliac spine to the medial epicondyle of the knee and centred on the junction of the upper and intermediate thirds of the thigh.

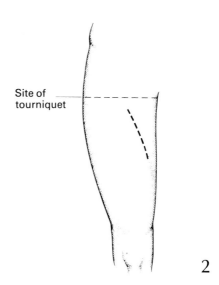

Site of tourniquet

2

Exposure

The fat and deep fascia are divided and the sartorius muscle reflected posteriorly. The femoral pulse is readily palpable in the subsartorial canal and the artery may be dissected from its sheath, from the veins which surround it and from the saphenous nerve. This dissection of the artery is usually easy, but small branches must be divided between fine ligatures, giving exposure of approximately 5 cm of the main artery. Dissection of the femoral vein at this point may be slightly more complicated as the vein may be multiple, in which case the larger vein should be dissected free for approximately 5 cm.

3

Both vein and artery are then snared with polyethylene tubing. The tubing is placed as a simple loop snare at the proximal extremity of the dissected vessel, but at the distal extremity it encircles the vessel twice and is then passed through a rubber tube, enabling this to be tightened with a pair of artery forceps when the cannulae have been sited.

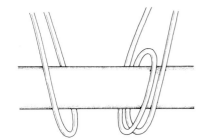

3

Perfusion

4

The completeness of the apparatus comprising the perfusion circuit is now checked. It is particularly important that 5000 units of heparin should have been added to the perfusion circuit (*see above*). Systemic anticoagulation is not necessary during this operation. The operating team's perfusion lines are assembled and connected to the main lines. The artery and vein are then controlled by arterial clamps and a transverse incision is made in both vessels, using Pott's scissors. This transverse incision does not cause stenosis when the vessels are sutured. A silk ligature is tied round each cannula, just proximal to the proposed point of its protrusion from the vessel, so it is possible to see whether it has accidentally changed its position during the operation. The cannulae are then inserted and snared in position distally using the polyethylene tubing. The distal clamps are removed. The proximal clamps remain for the duration of the perfusion. The tourniquet is then tightened, with an assistant carefully controlling the perfusion lines so that they are not dislodged during this procedure. The limb is then isolated and ready for perfusion.

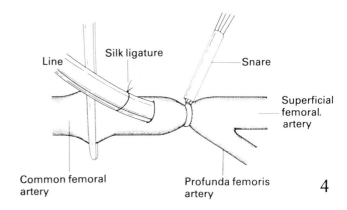

4

Perfusion is started and maintained at a flow rate between 100 and 200 ml/min. A careful watch is kept for distension of the femoral vein. Rapid distension of the vein indicates that the venous return is inadequate or that the tourniquet is not tight enough and the limb is filling with blood. Venous return can usually be improved by adjustment of the venous cannula, and the tourniquet must be tightened if necessary. Radioactive tracer and the first dose of Melphalan are then added to the *venous* side of the perfusion circuit. Injection of Melphalan into the arterial side may damage the artery. The dose is 1 mg/kg for the whole operation, divided into three doses; thus, for a 75 kg man 25 mg would be administered at this stage. We also administer 10 mg of thymoxamine which produces peripheral cutaneous vasodilation and increases

skin perfusion. The perfusing blood is warmed to at least 37 °C but kept below 45 °C and the limb is prevented from becoming cold, if necessary, by the application of towels. The first dose of systemic blood is sent for the measurement of a baseline of radioactivity and further samples are taken at 15 min intervals. Further doses of Melphalan are given every 15 min. Therefore, one-third of the total dose is given at 0 min and at 15 min. If the leak rate is acceptable, i.e. less than 10 per cent for this type of perfusion, a further full dose is given at 30 min. The total perfusion is then continued for 1 h. It is essential that the leak rate should have been determined on the first 30 min of perfusion by the time that the last dose of drug is given and, if it proves to be high, this last dose may be reduced.

Closure

At the end of 1 h the venous line is disconnected from the oxygenator and the limb is washed out with 2 litres of Ringer's lactate via the arterial line. There may be evidence of systemic hypotension and blood loss at this time because if the tourniquet is not completely effective, the low pressure in the 'isolated limb' allows bleeding from the systemic circulation into the limb. The anaesthetist must, therefore, be prepared to give blood if necessary to maintain the systemic blood pressure. Following this washout, the tourniquet is loosened and the arterial and venous lines removed.

5

The vessels are then sutured. The clamps are removed momentarily from the vein, allowing blood to flow from both proximal and distal ends, and if flow is not adequate, a Fogarty catheter should be passed in that direction to remove any thrombus. Thrombus is extremely rare at this stage in the procedure. The vein is then sutured, using a 4/0 Mersilene suture. A stay suture is placed at the proximal extremity of the transverse venotomy and tied to mark the end. Another suture is then tied at the far end of the venotomy and the vein closed with a running suture, approximately 1 mm apart and taking 1 mm bites of the vein wall. This is eventually tied to the first stay suture when the proximal end of the venotomy is reached. The venous clamps are again removed and venous bleeding is usually slight because the pressure is low.

The artery is tested for back- and downflow in a similar manner. Occasionally, there is a small amount of thrombus in the proximal artery at the end of the operation and if downflow is not good, it is essential that a Fogarty catheter be passed. Once good downflow is restored, the artery is sutured in exactly the same way as the vein. Bleeding from the artery is greater than from the vein and usually ceases with slight pressure for a few minutes. Once haemostasis is complete, the wound is insufflated with antibiotic powder and then closed in layers over a suction drain.

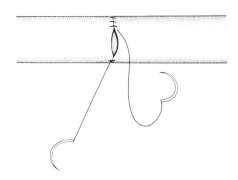

5

LOWER LIMB PERFUSION COMBINED WITH BLOCK DISSECTION

The major early complication of inguinal block dissection is necrosis of the skin flaps with lymph fistula and this is even more common when the block dissection is combined with a limb perfusion. The viability of the skin flaps is reduced, partly by the detrimental effect of spilt Melphalan in the tissues and partly because the increased duration of the operation allows the skin flaps to dry out.

For this reason it is best to perform the perfusion before completing the block dissection and before the major skin flap is cut. The position of the patient is the same as for simple perfusion, with preparation of the groin, the lower abdominal wall and the whole limb. The tourniquet is loosely placed round the root of the limb.

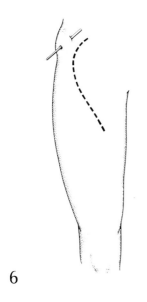

6

6

The incision

The incision is a curved one, based upon the proposed lateral margin of the block dissection. It is extended down through the deep fascia.

7

Exposure

The inguinal ligament and the sartorius muscle are identified and the whole subcutaneous tissue and deep fascia are dissected medially off the sartorius, the external oblique aponeurosis and, in succession, the femoral nerve, artery and vein. As the vein is reached, the termination of the saphenous vein is exposed, dissected distally for at least 1 cm and then ligated distally and clamped proximally. At this stage of the operation, the perfusion should be performed because the main flap of skin is still well nourished from its thick layer of subcutaneous tissue. A self-retaining Traver's retractor is placed in the wound to expose the femoral artery and vein. The artery and vein are then dissected on their deep surface in the following manner. A polyethylene tube is snared round the common femoral and the superficial femoral arteries. Gentle traction upwards upon these vessels exposes the origin of the profunda femoris artery which is separately controlled by a further polyethylene tube. A snaring tube is then placed to control the most distal common femoral artery. Great care must be taken not to damage small branches which may emerge from the junction of the superficial and the profunda femoris artery and which may cause very troublesome bleeding. The one snare controls reflux from superficial and profunda femoris. The common femoral, profunda femoris and superficial femoral veins are then dissected in the same way and controlled. A snare is placed above these vessels and below the termination of the common femoral vein.

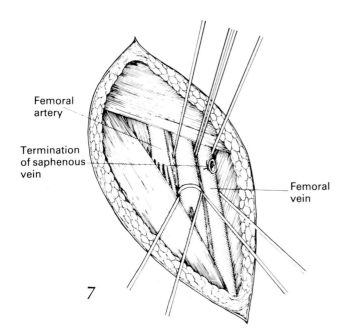

Femoral artery

Termination of saphenous vein

Femoral vein

7

8

In this operation the tourniquet must be above the site of the perfusion which necessitates it being placed obliquely across the groin. A Steinmann pin is passed through the wing of the ilium without transgressing the peritoneal cavity and the tourniquet is then looped over the Steinmann pin but not tightened.

The common femoral, superficial and profunda femoris arteries and their veins are then controlled separately with bulldog clamps and a transverse arteriotomy is made in the distal part of the common femoral artery. The common femoral vein may usually be entered via the termination of the saphenous vein, saving a venous suture line at this point. The vessels are then cannulated (*see above*), being certain that the cannulae pass down the superficial femoral artery and the superficial femoral vein, rather than into the profunda femoris vessels. The cannulae are snared and the clamps removed from the profunda femoris vessels. The proximal common femoral clamps remain *in situ*.

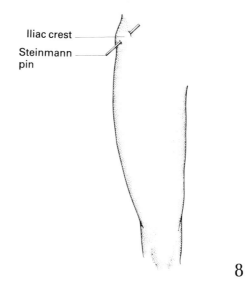

Iliac crest

Steinmann pin

8

Perfusion

The tourniquet is tightened and perfusion is conducted in the usual way. Flow rates are usually higher, ranging up to 300 ml/min.

Closure

The limb is washed out, the cannulae removed and the arteriotomy closed. The termination of the saphenous vein is ligated. The block dissection is then completed very simply by removing the block of glands and fat from the deep side of the skin flap, finishing at the pectineus muscle and the pubic tubercle, with division of the saphenous vein and lymphatics at the distal apex of the block. The wound is insufflated with antibiotic powder. A mass ligature which includes the lymphatics may lessen the incidence of lymph fistula. It is advisable at this stage to transpose the sartorius muscle to cover the femoral vessels because there may be necrosis of the skin with a risk of the vessels being exposed. If the sartorius has been transposed, this also makes it much easier to place a skin graft in the groin. The proximal origin of the sartorius is detached from the anterior superior iliac spine. It is freed from its fascial bed and swung medially to be sutured to the inguinal ligament, covering the femoral artery and vein. The flaps are then closed. The fat is loosely approximated with fine catgut sutures and the skin sutured with simple, interrupted nylon. Silk skin sutures are not satisfactory as healing may well be delayed and they become inflamed.

UPPER LIMB PERFUSION

The arm is shaved, including the axilla, and the skin is prepared over the whole arm, axilla and shoulder. The patient is placed supine with the arm extended on a rest. Axillary block dissection may be performed, but it is not possible to include the axilla in the isolated perfusion. The perfusion is carried out through the proximal part of the brachial vessels.

9

The incision

The incision of the axillary block dissection, or a separate incision, is carried along the medial border of the biceps brachii.

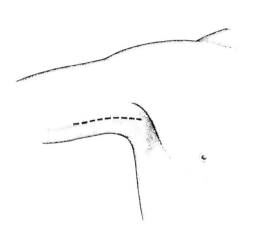

9

Exposure

The deep fascia is divided and the pulse of the brachial artery sought. The artery is dissected for approximately 5 cm and small branches are ligated and divided. Any larger branches are snared by a silk ligature but not divided. The brachial vein is then dissected at the same point. It may be multiple, in which case the largest vein must be selected.

Perfusion

The vessels are cannulated and the limb is perfused exactly as in a lower limb perfusion (*see above*), but the flow rate is usually 100 ml/min and the brachial vein does not give as good a venous return as the femoral vein, so adjustments of the venous cannulae are often necessary.

Closure

As before.

Postoperative care and complications

Early complications

Pain is not usually severe.

There is always a loss of some Melphalan from the perfusion circuit. It almost certainly sequestrates in the tissues of the limb and has an extended biological half life as it is normally metabolized by the liver. The Melphalan leaks back into the systemic circulation after the operation and may occasionally produce signs of systemic toxicity. Slight vomiting is very common in the first 24 h and must be controlled by antiemetics. Evidence of systemic toxicity caused by Melphalan is sought by daily white blood counts and platelet counts performed from the fifth post-operative day, the most severe depression usually occurring at around 14 days. If no depression is observed by the twelfth day, all is well.

Very careful watch must be kept on the arterial and venous circulation of the limb. It is our custom to record the ankle or radial pressures using Doppler ultrasound and a sphygmomanometer cuff at the end of the operation and again at daily intervals for the first 3 days. Pulses always return within 12 h if the artery has not been damaged and failure of the pulse to return by this time is an indication for exploration of the arteriotomy. However, the Doppler gives more precise information and allows one to explore earlier if necessary. Venous thrombosis is suprisingly uncommon considering that the main vein has been cannulated and perfused with an irritant substance. Sudden severe swelling of the limb is an indication for venous thrombectomy, but usually can be controlled by continuous intravenous heparin (10 000 u 8 hourly). Lymph fistula from the wound is uncommon unless the procedure has been combined with block dissection, but in these circumstances lymph usually collects under the flaps and must be aspirated promptly if it does not drain because it causes tension in the flaps with consequent necrosis. Reactionary haemorrhage may occur. It is essential that the arterial suture line be dry at the end of the operation and any further bright bleeding from the drain or wound during the first postoperative 24 h is an indication for re-exploration. Secondary haemorrhage has not occurred in our experience but is the consequence of sepsis, in which case an attempt to repair the artery is doomed to failure. Should a secondary haemorrhage occur, it is unfortunately essential that the main artery be ligated. In these circumstances, the circulation of the limb may be restored by routing a vein bypass around the infected field, e.g. from the iliac artery above to the superficial femoral artery below. Superficial sepsis is also uncommon and is treated by appropriate antibiotics. An overdose of Melphalan to the limb produces blistering and erythema of the skin plus neuropathy and, if suffi-ciently great, may cause massive necrosis of the limb which may necessitate amputation. It is essential for the dose to be carefully controlled, but a slight postoperative erythema, like sunburn, is an indication that a good, maximal dosage has been given.

Late complications

Failure to produce regression of tumour

In these circumstances the patient must be treated by excision of multiple tumours or, very, very rarely, by amputation of the limb. However, tumours should not be excised without some time lapse after perfusion because late regression is regularly observed following regional perfusion. It is reasonable that any tumours be left for at least 3 months unless they are growing, following the perfusion, and they may well regress over that time.

Failure to produce overall regression of tumour

Quite often some nodules of tumours will regress while others remain static or even grow, in which case the tumours that show evidence of activity should be excised or, if very numerous, should be treated by widespread excision of skin and subcutaneous tissue, with grafting. Cryosurgery may have a place in the control of dermal lesions which are widespread, in that it does produce relatively painless necrosis of the lesions with good early healing. Direct injection of BCG into unresponsive nodules is sometimes helpful.

Recurrence of tumour

A patient who has developed recurrent tumour after a response to regional perfusion or after a regional perfusion as part of adjuvant primary therapy must be fully re-assessed. Efforts are made to detect systemic metas-tases and the decision whether he should have a further perfusion must then be reached. It is probably not worth offering a further perfusion if the response to the first perfusion was transient or negligible, but if there has been a worthwhile remission following one perfusion, it is quite likely that there will be a second remission after another. It is important in performing a second perfusion that a new site be selected for arterial and venous cannulation, as re-exploration of previously perfused vessels is usually extremely difficult.

Oedema

Oedema following regional perfusion alone is not common and when it does occur is probably the result of venous thrombosis. Oedema following block dissection combined with regional perfusion is usual but seldom severe. Both respond to simple conservative measures and improve greatly over the months after the perfusion. Patients are advised to elevate their leg when possible, to wear firm, supporting elastic stockings, preferably a graded compression stocking such as the well tailored Sigvaris stockings. These graded compression stockings apply more pressure to the distal limb than to the thigh and therefore carry no risk of acting as a tourniquet and causing further venous or lymphatic obstruction. Patients who have severe and troublesome oedema may be helped by the use of intermittent compression, pneumatic leggings (such as are manufactured by Flowtron or by BOC) for 1 h/day. The intermittent pressure applied by these leggings helps to control oedema, which may then be maintained under control with elastic stockings.

References

1. Creech, O., Krementz, F. T., Ryan, R. F., Winblad, J. N. Chemotherapy of cancer: regional perfusion utilizing an extracorporeal circuit. Annals of Surgery 1958; 148: 616–632

2. McBride, C. M., Clark, R. L. Experience with L-phenylalanine mustard dihydrochloride in isolation-perfusion of extremities for malignant melanoma. Cancer 1971; 28: 1293–1296

3. Krementz, E. T., Ryan, R. F. Chemotherapy of melanoma of the extremities by perfusion: fourteen years' clinical experience. Annals of Surgery 1972; 175: 900–917

4. Stehlin, J. S., Giovanella, B. C., Ipolyi, P. D. de, Anderson, R. F. Results of eleven years' experience with heated perfusion for melanoma of the extremities. Cancer Research 1979; 39: 2255–2257

5. Polk, H. C. Adjunctive treatment for malignant melanoma. In: Varco, R. L., Delaney, J. P., eds. Controversy in surgery, p. 211. Philadelphia: W. B. Saunders, 1976

6. Davis, N. C., Herron, J. J., McLeod, G. R. Malignant melanoma in Queensland: analysis of 400 skin lesions. Lancet 1966; 2: 407–410

7. Bodenham, D. C. A study of 650 observed malignant melanomas in the south-west region. Annals of the Royal College of Surgeons of England 1968; 43: 218–239

8. Petersen, N. C., Bodenham, D. C., Lloyd, O. C. Malignant melanomas of the skin. A study of the origin, development, aetiology, spread, treatment and prognosis. British Journal of Plastic Surgery 1962; 15: 49–116

9. Weaver, P. C., Wright, J., Brander, W. L., Westbury, G. Salvage procedures for locally advanced malignant melanoma of the lower limb (with special reference to the role of isolated limb perfusion and radical lymphadenectomy). Clinical Oncology 1975; 1: 45–51

10. Bulman, A. S., Jamieson, C. W. Isolated limb perfusion with Melphalan in the treatment of malignant melanoma. British Journal of Surgery 1980; 67: 660–662

Illustrations by Frank Price and Robert Lane

Operations for benign breast disease

L. E. Hughes   DS, FRCS, FRACS
Professor of Surgery, Welsh National School of Medicine, Cardiff

Operations for benign breast disease fall into two broad groups: those necessary to allow a definitive tissue diagnosis to be made, and those necessary to control inflammatory conditions of the breast. Diagnostic procedures are dealt with first.

DIAGNOSTIC PROCEDURES FOR BREAST LUMPS

Plans of action are required for three clinical situations: a palpable breast lump, a subclinical lesion diagnosed on mammography and nipple discharge. For a palpable mass, the diagnostic process recommended is a sequence of needle aspiration (to exclude a cyst), needle biopsy and open biopsy.

Treatment of breast cysts

Simple cysts account for the majority of well-defined breast lumps in women of the 35–55 year age group, and most are satisfactorily dealt with by aspiration. There are two cardinal rules: the lump must disappear completely on aspiration, and the fluid must not contain blood. If either of these situations exist biopsy is mandatory: for a persistent mass because cysts and cancer are both common disorders and may coexist by chance; and for blood-stained fluid because this usually signifies the presence of a papillary tumour in the wall of the cyst. Most of these are benign, but a significant proportion, especially in older women, will be papillary carcinomas.

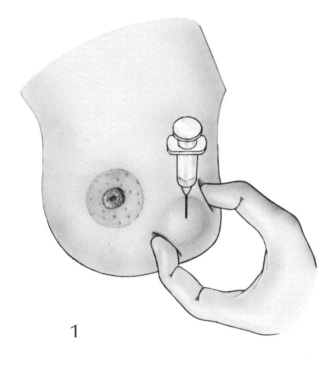

1

1

Technique of aspiration

The cyst should be steadied between two fingers, which also direct it towards the surface. A sharp 21 gauge needle is inserted (local anaesthetic is unnecessary), and there is a distinctive feel as the needle traverses the fibrous cyst wall and then suddenly penetrates into the cyst. The cyst may be deeper in the breast than appears on clinical examination, so deeper needling should be tried if no result is obtained from aspiration, before concluding that the mass is solid. Recurrence after aspiration is not infrequent, but a second or even third aspiration will usually give prolonged relief.

Pneumocystography

The procedure of pneumocystography is useful when the cyst fluid is found to be blood-stained or when a cyst recurs after two or three aspirations. The fluid is aspirated from the cyst and replaced with an equal volume of air. The patient then undergoes conventional mammography or xeromammography. The outline of the cyst is shown and any tumour in its wall is well demonstrated. We also have a strong clinical impression that persistent cysts are more likely to resolve after this procedure than after simple aspiration.

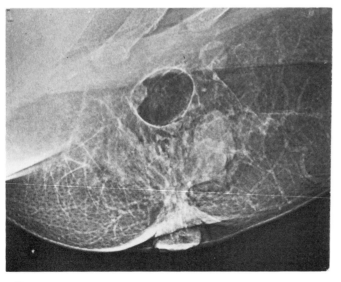

2

2

This pneumocystogram is from a patient whose cyst aspirate was blood-stained. It shows a benign papillary tumour in its wall. (The subareolar distortion is the result of an earlier biopsy.)

Needle biopsy

A definitive preoperative diagnosis of cancer is of great advantage both to the surgeon – in planning management and saving operating time – and to the patient by minimizing the psychological strain of going to theatre not knowing whether or not a mastectomy will be necessary. Three techniques are currently in use. Cytology from needle aspiration is favoured by some, but interpretation requires special expertise and the technique does not allow differentiation of preinvasive cytological malignancy from invasive cancer (see chapter on 'Fine needle aspiration of solid tumours of the breast', pp. 254–261). Drill biopsy is

highly effective in skilled hands, but requires apparatus better suited to a specialized unit. Needle biopsy using the Tru-cut needle (Travenol) will provide definitive histology in most cancers greater than 2 cm in diameter and in a substantial proportion of smaller cancers. Because of the rubbery nature of fibrocystic disease, the technique is less satisfactory for benign masses. The benefit lies only in obtaining a positive diagnosis of malignancy and it is wise to proceed to open biopsy in all cases where the needle biopsy report from a distinct mass is benign, because of possible sampling errors with this technique.

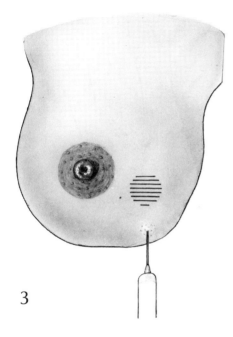

3

3, 4 & 5

Technique of needle biopsy

An intradermal weal of local anaesthetic is raised, avoiding any obvious subcutaneous veins. A stab incision is made with a disposable pointed scalpel blade and a 7.5 cm (3 inch) biopsy needle inserted into the breast in the closed position. The central needle is advanced into the mass and the cutting sheath then closed over it against gentle counterpressure from the opposite aspect of the breast. The closed needle is removed and any bleeding controlled by digital pressure. With practise the manipulation of the needle during insertion can be done with one hand, allowing the other hand to give direction and stability by holding the mass. The final cutting manoeuvre should be rapid, using both hands. It is helpful if an assistant steadies the mass and gives counterpressure at this time.

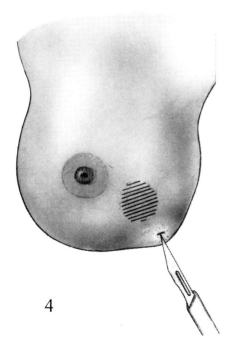

4

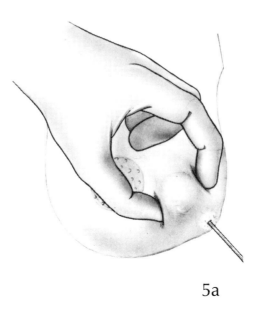

5a

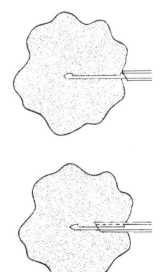

5b

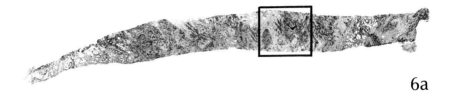

6a

6a & b

Typical biopsy specimens showing the quality of histological material provided.

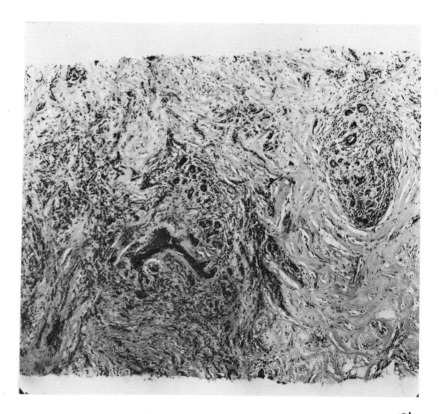

6b

Biopsy excision

Indications

There are four main indications for biopsy excision in benign breast disease: fibroadenoma, a discrete mass in the fibroadenosis/hyperplastic cystic disease complex, a subclinical lesion demonstrated on mammography, and for ductal discharge. Each requires a different technique. A simple cyst should always be excluded by needle aspiration as described above before subjecting a patient to open biopsy under anaesthesia.

Anaesthesia

General anaesthesia is recommended unless there is some special contraindication. Local anaesthesia for breast biopsy should not be undertaken lightly. Masses often lie deeper in the breast than they appear clinically, bleeding may be difficult to control and local tissue infiltration by the anaesthetic agent may obscure the mass that is being sought.

The incisions

7

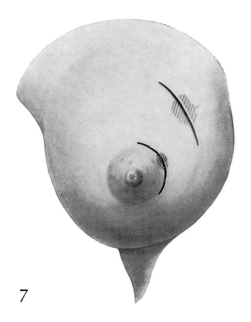

7

For lesions within about 5 cm of the nipple, a periareolar incision, extending no further than half the circumference, gives good access and an excellent scar. Otherwise, a curved incision sited over the mass and parallel to the areola is satisfactory. Cross-hatching helps accurate suturing of these curved incisions.

8

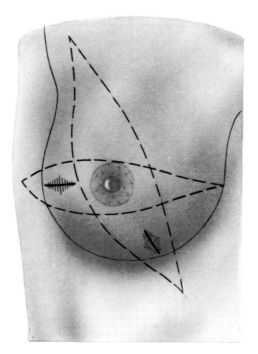

8

Radial incisions give a less satisfactory cosmetic result and a higher incidence of painful scars. However, where the mass may be malignant, the biopsy incision should be planned in relation to the possible mastectomy incision, so that the biopsy incision can be completely re-excised with a wide margin at mastectomy. This means that, for some peripheral masses, a radial incision lying in the line of the proposed mastectomy incision may be most suitable.

Excision of a fibroadenoma

Because fibroadenomas are usually found in young women a good cosmetic result is particularly desirable. Most are freely mobile and superficial and can be removed through a small incision lying in a skin crease. An occasional fibroadenoma is multifocal and merges with the surrounding breast tissue – this resembles fibroadenosis in its physical signs and should be removed as described for biopsy of this condition. 'Giant' fibroadenomas call for a special technique.

9

Surgical pathology of a fibroadenoma

The tumour is attached to the capsule by a stalk carrying its blood supply, and sometimes the adenomatous tissue extends into the capsule in the region of the stalk attachment.

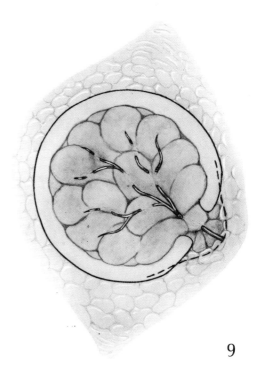

9

10

Technique

After incision through the skin and subcutaneous fat, the lesion is palpated and pushed into the incision, the capsule is opened and the fibroadenoma is shelled out. A piece of the capsule in the region of the stalk attachment should be removed to lessen the risk of recurrence, carefully securing the entering blood vessel, if necessary with a transfixion suture. The dissection should encounter few other vessels, so, if the wound is quite dry, it may be closed without drainage with a 4/0 chromic catgut suture to the subcutaneous tissue and 4/0 silk to the skin. If there is any tendency to oozing, the wound should be drained by a fine suction catheter, ensuring that the catheter lumen is not occluded by blood clot while the wound is being closed and before suction can be applied.

10

'GIANT' FIBROADENOMA

When a fibroadenoma is large, that is, more than 5 cm in diameter, it is likely to be deeper in the breast than is clinically apparent, and is best approached from behind. Such lesions are almost always benign, but histological examination will occasionally show them to be of borderline or even frank malignancy.

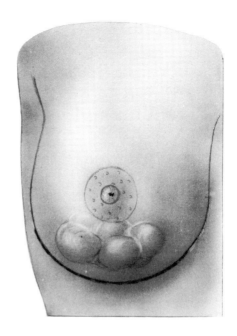

11

11 & 12

An appropriate circumferential incision at the edge of the breast disc, and usually in the submammary fold, is deepened to the fascia overlying pectoralis major or serratus anterior. Blunt dissection is readily developed in this almost bloodless plane between breast tissue and fascia. The fibroadenoma is then pushed into the wound and removed as described earlier. Suction drainage is used routinely, and the wound closed with 4/0 chromic catgut to the subcutaneous tissues and 4/0 silk to the skin.

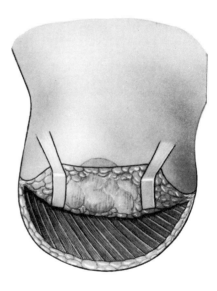

12

Biopsy excision of a discrete mass of fibroadenosis

Biopsy of a dominant mass in a fibroadenotic breast differs considerably from removal of a fibroadenoma for a number of reasons. First, the possibility that the mass will prove to be malignant must be considered from the outset. Second, the lump under suspicion may be more difficult to detect at operation than to palpate before operation. Third, control of bleeding is much more difficult because the blood vessels lie in the tough rubbery stroma of fibroadenosis, into which they tend to retract on division.

The incision

The incision should be more generous than with fibroadenoma, to ensure that the lump in question is completely excised and to facilitate control of bleeding points. A direction parallel to the areola is suitable in most cases, with the proviso related to a possible mastectomy incision discussed earlier.

Localizing the mass

It is helpful to mark the site of the lesion preoperatively, with the arm abducted in the position it will occupy on the operating table. When the patient has been prepared and towelled up in theatre, if the mass is not very obvious, it is useful to insert a needle through the skin into the mass leaving it there as a guide while the incision is deepened through the breast tissue.

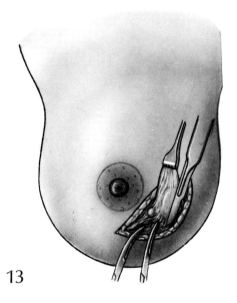

13

13

Removing the mass

After dividing the skin and ligating any subcutaneous veins, the lump is located by palpation and held with an Allis tissue forceps, which is used to draw the mass to the surface. The extent of the lump is then defined by palpation and that area of tissue excised by a scalpel. In the markedly fibroadenotic breast the appearance of the tissue cannot be used to define the extent of the lesion in that fibroadenosis is a diffuse disease with a uniform macroscopic appearance. Any attempt to remove all the macroscopically abnormal tissue must be resisted, because this will lead to an excessively large excision and even to inadvertent simple mastectomy in a small breast. As each vessel is divided, it must be caught with a fine mosquito forceps before it retracts into the rubbery tissue. It may be cauterized, ligated or under-run with fine chromic catgut on a stout needle.

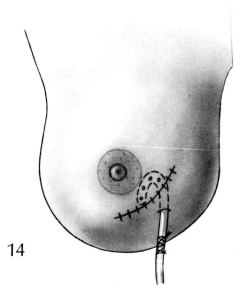

14

14

Drainage and closure

If the incision has been made as large as the underlying cavity and the vessels caught as they have been divided, there should be no major bleeding at the end of the procedure, but small bleeding points ooze from the fibrous tissue and attempts to stop these tend to be unproductive. The cavity may be obliterated but the tough fibrous tissue can only be sewn with a stout trocar pointed needle and strong catgut, and such manoeuvres tend to exacerbate bleeding. Once the major bleeding points are secured it is best to ignore the cavity and to insert a suction drain, suturing skin and subcutaneous tissues only. The drain can be removed at 24 h.

Biopsy of a subclinical lesion

Mammography may demonstrate a lesion suggestive of malignancy in a region where no abnormality can be detected clinically. Such lesions are likely to prove to be either invasive cancer, intraduct cancer or sclerosing adenosis[1]. A particular area of the breast may change its position relative to external markers when the patient assumes different positions, especially abnormal positions such as those used for mammography and surgery. This makes localization of a mammographic lesion difficult at operation. Since at least half these lesions will prove to be benign, a technique should be used which allows definite excision of the radiological abnormality while removing a minimal amount of normal breast tissue.

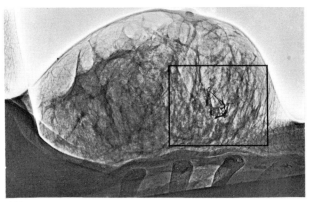

15a

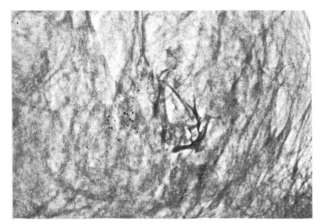

15b

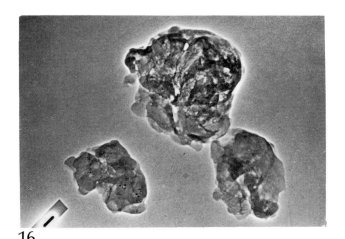

16

15a & b

Radiological localization

On the morning of operation the patient is taken to the X-ray department and placed on the X-ray table in the position of the lateral film. After consideration of the mammograms, the radiologist injects 0.5 ml of a dye mixture into the site at which he considers the mass to be. The mixture contains 1 ml of 25 per cent Hypaque (to give radiological localization) and two drops of patent blue violet (to allow recognition at operation). Repeat mammograms are then taken in the two conventional planes and the radiologist reports the relationship of the radiological abnormality to the dye. An alternative practice is to leave the needle *in situ*.

16

Operative procedure

The patient is taken to theatre, the site of the dye is exposed and the appropriate area excised. While the patient remains anaesthetized, the specimen is returned to X-ray for specimen radiography to ensure that the radiological abnormality is included and to localize the exact site under suspicion for the pathologist. (Specimen radiography is less certain in the absence of microcalcification.) The specimen radiograph illustrated here shows the microcalcification to be confined to the smallest of the three specimens.

If the specimen removed has classic macroscopic features of a carcinoma it is submitted to frozen section, proceeding to mastectomy if indicated. Otherwise, and in the majority of cases, the author prefers to await urgent paraffin section so that the management can proceed after full evaluation.

Biopsy procedures for nipple discharge

General management of nipple discharge

A blood-stained or clear serous nipple discharge is most frequently caused by benign papilloma, single or multiple. The commonest entity is a solitary papilloma giving discharge from a single duct and this is treated by microdochotomy (excision of a single duct and its drainage system). Occasionally papillomatosis leads to discharge from multiple ducts, usually in women near the menopause and total duct excision is the preferred operation. Rarely a duct carcinoma will be found on histology. (Blood discharge from multiple ducts, and commonly from both nipples, may also be seen during pregnancy when it is due to a physiological hyperplasia of the duct epithelium.)

Discharges other than blood-stained or serous are causally associated with cancer so rarely that operation is not necessary as a diagnostic procedure. But such discharges (usually yellowish or green and due to duct ectasia) may be sufficiently profuse for inconvenience to indicate the operation of total duct excision.

The presence of dilated ducts, as detected on mammography, is not in itself an indication for total duct excision. Likewise, when some duct dilatation is seen during biopsy of a mass behind the nipple, the mass should be removed in the usual way and the ducts left undisturbed. Healing is usually uneventful despite the transected dilated ducts, and it should be remembered that some duct dilatation is present in a majority of women at or near the menopause. Total duct excision is associated with higher morbidity and a less satisfactory cosmetic result than simple biopsy.

MICRODOCHOTOMY

This operation is indicated for blood-stained or serous discharge from a single duct whose orifice can be identified. Where the discharge has ceased by the time the patient is seen, so that the duct cannot be identified, the patient may be observed if she is under the age of 40 years since duct papillomas commonly slough spontaneously. In all patients over this age we would carry out a total duct excision operation because of an increased risk of multiple papillomas or intraduct cancer.

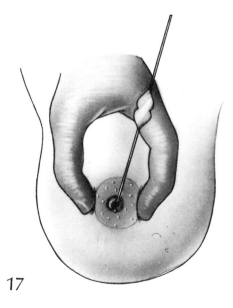

17

17

Technique

The nipple is first squeezed to produce some discharge to identify the affected duct. A lacrimal probe is then gently inserted as far as possible, without forming a false passage. Frequently this is only for 1 or 2 cm because dilated ducts may be tortuous or blocked by papillomas which form little pockets in their walls, but the probe can be passed far enough to show the general direction of the duct and indicate in which direction the excision should be made.

18 & 19

A radial incision is made in a racquet shape to include the terminal part of the duct, then crosses the areola to extend into the breast for about 5 cm. The two flaps are dissected in the level between the deep fascia and the breast lobules – this plane is easiest to develop in the region of the margin of the areola. In the central portion of the duct the incision should be kept as close to the probe as possible, to avoid removing adjacent ducts. The duct system is then dissected peripherally for about 5 cm; this is normally sufficient to remove all the major duct system of the affected segment. Haemostasis is ensured and a suction drain is inserted before closing the wound with 4/0 chromic catgut to the deep fascia and 4/0 silk to the skin. This radial incision heals with a surprisingly good cosmetic result. Where the duct to be removed opens on to the central portion of the nipple, some trauma to adjacent ducts is inevitable, but this does not give long-term problems.

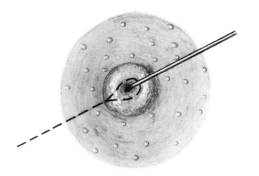

18

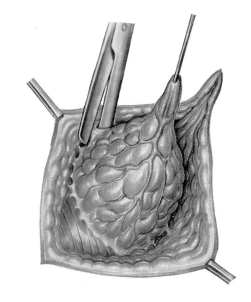

19

EXCISION OF THE DUCT SYSTEM OF THE BREAST

This operation is indicated for blood-stained or serous discharge from one or more ducts in women over the age of 40; and for nipple discharge from duct ectasia sufficient to embarrass or seriously inconvenience the patient[2]. With milky discharges, galactorrhoea of pituitary origin should be excluded before proceeding to duct excision.

20

The incision

The ducts may be approached by periareolar or radial incisions. The former has the advantages of a better cosmetic result, and of allowing easier access to the correct plane for dissection of the ducts. The incision is deepened through the skin and the subcutaneous fascia until the subcutaneous veins are reached. These are carefully ligated with 4/0 chromic catgut and serve as a guide to the plane of dissection which lies immediately deep to them. This plane is between the fat lobules of the breast and the fascia underlying the areola and preserves the subdermal vascular plexus of the areola, and with it the viability of the nipple.

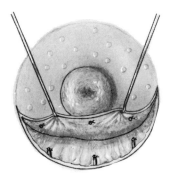

20

21 & 22

The nipple is elevated with hooks and mobilized until the main duct system has been exposed. Keeping in the same plane, further dissection of the areola is carried out on both sides, using blunt curved artery forceps such as Kelly-Halsted. In this way, a subareolar tunnel is produced in the subcutaneous plane right around the ducts, which are then grasped at their termination by a small Kocher forceps and the ducts divided just below the nipple. The duct system is dissected back into the breast for a distance of 2–3 cm and again divided with a scalpel. Bleeding vessels are immediately caught with mosquito forceps and ligated with 4/0 chromic catgut before they are lost through retraction into the breast tissue. In most cases dilated ducts are not detectable more than 2–3 cm into the breast tissue. When they are still dilated at the point of transection, an attempt should be made to catch them with forceps and ligate them with fine catgut, although this is not always possible, and failure to do so seems to cause no trouble.

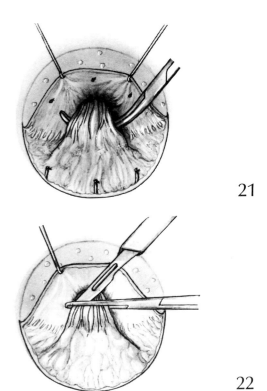

21

22

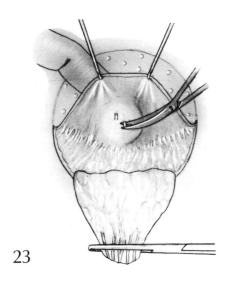

23

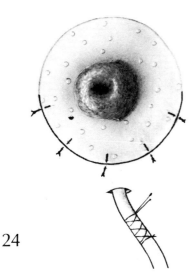

24

23

The completeness of excision of the terminal ducts is checked by inverting the nipple and trimming any residual duct with scissors and, second, by ensuring that the subareolar dissection has encompassed the complete duct system.

The nipple will usually remain everted after excision of the duct system, but if it tends to reinvert, a fine catgut suture can be placed in the deep fascia to maintain eversion.

24

Closure

Provided there is no evidence of active infection, the skin is closed with 4/0 silk and suction drainage instituted. Some epidermal necrosis of the lower flap may be seen if dissection too superficially has compromised the subdermal plexus, but this usually separates spontaneously.

PROCEDURES FOR INFLAMMATORY LESIONS OF THE BREAST

Operations for inflammatory conditions fall into two broad groups: the well-defined breast abscess associated with lactation, and a much less well-defined group of conditions of subacute chronic suppuration of the breast.

Drainage of a lactational breast abscess

Acute mastitis in the lactation period is usually the result of a staphylococcal infection associated with a cracked nipple and can sometimes be obviated by control of breast engorgement and antibiotics. But unless resolution is clearly rapid and complete within 48 h, drainage should be undertaken early, because excessive destruction of breast tissue will occur by the time the abscess shows obvious fluctuation or skin involvement. Where the patient is afebrile and throbbing pain absent, the possibility of inflammatory carcinoma should be considered; needle biopsy rather than open biopsy is preferred in this situation.

25 – 28

Technique

A skin-crease incision is used, slightly below the point of maximal swelling and tenderness.

A finger is then inserted into the cavity to ensure that all loculations are broken down, so that no undrained areas persist. If the resulting cavity is found to be centred behind the incision, counterdrainage is not necessary.

The incision should extend to at least three-quarters of the diameter of the cavity, which is then gently packed – gauze soaked in acriflavine emulsion is suitable.

Where the cavity is obviously dependent in relation to the incision, it is best to use counterdrainage at the lowest point, inserting a wide plastic corrugated drain. The initial incision should be loosely sutured only if the margins are healthy. Where the abscess cavity has already reached the surface, primary healing of the edges will not occur.

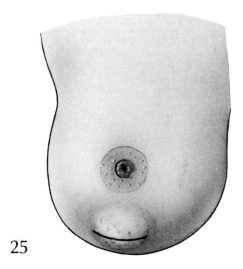

25

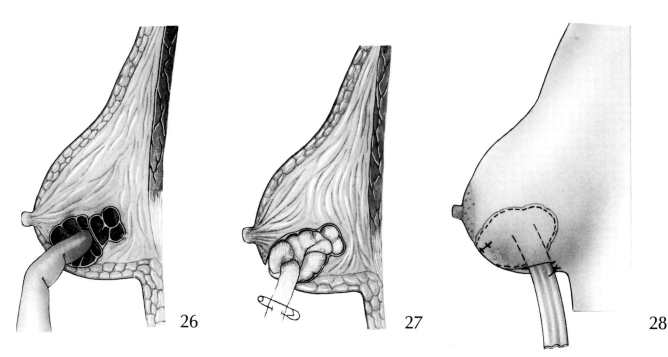

26   27   28

Subacute and recurrent abscesses of the breast

Most breast abscesses unrelated to lactation are associated with duct ectasia and its complication, periductal mastitis. This is a reaction to irritating duct contents which have escaped into periductal tissues and is initially sterile, although secondary bacterial invasion, especially with anaerobic organisms, may occur later or after drainage. The hallmarks of these abscesses are their periareolar location, frequent association with nipple inversion, relatively chronic or relapsing course and a lesser degree of pain than is seen with lactational abscesses. In addition it is not rare for both breasts to be affected, with an interval of several years between the two sides. Patients with these abscesses tend to fall into two main groups which are associated with a single or with multiple duct involvement. This distinction is clinical rather than pathological, since the 'single duct' variety may show a number of dilated ducts. Hence it is not surprising that the distinction is sometimes blurred. However, most cases fall clearly into one or other clinical pattern and are managed satisfactorily by the appropriate surgical approach.

The single duct entity, the mammillary duct fistula of Atkins, is diagnosed when recurrent abscesses always appear at the one site, usually a point on the medial edge of the areola, and when a fistula can be demonstrated in between acute episodes by passing a probe from the site of the abscess discharge through to the nipple. It is satisfactorily treated by the fistula excision operation first described by Atkins[3].

The multiple duct entity, when retroareolar infection is less well localized, is seen more commonly close to the menopause but may on occasions be found even in young nulliparous girls. Where there is extensive and poorly localized retroareolar infection, excision of the whole duct system is necessary to control the infection. This type also differs from the first group in that some cases show dilatation of ducts extending well out into the peripheral breast tissue, the ducts being filled with toothpaste-like material. Recurrent subareolar abscess from a single duct mammillary fistula is not associated with peripheral dilatation.

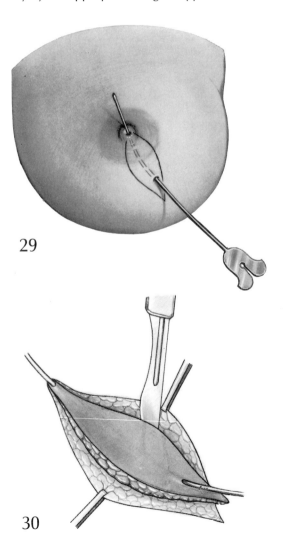

29

30

EXCISION OF MAMMILLARY DUCT FISTULA

29 & 30

A probe is passed through the opening and will be found to emerge from the nipple through the affected duct, which is always dilated. The skin incision encompasses the fistulous track, encircles the affected duct and is continued for 2 cm distal to the opening of a fistula. It is unnecessary to remove more than 0.5 cm of skin on either side of the track. The incision is deepened to expose the underlying tissues, and the fistula excised as a formal operation. It is essential to excise the central portion of the duct; if it is left behind recurrence is certain.

31

The wound is best left open and packed to allow healing by granulation. Primary closure is followed by wound breakdown in a considerable number of cases, and may lead to further chronic infection.

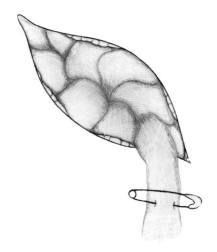

31

TOTAL DUCT EXCISION FOR SUBAREOLAR SEPSIS

This follows the same general principles as described under 'Total duct excision for discharge'. Development of the correct plane may be difficult if persistent inflammation is present. It may then be better to use a radial incision as first described by Urban[4] to excise the most badly affected skin.

If dilated ducts containing cheesy contents are found to extend into the breast tissue beyond the 3 cm normally removed, an attempt should be made to catch the transected ducts with artery forceps and ligate them with fine chromic catgut. The wound is packed and allowed to heal by granulation. Attempts at primary closure, even with drainage, are likely to be followed by persistent sepsis and possible necrosis of the overlying nipple.

Most patients will have no further trouble, but in some, more peripheral inflammation will subsequently develop. This will usually localize to a segment of the breast, so that subsequent excision of perhaps one-third of the breast is necessary. Less commonly, inflammation is so extensive that the condition will only be eradicated by total sub-cutaneous mastectomy. Perioperative use of an agent active against anaerobic organisms, such as metronidazole, may reduce the incidence of postoperative or recurrent sepsis, but clear evidence to support this is not available at present.

References

1. Preece, P. E., Gravelle, I. H., Hughes, L. E., Baum, M., Fortt, R. W., Leopold, J. G. The operative management of subclinical breast cancer. Clinical Oncology 1977; 3: 165–169

2. Hadfield, G. J. The pathological lesions underlying discharges from the nipple in women. Annals of the Royal College of Surgeons of England 1969; 44: 323–333

3. Atkins, H. B. Mammillary fistula. British Medical Journal 1955; 2: 1473–1474

4. Urban, J. A. Excision of the major duct system of the breast. Cancer 1963; 16: 516–520

Fine needle aspiration of solid tumours of the breast

Dulcie V. Coleman MB BS, MD, MRCPath

Senior Lecturer in Cytology, Department of Pathology, St Mary's Hospital, London

Introduction

Numerous studies have shown that cytological examination of cells obtained by aspiration through a fine needle is a rapid and reliable method of diagnosing malignant disease of the breast[1-8]. This method of investigation is widely used in Scandinavian countries for the pre-operative diagnosis of breast cancer, and surgeons in the United Kingdom who have clinical experience of the technique have found that it can be included with advantage in the routine investigation of all patients presenting with a discrete palpable lump in the breast. Cytological assessment of these patients by fine needle aspiration shortly after their initial consultation with the surgeon in the breast clinic enables the surgeon to make a definitive diagnosis of cancer in patients with clinical features of the disease, and to identify malignant disease in patients where clinically none was suspected.

The technique of fine needle aspiration is familiar to most surgeons. It is already established as the method of choice for the diagnosis and treatment of benign breast cysts (see p. 240). Some modification of the technique is necessary for the successful cell sampling of solid tumours and special attention must be paid to the preparation of the aspirate before its transfer to the laboratory if it is to be suitable for cytological analysis.

Aspiration technique

1

Satisfactory aspirates can be obtained using a disposable 10 ml Luer-Lok syringe fitted with a 40 mm 8/10 (No. 21) gauge needle. The skin over the lump is wiped with antiseptic solution and the lump fixed between the finger and thumb and held steady for needling. The needle is guided through the skin into the tumour. Local anaesthetic is generally not necessary; it is usually painful and may obscure the mass.

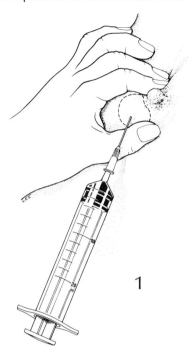

1

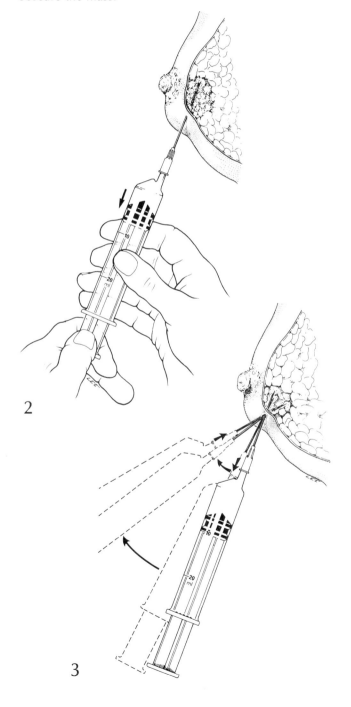

2

3

2

Once the needle is felt to enter the tumour, the plunger of the syringe is retracted to create a vacuum. Should the lesion prove to be cystic, the fluid should be aspirated in its entirety, expressed into a universal container and sent for cytological examination.

3

If the lump is found to be solid, the needle is gently moved back and forth in the substance of the tumour three or four times and inserted into a different part of the tumour mass each time to dislodge the cells from the tumour so that the aspirate will contain sufficient material for cytological studies.

Throughout this manipulation a negative pressure must be sustained in the syringe. Only after the tumour has been repeatedly probed should suction be released, the pressure in the syringe allowed to return slowly to atmospheric pressure and the needle withdrawn from the breast. The pressure in the syringe must be adjusted in this way so that the aspirated cells are retained in the lumen of the needle. Sustained suction as the needle is being withdrawn may result in the cells being drawn into the barrel of the syringe, rendering them inaccessible for processing.

Preparation of the aspirates

It is possible to make smears directly from the aspirate in the outpatient clinic. Alternatively the aspirated cells can be suspended in fixative and transferred to the cytology laboratory for processing. Whichever course is adopted, a cytological report on the specimen can be given within a few hours.

Preparation of the smear

4

After aspiration the syringe and needle are disconnected and the syringe filled with air.

5

A clean glass slide with a frosted end should be marked clearly in pencil with the patient's name. The needle is reconnected and the aspirated material is expressed onto the slide, taking care to deposit it as a single drop at one end of the slide.

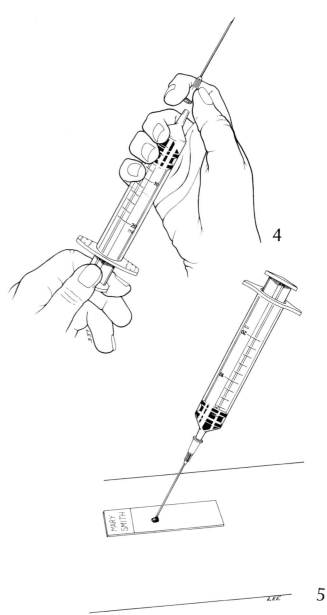

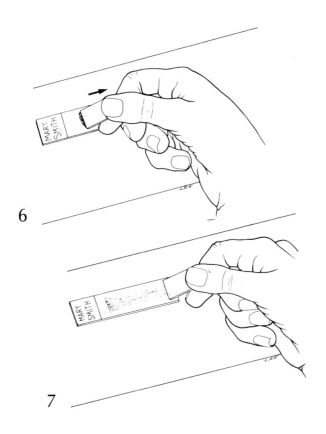

6 & 7

A thick glass coverslip is drawn across the slide to spread the aspirate so that a thin even layer of cells is formed on the slide. Any large tissue fragments which do not spread easily should be squashed between the coverslip and the slide. The smear is air-dried in preparation for staining by the May-Grunwald-Giemsa method.

8

Some cytopathologists prefer to interpret slides stained by the Papanicolaou method. For successful Papanicolaou staining, smears must be fixed before air-drying can occur. As this is very difficult to achieve when slides are thinly spread, thicker smears should be made when this type of staining is contemplated. Immediately after preparation, the smears should be placed in a Coplin jar containing 74 OP industrial alcohol. The smears can be removed from the fixative solution after 15 min and dispatched to the laboratory for staining.

Preparation of cell suspension

9

As soon as the aspirate has been collected, the syringe and needle are rinsed out with 3 ml of a fixative solution made up of equal parts of 74 OP industrial alcohol and normal saline. The washings are expelled into a universal container and dispatched to the cytology laboratory for processing. The cells in the suspension are harvested either by the technique of cytocentrifugation or by membrane filtration.

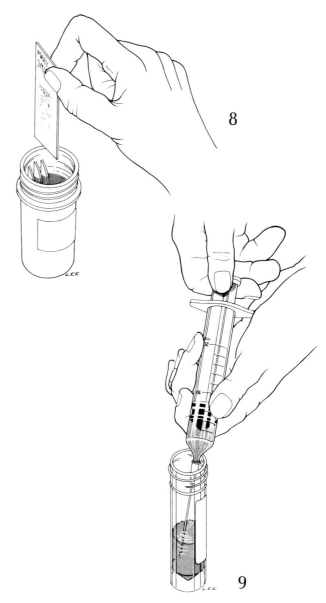

8

9

Factors influencing success of method

The surgeon's decision to adopt one or another of the preparatory techniques described above for solid lesions should be influenced by the speed and dexterity with which he learns to prepare smears from the aspirated cells. Good smear-making demands skill and attention to detail and can only be perfected if combined with microscope analysis. The amount of blood and mucus in the sample and the cellularity of the aspirate affects the quality of the smears. The cell yield from a fibroadenoma, medullary carcinoma and colloid or mucinous carcinoma is usually quite adequate for the preparation of two or more smears. In contrast, aspirates from fibrotic lesions, particularly scirrhous carcinomas, contain very few cells and smears prepared from these samples are frequently too scanty for reliable cytological analysis. As not all the cells in the lumen of the needle can be expelled onto the slide, cell loss is inevitable and up to 17 per cent of aspirates prepared by the smear method have been found to be unsatisfactory for reporting because they contain too few cells. This is a serious limitation of the smear technique.

It has been found that the alternative method of making membrane filter preparations from a cell suspension of the aspirate has an advantage over the conventional smear technique in this respect. The number of unsatisfactory samples is reduced to 5 per cent as none of the cells are lost in processing. It is frequently possible for the surgeon to estimate the cellularity of the aspirate while needling the lesion and adapt his preparatory technique accordingly. Those solid lesions which have a soft consistency generally yield reasonably cellular aspirates which make satisfactory smears. Lesions which feel hard and gritty to the needle frequently prove to be scirrhous carcinomas, and these are better prepared as cell suspensions.

The preparation of cell suspensions from breast aspirates offers other advantages over the smear technique. It is often possible to tell from a cell suspension whether aspiration is successful by holding the container up to the light. The presence of small fragments of tissue floating in the fixative is indicative of an adequate sample. If no fragments are seen the aspiration can be repeated. In addition, filter preparations made from the cell suspension are frequently easier for the pathologist to interpret than air-dried smears. Membrane filters prepared from the cell suspension can be stained by the haematoxylin and eosin method, enabling duct-lining cells, apocrine cells and adipose cells to be identified and correlated with their histological counterparts.

Assessment of fine needle aspiration

Practical advantages and safety of the technique

10

Fine needle aspiration is particularly appropriate for the investigation of the patient in an outpatient setting as the technique is well tolerated by the patient and no anaesthetic is required. No skin incision or obturator is necessary when a fine needle is used. Nor is any special apparatus required, although some surgeons recommend the use of a Cameco Syringe holder (Cameco A6 Tabyvagen 71–180 Enebybang, Sweden) to facilitate the manipulation of the syringe during aspiration. This special handle can be adapted to fit the barrel of the syringe to hold it steady while continuous traction is applied to the plunger to sustain the negative pressure essential for successful aspiration.

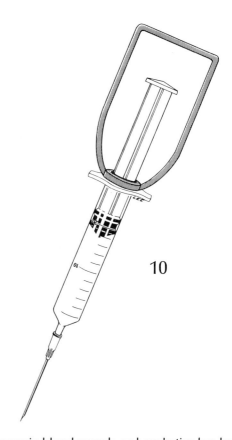

10

The technique of fine needle aspiration causes little or no damage to breast tissue; and none of the serious complications associated with surgical biopsy or needle biopsy have been observed in large numbers of patients investigated by this method. Neither haemorrhage nor sepsis has been encountered and small haematomas have been noted only occasionally.

Following reports of dissemination of tumour along the needle tract after aspiration with a large bore needle the safety of fine needle aspiration in this respect has been thoroughly investigated. Five year follow-up of 656 patients who had fine needle aspiration at the Karolinska Hospital has revealed no local seeding of tumour in the path of the needle[9]. The possibility of distant spread of tumour via blood vessels or lymphatics has been investigated by Berg and Robbins[10], who examined the effect of fine needle aspiration on the survival of 1046 patients with mammary carcinoma and found that the 10 year survival rate of patients who had been subjected to aspiration was no different from that of patients who had not been investigated by this method. There is also experimental evidence that the risk of tumour dissemination is not increased after fine needle aspiration. Engzell et al.[9] cannulated the lymphatics and efferent veins draining malignant lymph nodes of rabbits but were unable to detect tumour cells in the blood or lymph after fine needle aspiration of the malignant nodes. There is, therefore, ample clinical and experimental evidence to indicate that the risks of fine needle aspiration are very small indeed.

Accuracy of cytological reporting

When fine needle aspiration is adopted for routine use in the preoperative diagnosis of mammary cancer, heavy demands are made on the cytologist formulating the report and on the clinician evaluating it. Both need to be fully aware of the reliability of a cytodiagnosis as well as the limitations of this method of investigation.

The specificity of the technique has been shown in many large surveys to be very high and in skilled hands over 99 per cent of breast cancers are reported correctly. False positive reporting is rare and with experience may be as low as 1 in 1000 cases (*Table 1*). The tumours that may present pitfalls of diagnosis to the cytologist are usually characterized by widespread epitheliosis and papillomatosis and are the very same lesions that pose diagnostic problems for the histopathologist as well. Fibroadenomas which rarely present problems to the histologist may be erroneously reported as malignant by an inexperienced cytopathologist. False positive diagnoses can be minimized if a cytodiagnosis of malignancy is made only when numerous cells in the aspirate display unmistakable characteristics of malignancy.

One of the limitations of fine needle aspiration is the frequency with which a negative cytology report may be given in a patient with breast cancer (*Table 2*). False negative reporting is almost always a consequence of inadequate sampling and is most likely to occur if the tumour is small (less tham 1 cm diameter) or sclerotic. Occasionally a false negative report is given if the tumour is sited deep in a large pendulous breast and the regular 21 gauge needle fails to penetrate the tumour. When aspirating tumours of this type, it may be advisable to select a larger needle. The risk of obtaining an unrepresentative sample from a malignant lesion of the breast is approximately 10 per cent and can only be kept to this minimum by careful attention to the collection and preparation of the aspirates and to the judicious taking of repeated samples when few fragments are seen in the alcohol/saline suspension of the aspirate.

The overall diagnostic accuracy of cytological reporting by an experienced cytopathologist is known to be very high. The benign or malignant nature of a breast lump can be correctly diagnosed from fine needle aspirates in over 95 per cent of cases. Several comparative studies have shown that cytological investigation is more likely to provide accurate information about the character of a breast lump than either clinical examination or mammography alone. A combined clinical and cytological approach to the diagnosis of a breast lump can achieve an accurate diagnosis in 98 per cent of cases. Contrary to expectation, routine investigation of patients with a breast lump by a triplet of investigative techniques – clinical examination, cytology and mammography – does not improve the accuracy of the preoperative diagnosis of the patient, because mammography increases the number of false positive diagnoses[5].

Table 1 Frequency of false positive reports on samples obtained by fine needle aspiration

Series	No. of cases with benign breast disease	Fine needle aspiration	
		Correct cytodiagnosis (%)	False positive report (%)
Zajicek[8]	1009	1008 (99.9)	1 (0.1)
Zajdela et al.[7]	878	875 (99.7)	3 (0.3)
Coleman[11]	244	240 (98.3)	4 (1.7)
Kline, Joshi and Neal[4]	3177	3117 (98.2)	60 (1.8)

Table 2 Frequency of false negative reports on samples obtained by fine needle aspiration

Series	No. of cases with clinically or histologically proven carcinoma	Fine needle aspiration	
		Correct cytodiagnosis (%)	False negative report (%)
Zajicek[8]	1068	962 (90.1)	106 (9.9)
Zajdela et al.[7]	1745	1593 (91.2)	152 (8.7)
Coleman[11]	103	94 (91.3)	9 (8.7)
Kline, Joshi and Neal[4]	368	333 (90.4)	35 (9.6)

The place of fine needle aspiration in the management of the patient

On the strength of our experience with fine needle aspiration, it is now the practice at this hospital to include cytological assessment in the routine investigation of all women with a discrete palpable breast lump seen in the outpatient clinic. The lump is first graded by the surgeon as clinically benign, clinically malignant or of doubtful malignancy. Needle aspiration is then performed and a cytology result obtained within 24 h. Correlation of the clinical and cytological opinion permits the surgeon to decide upon a rational plan of management for each patient. The plan of investigation adopted at this hospital is shown in the flow chart below.

If the lump is found to be cystic the fluid is sent for routine cytological examination. This is a particularly useful precaution if the fluid is blood-stained or if the mass does not disappear completely after aspiration, as both these signs may indicate the development of an adenocarcinoma in the wall of the cyst or the presence of pseudocystic spaces in a solid malignant tumour[12].

A positive cytology report enables the surgeon to select with confidence those cases requiring further preoperative tests or urgent biopsy. In those cases where the cytological diagnosis confirms the clinical impression of malignancy, the patient can be informed of the very real possibility of mastectomy and prepared psychologically for this traumatic event. It must be stressed that in view of the frequency with which false negative cytology reports

may be given, a clinical diagnosis of malignancy must always override a benign cytological statement. In consequence, the contribution of cytology to the management of patients whose lesions are clinically considered to be of doubtful malignancy is necessarily limited. All such cases are candidates for mammography and urgent biopsy.

There has been considerable controversy about the need for a needle biopsy or a frozen section when a confident clinical and cytological diagnosis of malignancy has been obtained. In view of the faint but real possibility of a false positive cytology report it would seem sensible to obtain histological confirmation of the diagnosis whenever possible. Moreover, a distinction between preinvasive cancer and invasive cancer cannot be made from the cytological smear, nor can the tumour be precisely classified as to its cell type. Most surgeons agree that biopsy is mandatory prior to mastectomy except where it is contraindicated on the grounds of age or extent of the tumour. In those cases it is reasonable to accept the report of an experienced cytopathologist and proceed to ablative therapy without histological confirmation of malignancy.

Cytology is perhaps of greatest value in detecting malignant disease in patients where none was clinically suspected. Only by the routine cytological investigation of all patients with breast lumps can mismanagement of this small but important group of patients be eliminated.

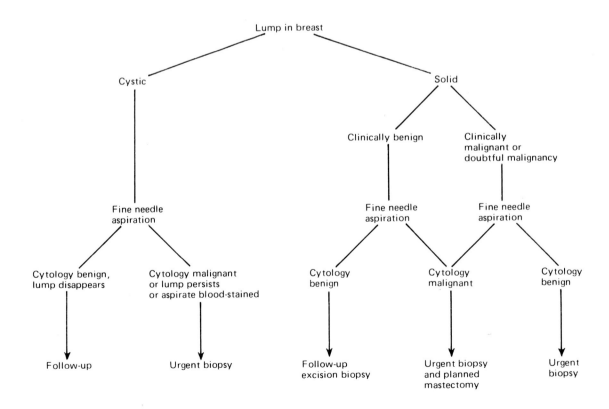

Alternative techniques

Alternative techniques for making a preoperative diagnosis of breast cancer have been developed, but none is quite such a simple or safe procedure as fine needle aspiration. Both needle biopsy and drill biopsy have an advantage over fine needle aspiration in that the core of tissue obtained can be processed for histological examination, but both techniques demand considerable skill in their execution and may damage breast tissue. Haemorrhage and sepsis are not uncommon complications. Moreover, satisfactory samples cannot be obtained from lesions less than 3 cm diameter and a reliable diagnosis can be made in only 75 per cent of cases[4, 13].

The various techniques available to the surgeon seeking to make a preoperative tissue diagnosis of breast cancer all have their advocates and the protocols adopted will vary from one clinic to another. Fine needle aspiration has the advantage of simplicity, safety and accuracy which ensures it a firm place in the sequence of investigations carried out on the patient presenting with a palpable breast lump.

References

1. Coleman, D., Desai, S., Dudley, H., Hollowell, S., Hulbert, M. Needle aspiration of palpable breast lesions: a new application of the membrane filter technique and its results. Clinical Oncology 1975; 1: 27–32

2. Franzén, S., Zajicek, J. Aspiration biopsy in diagnosis of palpable lesions of the breast. Clinical review of 3479 consecutive biopsies. Acta Radiologica Therapy 1968; 7: 241–262

3. Furnival, C. M., Hughes, H. E., Hocking, M. A., Reid, M. M. W., Blumgart, L. H. Aspiration cytology in breast cancer: its relevance to diagnosis. Lancet 1975; 2: 446–449

4. Kline, T. S., Joshi, L. P., Neal, H. S. Fine needle aspiration of the breast: diagnoses and pitfalls. A review of 3545 cases. Cancer 1979; 44: 1458–1464

5. Thomas, J. M., Fitzharris, B. M., Redding, W. H., Williams, J. E., Trott, P. A., Powles, T. J., Ford, H. T., Gazet, J. C. Clinical examination, xeromammography, and fine-needle aspiration cytology in diagnosis of breast tumours. British Medical Journal 1978; 2: 1139–1141

6. Webb, A. J. The diagnostic cytology of breast carcinoma. British Journal of Surgery 1970; 57: 259–264

7. Zajdela, A., Ghossein, N. A., Pilleron, J. P., Ennuyer, A. The value of aspiration cytology in the diagnosis of breast cancer, Experience at the Fondation Curie. Cancer 1975; 35: 499–506

8. Zajicek, J. Aspiration, biopsy, cytology. Part I: Cytology of supradiaphragmatic organs. In: Wied, G. L., ed. Monographs on clinical cytology, Vol. 4. Basel: S. Karger, 1974

9. Engzell, U., Esposti, P. L., Rubio, C., Sigurdson, A., Zajicek, J. Investigation of tumour spread in connection with aspiration biopsy. Acta Radiologica Therapy 1971; 10: 385–398

10. Berg, J. W., Robbins, G. F. A late look at the safety of aspiration biopsy. Cancer 1962; 15: 826–827

11. Coleman, D. V. Cytological screening for cancer of the breast. Journal of the Royal Society of Medicine 1976; 69: 494–496

12. Forrest, A. P. M., Kirkpatrick, J. R., Roberts, M. M. Needle aspiration of breast cysts. British Medical Journal 1975; 3: 30–31

13. Davies, C. J., Elston, C. W., Cotton, R. W., Blamey, R. W. Preoperative diagnosis in carcinoma of the breast. British Journal of Surgery 1977; 64: 326–328

Modified-radical and radical mastectomy

Hugh Dudley ChM, FRCS(Ed.), FRACS, FRCS
Professor of Surgery, St Mary's Hospital, London

Introduction

The recognition that breast cancer is often widely disseminated at an early stage, the knowledge that local spread is centrifugal – to both axillary and internal mammary nodes – and the desire to avoid mutilation have all contributed to a drift away from classical radical mastectomy. This was the operation developed by Halsted in the USA, and Stiles and others in the UK and brought to technical perfection by Haagenson. It still enjoys considerable popularity but there is little evidence to support the idea that in terms of either outcome or local recurrence it confers any greater benefit than muscle-preserving procedures practised alone or in combination with radiotherapy when regional lymph nodes are found to be involved. The argument in favour of clearing the axilla is much more on the lines that it gives useful information on pathological stage and thus prognosis. For this purpose the ability to remove the last scrap of tissue beyond the pectoralis minor is not vital though in my experience it is usually possible to achieve this.

This chapter describes the steps of radical mastectomy with and without muscle preservation.

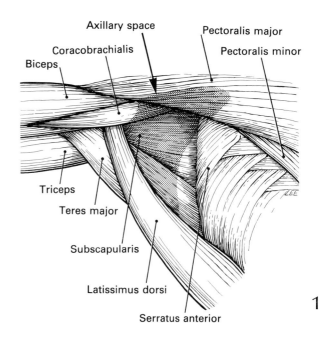

Anatomy

1

The objective is to clear the triangular mass of fibrofatty tissue bounded by the serratus anterior below, the latissimus dorsi posteriorly and laterally, the coracobrachialis above and the axillary apex medially. The axillary contents are shielded medially and in front by the pectoral muscles which must either be retracted forwards so that the surgeon can see under them or detached from their insertions so that the whole fatty mass is clearly seen.

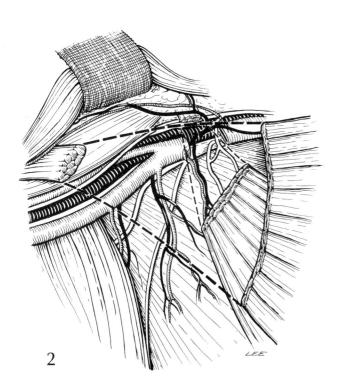

2

The anatomical keys to axillary dissection are the plane anterior to the subscapular vessels and nerve to latissimus dorsi which is found by exposing the anterolateral edge of that muscle and which passes medially across the chest wall anterior to the long thoracic nerve; and the attenuated lateral clavipectoral fascia on the coracobrachialis.

The operations

Excisional biopsy

It is now rarely necessary to carry out excisional biopsy as a preliminary to mastectomy. If it is done, it can either be as a separate procedure under local or general anaesthesia or for confirmation at the time mastectomy is contemplated.

3

The operation is performed through an appropriate radial incision which can be encompassed by the subsequent mastectomy incision.

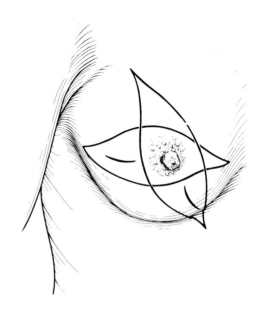

3

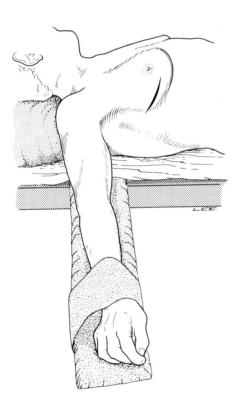

4

4

The patient lies prone, with arm outstretched upon an arm board to which the wrist is secured by a bandage; the forearm is supinated so that the palm faces the floor, in order to avoid nerve damage at the root of the limb. The scrub nurse may stand either on the opposite side or at the head of the table in order to get an uninterrupted view of the operative field.

The biopsy is quite separate from the definitive procedure. A separate trolley and completely different instruments are used for incision and closure. Though we do not know of conclusive evidence that inoculation can occur, every effort should be made towards its prevention.

5a–d

Principles of biopsy

(a) Excision of the tumour, provided that this does not require dissection down to the pectoral fascia, in which case incisional biopsy is preferred.

(b) Absolute haemostasis to prevent tumour cells contaminating the field by being washed out in a bloody exudate.

(c) Lavage of the wound area before closure with a tumoricidal agent – 1/5000 perchloride of mercury or 2 per cent cetyltrimethylammonium bromide are appropriate.

(d) Continuous skin closure – the author finds a continuous nylon or polypropylene suture appropriate – in order to reduce further the likelihood of tumour inoculation.

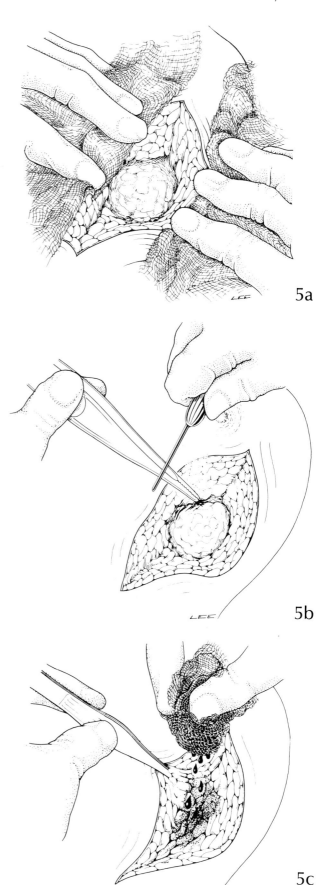

5a

5b

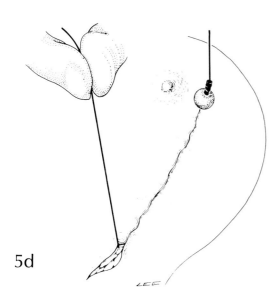

5d

5c

Frozen section biopsy

6

Frozen section biopsy gives the surgeon almost absolute certainty that he is on the right path though there is little doubt that the experienced operator can give almost as reliable a diagnostic opinion from gross inspection and the feel of the cut surface. The biopsy must not be touched with the gloved hand and the knife is discarded. However, where facilities are available the frozen section technique should be used. The time taken to close the biopsy wound is about the same as that for a cryostat section.

If there is doubt on frozen section, nothing is lost by closing the wound as described and awaiting the result of a paraffin-embedded specimen. There is no evidence that this in any way affects mortality in the long term provided the ablation is carried out within a week.

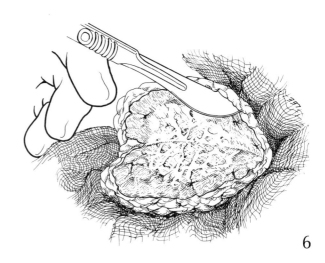

6

Towelling

If the diagnosis is confirmed then formal towelling is the next step.

7a & b

(a) The patient can be sat up and supported from the unaffected side in the position shown. (b) Alternatively the arm and shoulder girdle can be elevated well clear of the table. The back and flank on the affected side are painted with the skin preparation material. An impervious sheet covered with a sterile towel is laid behind the back as far down as the buttocks. The patient is gently lowered back into the horizontal position. This method of towelling is necessary or the posterior part of the flank on the affected side will not remain sterile throughout the operation.

The towelling is completed as shown in *Illustration 8*. The author finds it convenient to towel the arm so that the muscles of the shoulder girdle may be tensed or relaxed at will by positioning the arm appropriately.

The donor area

In all cases in which there is a *possibility* of a skin graft it is time-saving to prepare and towel a donor area – usually the thigh – before beginning the operation. A sandbag placed behind the knee flexes the thigh and eases the cutting of the graft. However, unless they require very extensive mobilization, flap procedures where possible are preferred to split-skin grafts.

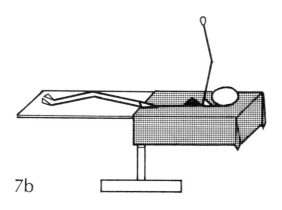

7a

7b

The incision

The incision is planned preoperatively. It should *never be made on the spur of the moment* on the operating table. An unplanned incision may find the operator unprepared for a skin graft or may result in a badly sited scar which restricts postoperative movement. The cut is marked out in indelible ink as the first step of the operation and should be so placed that the growth is in the centre of an elliptical island of skin. The incision should never be less than 4 cm from the palpable edge of the tumour.

8

By far the best incision for central tumours is the transverse or slightly oblique incision as shown. For mastectomy with preservation of the pectoral muscles it is only rarely necessary to vary this in order to produce a more oblique line. Full access to the axillary contents is facilitated and there are two other substantial advantages: the anterior border of the latissimus dorsi is surely and quickly defined; and the postoperative cosmetic effect is much more pleasing without sacrificing anything in the way of the thoroughness of the dissection.

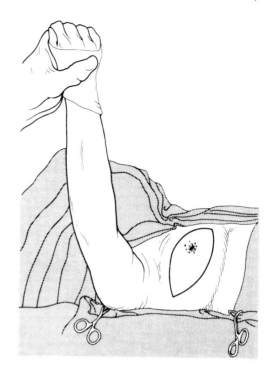

8

9

For classical radical mastectomy the incision is better oblique so as to permit easy access to the insertion of pectoralis major. It extends from the base of the xiphoid process below to just beyond the tip of the coracoid process above. The axillary end of the incision should be placed well to the medial side of the outer border of the pectoralis major (anterior axillary fold). It should *never* be turned down on to the arm over the front of the shoulder. Thus curved extension is unnecessary and results in a scar which cannot be concealed or disguised.

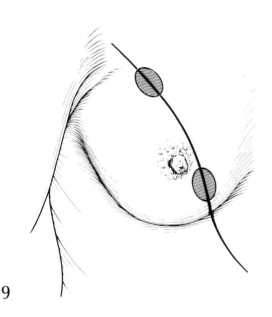

9

10

A vertical incision can be used for a tumour in the upper and inner or lower and outer quadrant.

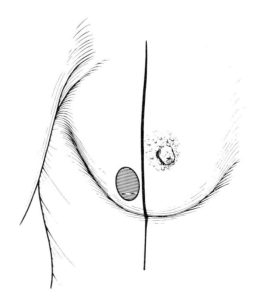

10

Elevation of flaps

11a, b & c

The objective is to dissect in the plane between sub-cutaneous and breast fat, the latter being easily recognized by the veins that course over its surface. The plane is entered by stretching the skin as it is incised and then using the flat of the knife blade (a). Superiorly the flap is raised to the limit of the breast and the dissection taken down to muscle (b). Inferiorly the flap is raised to a similar extent (c).

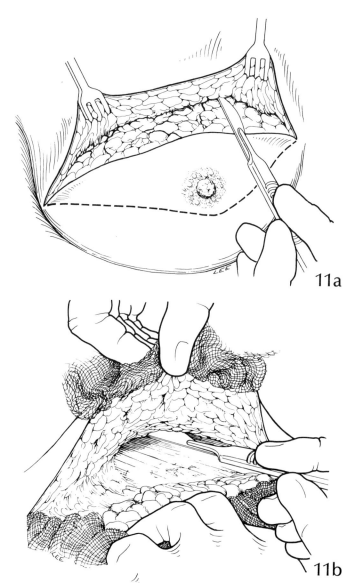

11a

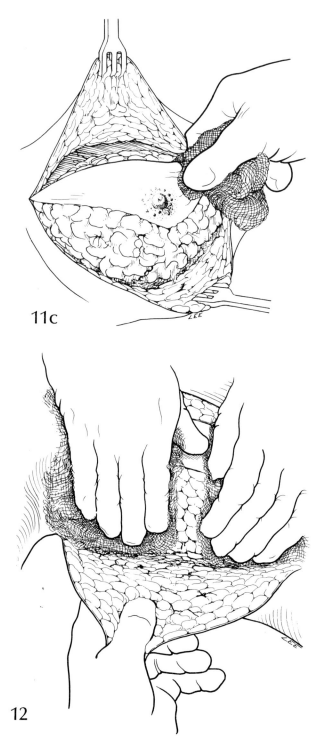

11c

11b

12

12

As the flap is raised it can be stretched by being grasped between the operator's fingers and thumb. Haemostasis should at this stage be by firm gauze pressure and the occasional use of electrocoagulation. Forceps in the wound obscure the view. As the elevation of the flap proceeds, the assistant advances with the gauze, keeping close to the point of the knife as it works its way under the flap. He suppresses all bleeding by pressure the instant it occurs. With practice and the *determination not to use haemostats*, the method will be found to reduce blood loss to a minimum.

13

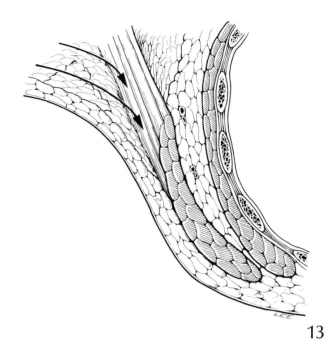

13

Correct lateral elevation of the lower flap

The aim is to raise a flap of even thickness. The elevation should be carried back to just beyond the anterior border of the latissimus dorsi. Dissection on too deep a plane results in too thick a flap being cut: the disadvantage of this is that pieces of breast tissue may be left attached to the centre of the flap or lymph nodes left embedded in the fat at its axillary end; in addition, by cutting too thick a flap the operator may be led into continuing the later part of the dissection on the deep face of the latissimus dorsi instead of just medial to it. In these circumstances, as well as failing to find the anterior edge of the latissimus dorsi for which he is searching, he is likely to be embarrassed by entering the plexus of large veins which drain into the subscapular vessels.

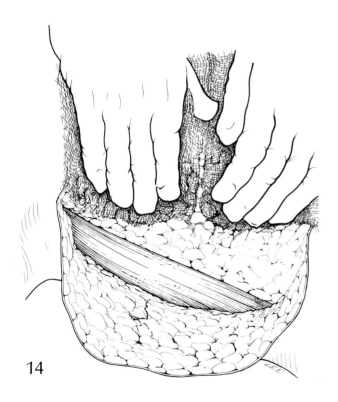

14

14

A correctly placed dissection will now expose the latissimus dorsi as shown.

Up to this point the procedures for muscle preservation and classical mastectomy are the same. From here they diverge. The muscle-preserving technique will be described first.

MUSCLE-PRESERVING TECHNIQUE

15 & 16

Completion of the flaps above and medially allows the angle at their medial end to be entered. By turning the breast laterally it can be peeled from the fascia overlying the pectoralis muscles. The dissection begins at the intercostal spaces (hidden medially in the illustration) and proceeds laterally. At this point a variable number of perforating vessels is dealt with by diathermy coagulation.

By this process the whole of the pectoralis major is cleared to its lateral edge. A few small vessels projecting from the cut edge are next encountered and may be clipped or coagulated. The breast has now been turned over on itself and traction on it downwards and laterally prepares for the next stage of the procedure.

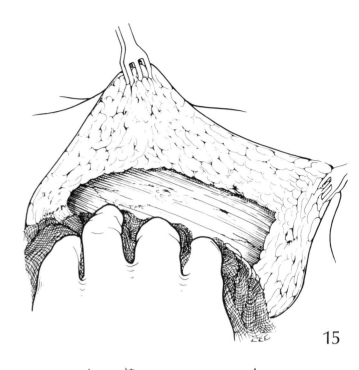

15

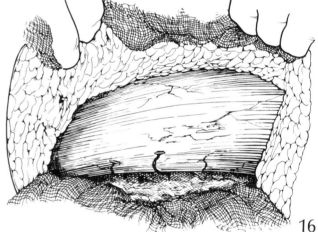

16

17

This is to enter the axilla by dissecting along the chest wall posterior to the pectoralis major muscle, continuing to mobilize the axillary tail. To facilitate this the pectoralis major is lifted up (hence its curved aspect in the illustration).

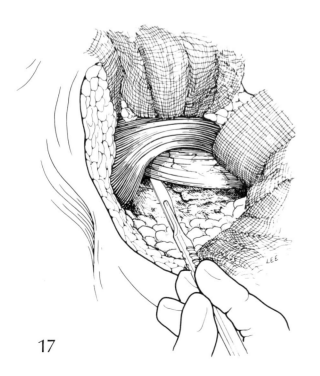

17

18

As this mobilization takes place the edge of the pectoralis minor comes into view, the dissection proceeding backwards across it, dividing small vessels and (usually) the lateral pectoral nerve. As the pectoralis minor is traced superiorly, the fascia overlying the axillary vessels begins to become obvious at the apex of the wound.

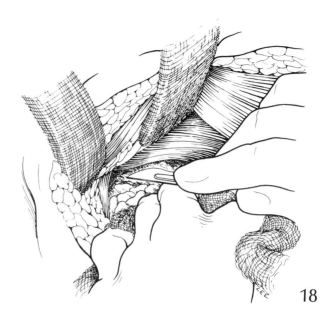

18

19

Attention is then directed laterally and inferiorly. Laterally, the fascia in front of the vessels is divided and all fat and lymph nodes are mobilized downwards from the junction of the axillary and brachial arteries. This process gradually converts the axillary tail of the breast and the contents of the axilla into a 'tongue' of tissue and permits the posterior aspect of the tail to be raised more easily from the anterior edge of the latissimus dorsi behind.

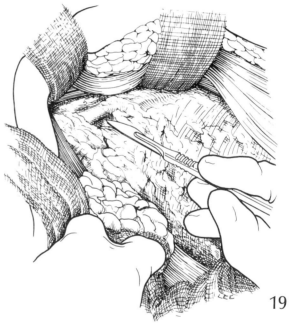

19

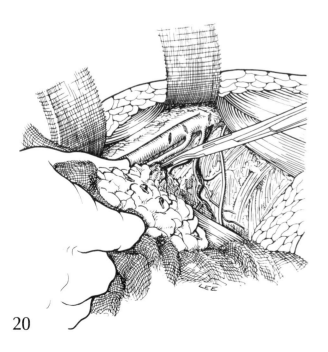

20

20

Both dissections are now continued. Superiorly, the pectoralis minor is lifted by a narrow retractor and all tissues over the vessels are swept downwards and laterally from the axillary apex, vessels being clipped or ligated seriatim. In the floor of the dissection, this exposes the infrascapular trunks and the nerve to the latissimus dorsi. More laterally, the latissimus dorsi is cleared.

Rarely, it may be necessary to divide the pectoralis minor tendon from the coracoid process, but as long as the first rib can be palpated at the point where the dissection begins axillary node removal will be complete.

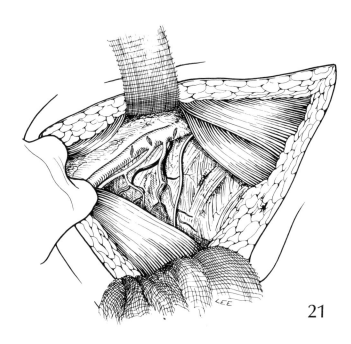

21

21

The completed dissection is carried back to, but does not always expose, the nerve to the serratus anterior.

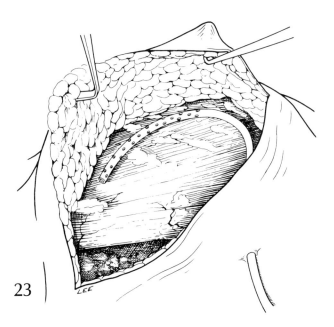

22

22, 23 & 24

Suction drains are inserted to lie over the pectoralis major and in the axilla.

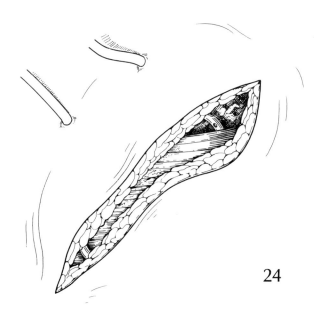

23

24

CLASSICAL RADICAL MASTECTOMY

25

For classical radical mastectomy the flaps have been raised medially and laterally. Two options can then be taken – to raise the pectoral muscles and turn them laterally, dividing the perforating branches of the internal mammary, or preferably, to delay the mobilization of the muscles medially and open the axilla by severing the attachment of the pectoralis major to the humerus and of the pectoralis minor to the coracoid process. To achieve this, the upper lateral flap is raised and the line of separation between the pectoral and clavicular heads of the pectoralis major is identified. The line is followed laterally, the insertion mobilized over a director and the now deeper pectoralis fibres divided as close to the bone as possible. Care must be taken not to injure the underlying brachial plexus.

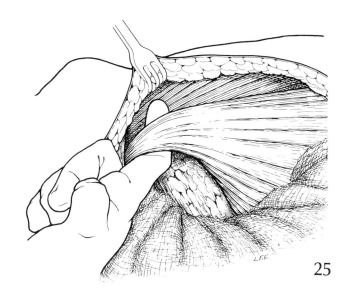

25

26

26

Deep to the muscle one next encounters the attenuated lateral aspect of the clavipectoral fascia and the coraco-brachialis muscle. Working downward, this thin fascial sheet is divided and the distal axillary vessels are now exposed.

27

Before proceeding further with that direction of dissection which would free the lateral axillary contents, the knife runs medially along the face of the coracobrachialis to the coracoid process and detaches the insertion of pectoralis minor. Sharp dissection is now continued in the same line to divide the costocoracoid membrane and secure the acromiothoracic vessels which pierce it to enter the posterior face of the pectoralis muscle.

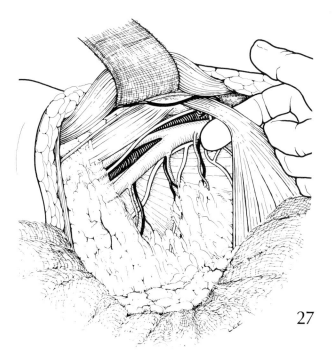

27

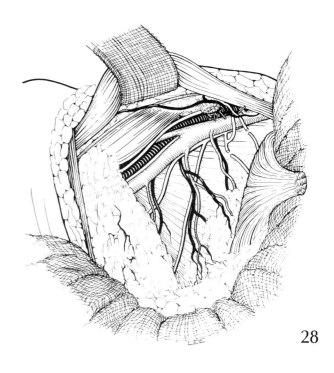

28

The apex of the axilla is now exposed and the vessels and nerves which course forward into and round the pectoral muscles – principally the medial and lateral nerves and the lateral thoracic artery and vein – are divided to expose the axillary vessels in their entire length.

28

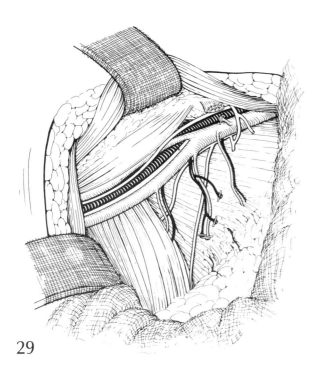

29

29

Attention is now directed laterally to complete the dissection on the anterior edge of the latissimus dorsi between where the vessels were exposed after severing the pectoralis major tendon and the edge of the latissimus dorsi, exposed when the lateral flap was raised.

30

The axillary contents are swept medially anterior to the subscapular vessels and the nerve to the latissimus dorsi. The dissection then proceeds towards the medial wall of the axilla to clear the anterior face of the subscapularis and the angle between this muscle and the serratus anterior, exposing but of course sparing its nerve.

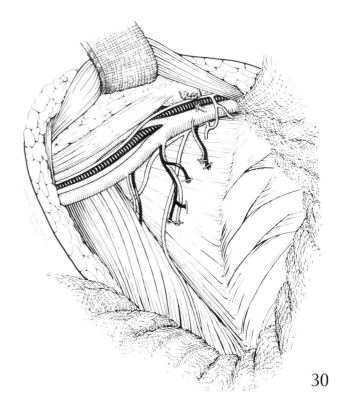

30

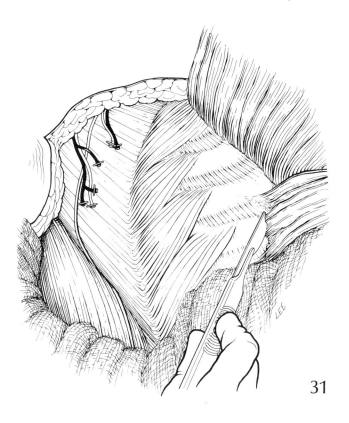

31

31 & 32

The whole mass of axillary contents can now be turned downwards and medially so that the undersurface of first the pectoralis minor and next the pectoralis major is exposed. Sharp dissection is taken medially to raise the pectoral muscles. The perforating vessels from the internal mammary are preferably identified before they are clipped and ligated. The pectoralis major muscle having been divided medially, all that remains is final detachment from the medial skin flap.

Closure and postoperative care are as for ordinary muscle-preserving mastectomy.

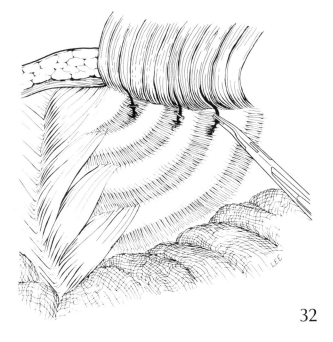

32

Surgery combined with other techniques

This is a book about operations and operative technique. However, in some cancer therapy, surgery must work in harness with other techniques – ionizing radiation, hormone manipulation and chemotherapy. This is particularly true of breast cancer. Therefore we include here a brief account of the supplementary measures which are applicable in this disease.

Current axioms in management which will doubtless change before long are as follows.

1. Surgery can only cure local disease. There is upwards of a 90 per cent chance that a patient with a tumour in the lateral half of the breast whose axilla does not contain malignant disease is cured. Adjuvant treatment is thus not currently indicated if the axillary nodes have been removed and proven innocent.
2. By contrast, a patient with a medial-half tumour (which is relatively uncommon) cannot be guaranteed to be free of internal mammary node metastases, in spite of the absence of axillary metastases. Radiotherapy to the internal mammary chain is often used though there is no statistic to support its efficacy.
3. If patients have involved axillary lymph nodes, whatever the position of the tumour in the breast, then *ipso facto* their disease is more advanced and only 45–55 per cent will survive 5 years. Furthermore, after radical or modified radical mastectomy local recurrence rates in such patients may reach 20 per cent. Thus two modalities may be used: systemic chemotherapy to attack distant micrometastases and local irradiation to reduce recurrence in the operative field. As to the former, two regimens have been shown to be effective – phenylalanine mustard[1] and cyclophosphamide-5FU-methotrexate[2, 3]. Both are used for a year. Selective scalp cooling should be employed to minimize hair loss. As to the latter, controlled trials[4, 5] have shown a significant reduction in local recurrence though the technique is not as widely used in the USA as in the UK.

4. The response to chemotherapy is to some extent governed by whether the patient is pre- or postmenopausal, the former being associated with better results; the oestrogen receptor status of the tumour (which correlates with degree of differentiation) is also of some significance, better differentiated or oestrogen receptor positive tumours showing a better response.
5. Oophorectomy and the use of oestrogen analogues (e.g. tamoxifen) which block the action of oestrogen at cell nuclear level have not as yet been shown to influence 5 year survival; this may change.

References

1. Fisher, B., Carbone, P., Economou, S. G. *et al.* L-phenylalanine mustard (L-PAM) in the management of primaty breast cancer: a report of early findings. New England Journal of Medicine 1975; 292: 117–122

2. Cooper, R. G., Holland, J. F., Glidewell, O. Adjuvant chemotherapy of breast cancer. Cancer 1974; 44: 793–798

3. Bonnadonna, G., Brusamolino, E., Valagussa, P. *et al.* Combination chemotherapy as an adjuvant treatment in operable breast cancer. New England Journal of Medicine 1976; 294: 405–410

4. Fisher, B., Slack, N. H., Cavanagh, P. J., Gardener, B., Ravdin, R. G. Post-operative radiotherapy in the treatment of breast cancer. Results of the NSABP clinical trial. Annals of Surgery 1970; 172: 711–729

5. McWhirter, R., The position of radiotherapy in the treatment of breast carcinoma. Strahlentherapie (Munchen) 1957; 102: 451–455

Illustrations by Ann McNeill

Total mastectomy and axillary node sample

A. P. M. Forrest MD, ChM, DSc, FRCS, HonFACS
Regius Professor of Clinical Surgery, University of Edinburgh

Preoperative

Indications and objectives

Histological staging of the axillary lymph nodes is now an accepted part of the treatment of breast cancer. The objective of the operation of total mastectomy and axillary node sample is to remove all breast tissue including the axillary tail of the breast and its contained nodes and to identify and excise, for histological examination, one or more of the lymph nodes of the pectoral group which lie close to the upper medial aspect of the tail. This can be regarded as one of the standard operations for treating the disease.

In all cases a histopathological diagnosis is made preoperatively either by Trucut biopsy (*see* p. 241) or, if the tumour is small (<1 cm), by local excision (*see* p. 243). Preliminary frozen section examination (*see* p. 247) is now rarely used.

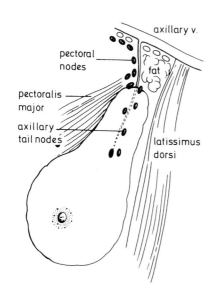

1

1

Diagram of relationships.

The operation

2

Position of patient

A general anaesthetic is used and the patient lies supine with the arm outstretched. A long rubber wedge placed on an arm board supports the arm forward of horizontal and slightly raises the scapula. A 'terry towel' or pack is placed on the operating table alongside the posterior axillary fold and the affected side is towelled off.

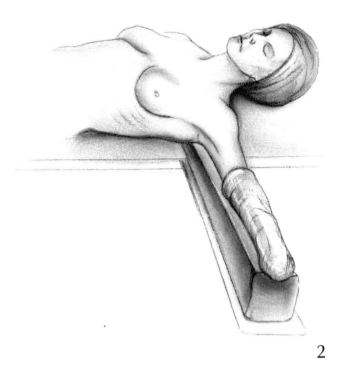

2

3

The incisions

Elliptical incisions to include the nipple and the tumour are planned to leave a scar which will lie as nearly transverse as possible. The margin of skin around the tumour is variable and depends on its size compared to that of the breast. In general, it should not be less than 3 cm from the outer border of the tumour in any direction. The incision should not extend further than the midline anteriorly or posterior to the anterior axillary fold.

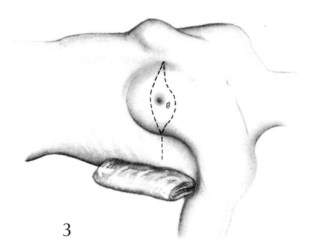

3

Upper skin flap

4

Raising of upper flap

The upper incision is made first and the upper flap mobilized to the level of the second rib. The raising of the flap is started with a knife, but as the dissection extends upwards, curved scissors allow easier definition of the plane of separation of the skin flap which is between the superficial fascia of the breast and the subdermal fat. This plane is wider and easier to define in a stout patient.

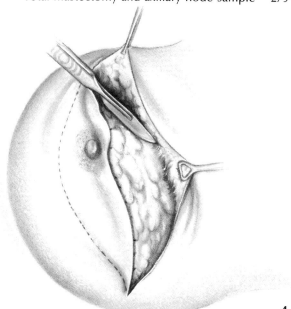

4

(Courtesy of British Journal of Surgery; 73: 569)

5

Dissection at upper margin of breast

As the upper limits of the flap dissection are reached, the scissors are used to divide the superficial fascia at the upper margin of the breast and to define the underlying pectoral fascia.

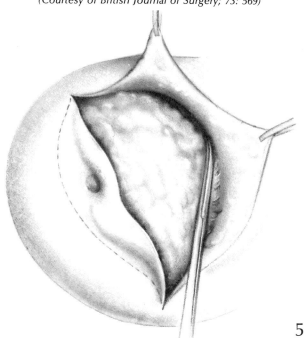

5

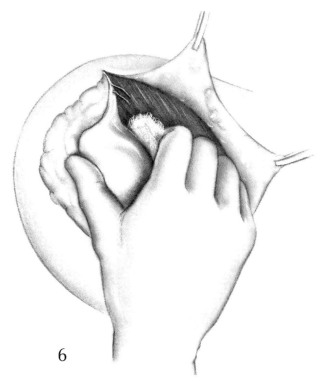

6

(Courtesy of British Journal of Surgery; 73: 569)

6

Mobilization of breast

The breast is mobilized from the pectoral fascia and underlying muscle and chest wall by burrowing from above downwards between the breast and the pectoral fascia using the fingers or a gauze swab. This separates the medial two-thirds of the breast from the chest wall except for its medial attachment to the sternum and its inferior attachment to the pectoral fascia. By pulling the breast forwards and downwards, the perforating branches of the internal mammary vessels may be seen and can be ligated and divided before they enter the deep surface of the breast.

Lower skin flap

7

Completion of incision and mobilization of lower skin flap

The lower skin incision is now made and the lower flap separated from underlying breast tissue first with the knife and then with scissors.

8

Completion of mobilization of breast from chest wall

In a thin person, the breast parenchyma may be close to the skin from which it must carefully be dissected.

The medial border of the breast is dissected from the sternum and costal cartilages, the remaining perforating vessels being ligated and divided in turn. The breast is drawn medially and its remaining attachment to the pectoral fascia divided from medial to lateral so that the breast is completely mobilized as far as the outer border of the pectoralis major muscle.

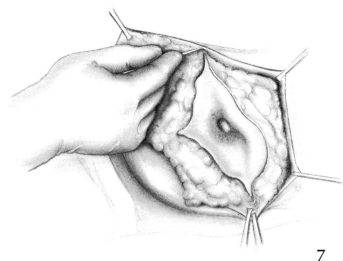

7

(Courtesy of British Journal of Surgery; 73: 569)

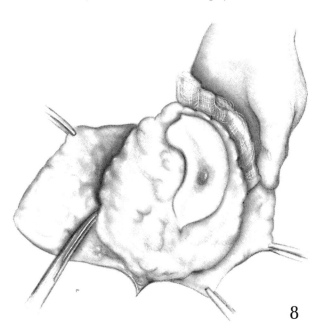

8

(Courtesy of British Journal of Surgery; 73: 569)

Lateral dissection

9

The lateral skin flap is undermined for 2.5 cm to facilitate lateral retraction of the breast. The outer border of the pectoralis major muscle is exposed by sharp dissection and the deep aspect of the breast swept laterally from the fascia overlying the serratus anterior muscle on the lateral chest wall by gauze dissection. The external mammary branches of the lateral thoracic artery and the lateral perforating branches of the intercostal vessels are put on the stretch and can be ligated and divided. Small lymph nodes may be associated with these vessels and should be removed for histological examination.

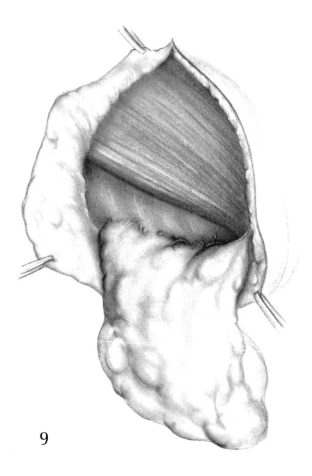

9

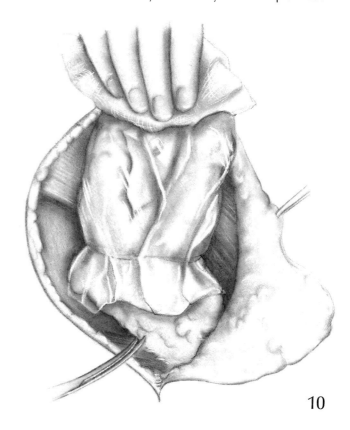

10

10 & 11

The fascia overlying the breast is attached laterally to the latissimus dorsi. The breast is drawn medially and the skin flaps elevated laterally until the anterolateral border of this muscle is reached. The fascial connections of the breast are divided from below upwards. The breast is completely mobilized except for its axillary tail.

The breast is enclosed in a polythene bag secured by a ligature. This facilitates its handling and protects the wound from contamination with fat and shed cells.

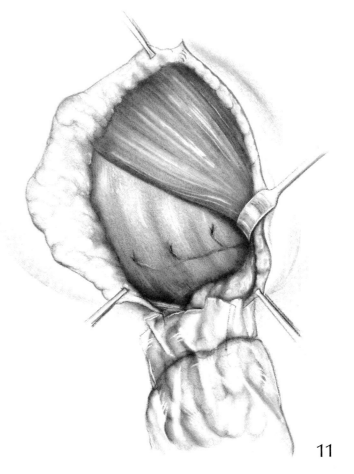

11

Dissection of axillary tail

12

Reflection of skin off tail

The skin and subcutaneous fat of the upper flap is elevated off the anterior surface of the axillary tail of the breast using curved scissors. The dissection is kept close to the breast tissue, particularly as one approaches the axilla, so that the skin is not penetrated.

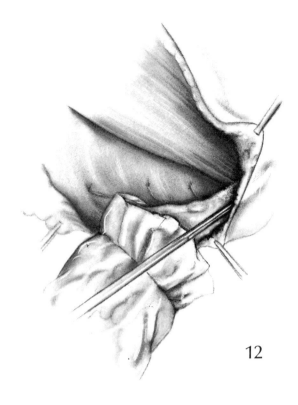

12

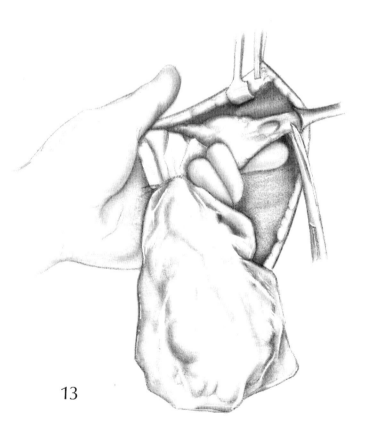

13

13

Final separation of tail

The axillary tail is then separated in front from the pectoralis major and behind from the latissimus dorsi and stripped upwards towards the axilla.

The anterior layer of the axillary fascia is divided with scissors to expose the axillary fat. The level at which the parenchymatous tissue of the axillary tail merges into this fat can be felt between finger and thumb.

It is at this point that lymph nodes of the pectoral group may be seen or felt and three or four nodes should be teased out for histological examination. Separation of the axillary tail from the axillary fat is best performed with scissors. The 'axillary tail' vein which runs into the axillary fat towards the axillary vein and is constantly present requires ligation before it is divided. The intercostobrachial nerve may run in close apposition to the top of the tail and may also be divided.

Careful palpation of the axilla is now performed. The axillary vein may be seen shining through the axillary fat but is not exposed. The fingers should be run up the line of the vein under the pectoral muscles and the findings recorded.

14

Examination of specimen

The surgeon must ensure that three to four lymph nodes have been removed with the specimen and should dissect these out and place them in fixative. Should no nodes be present he should repalpate the axilla and, if necessary, remove a block of axillary fat from the subscapularis medial to the subscapular vessels and nerve to the latissimus dorsi, in which nodes are always present. It cannot be sufficiently stressed that it is the *surgeon's* responsibility to provide the pathologist with nodes for histological examination.

At this stage it is a simple matter to extend the operation into a formal total axillary clearance (*see* p. 270) by retracting the pectoralis major, detaching the pectoralis minor from the coracoid process, defining the axillary vein and dissecting lymph nodes and fat from above down. If this is contemplated the arm must be separately towelled so that it can be elevated during the dissection (*see* p. 267).

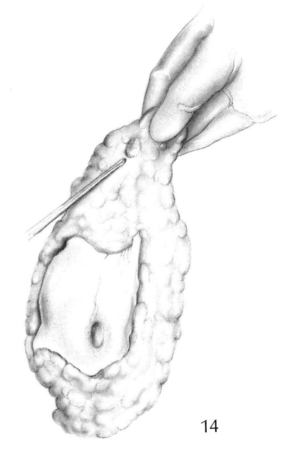

14

15–18

Internal mammary node biopsy

If the tumour is medially placed, the internal mammary vessels can be exposed through the medial aspect of the second, third or fourth intercostal spaces. The pectoralis major muscle is divided in the line of the sternum and the intercostal muscle, parallel to the ribs. A thin layer of fascia roofs over the fatty tissue in which the internal mammary vessels and the lymph trunks and nodes lie and this is divided with fine scissors. The nodes, which may be tiny, lie on the lateral side of the vessels.

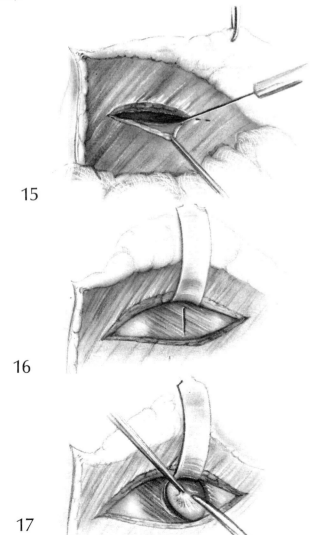

15

16

17

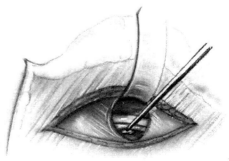

18

Insertion of prosthesis

19

If the patient wishes it, a silicone-containing prosthesis can be inserted. This is best placed in a subpectoral pocket so that healing of the skin wound is undisturbed and encapsulation of the prosthesis avoided. Access to the subpectoral region is by an incision in the serratus anterior and a tunnel under the muscle.

Alternatively, insertion may be from above, splitting the pectoralis over the second interspace in the line of its fibres.

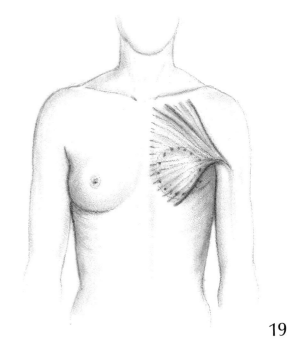

19

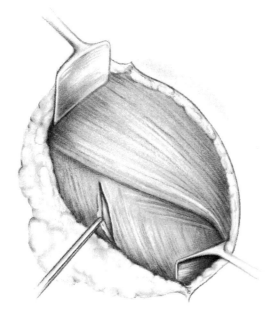

20

Formation of pocket

20

The incision in the serratus anterior is over the sixth or seventh rib and 3–5 cm in length. A finger is used to tunnel forwards under the serratus detaching its fibres from the ribs with scissors and entering the subpectoral space.

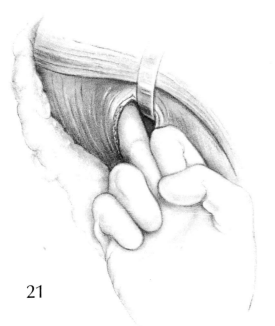

21

21

A pocket is formed under the pectoralis major by sweeping a finger between it and the chest wall and between the pectoralis major and minor muscles superiorly.

22

As the pectoralis major is attached to the anterior rectus sheath and/or ribs at a higher level than the inframammary fold it may be necessary to extend the pocket inferiorly. This can be done by burrowing under the rectus sheath from the lateral to the medial side. In some patients it is necessary to detach the lower medial fibres of the pectoralis major from the ribs and suture these to the anterior rectus sheath or the undersurface of the skin flap.

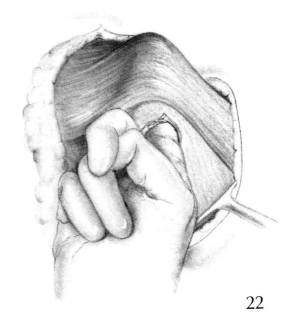

22

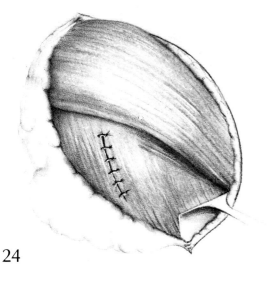

23

23

Placement of prosthesis in pocket

The prosthesis is inserted into the pocket and flattened out onto the chest wall. A 'sizing set' of prostheses is convenient as it allows a better estimate of the most suitable size. Normally a prosthesis of 150–250 ml is used.

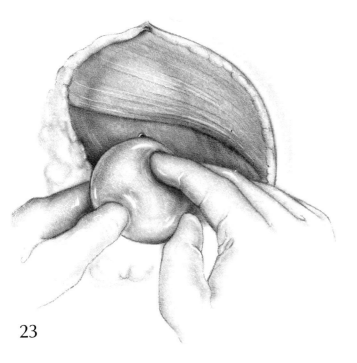

24

24

Closure of serratus anterior

The serratus anterior is closed with interrupted 2/0 Dexon sutures.

25

Wound drainage and closure

The wound is irrigated with 600 ml 1:120 cetrimide (prepared by diluting 100 ml 1:20 solution with 500 ml saline) and two suction drains of small diameter are inserted.

The wound is closed in two layers: a subcutaneous suture of interrupted 2/0 Dexon and a continuous subcuticular suture of Prolene, fixed at either end with a bead and cuff.

Suction drainage bottles (Redivac or Steritex) are attached to the drains and the wound dressed with a strip of gauze fixed with skin adhesive (Nobecutane). No bandages or other dressings are used.

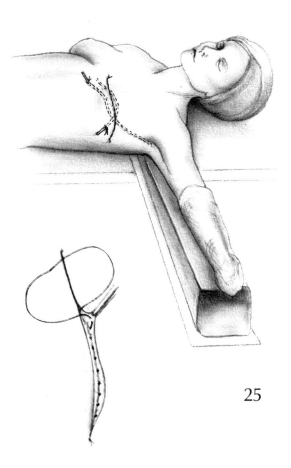

25

Postoperative care and complications

If a silicone prosthesis has been inserted penicillin therapy (penicillin V 250 mg and flucloxacillin 250 mg four times a day) is given for 5 days, starting preoperatively.

The small suction drains are removed when drainage ceases, usually after 2–3 days. Full mobility is encouraged from the day after operation and the patient should wear her normal brassiere as soon as possible. If a silicone prosthesis has been inserted a soft wool pad may be required as a filler. If a subpectoral prosthesis has not been inserted a soft external prosthesis is used.

A collection of serum, most common laterally, may complicate the operation but this is rare. Aspiration is performed. The subcuticular suture is removed in 7–10 days.

A decision regarding additional postoperative treatment, either locally with radiotherapy or systemically with chemotherapy or endocrine means, is dependent upon the results of the node biopsy. Provided nodes have been examined and shown to be free of metastases local recurrence rates are low and it is safe to withhold radiotherapy.

Illustrations by Robert M. Reed

Partial mastectomy for carcinoma of the breast

Robert E. Hermann MD
Department of General Surgery, The Cleveland Clinic Foundation, Cleveland, Ohio

Caldwell B. Esselstyn, Jr MD
Department of General Surgery, The Cleveland Clinic Foundation, Cleveland, Ohio

Introduction

Many of the earliest operations performed for the treatment of breast cancer were local excisions, cauterization of the tumour, or partial mastectomy. Cancers of the breast at that time were predominantly large tumour masses for which local excision or partial mastectomy was clearly inadequate. These procedures were performed without regard for any of the principles of cancer surgery as we now understand it – complete excision of the tumour mass with a surrounding area of adjacent, normal breast tissue. The unfortunate results of these early operations, ulceration and breakdown of the operative wound and early, often massive recurrence of the tumour in the breast or chest wall, gave these limited operative procedures a deservedly bad reputation. With the introduction of radical mastectomy in the 1800s, lesser procedures were no longer performed.

As physicians and patients became educated to the importance of a mass in the breast and as breast cancer detection developed throughout the twentieth century, more and more women were seen with small breast masses – frequently smaller than 2 cm – and without clinical evidence of axillary metastases. The standard radical mastectomy as the only operative therapy for these smaller or earlier breast cancers began to seem inappropriate to many surgeons.

In addition, during the past two or three decades, the fear of radical mastectomy and the emotional importance of breast preservation to women has become appreciated by many physicians and surgeons. Thus, in the past 25 years, partial mastectomy with or without axillary dissection or postoperative radiation therapy or both has been reintroduced for the treatment of carcinoma of the breast in selected patients.

Preoperative

Selection

We believe that partial mastectomy is appropriate in patients whose breast cancer is smaller than 2 cm, peripheral in the breast tissue, not lobular or intraductal (because of the higher incidence of multicentricity of these types), in whom the preoperative xeromammogram shows no other suspicious lesions of the breast, and who wish to have an operation that preserves breast tissue for the cosmetic advantages[1].

All patients should have a xeromammogram preoperatively. Unless there is evidence of a large tumour, involved axillary lymph nodes, or other signs of unfavourable disease, a bone scan or liver scan is not performed preoperatively.

Choice of operation

It is important that both the patient and her husband understand preoperatively that there is a choice of operative procedures for the treatment of individual breast cancer: radical mastectomy, modified radical mastectomy, total (simple) mastectomy with or without radiation therapy, partial mastectomy with or without radiation therapy, and excision of the tumour mass with radiation therapy. These procedures all may achieve local control of the disease. Therefore it is important that the diagnosis be established precisely, usually by excision biopsy.

The operation

1

For partial mastectomy a number of incisions are acceptable, depending on the site and location of the lesion. We prefer axillary dissection with all partial mastectomies. The axillary dissection is discontinuous for lesions of other than the upper outer quadrant, where a dissection in continuity is appropriate.

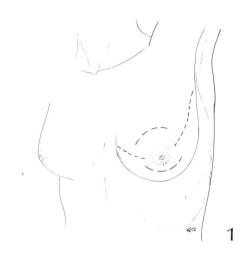

1

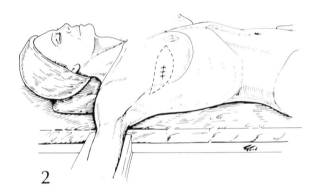

2

2

After the patient is properly positioned, the skin is marked elliptically to achieve 1.5–2.0 cm of skin clearance from the biopsy site.

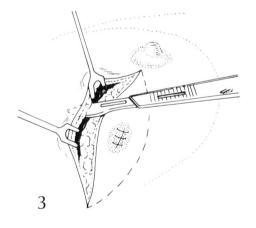

3

3

The initial incision through the superior flap is limited to skin depth at which point the scalpel is beveled in a lateral direction from the lesion to ensure an adequate or wide margin (2.5–3.0 cm) of normal breast tissue beyond the tumour. The dissection is completed down to the pectoralis major fascia.

4

Separation of the pectoralis major muscle from the specimen is continued inferiorly.

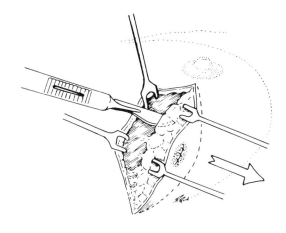

4

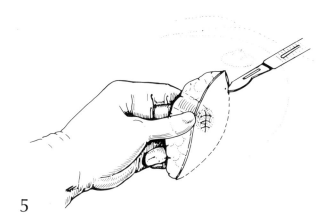

5

5

Dissection is continued until the surgeon's finger can be placed beneath the entire specimen. For deep-lying tumours, a segment of pectoralis muscle may be included with the specimen removed to ensure a clear inferior margin.

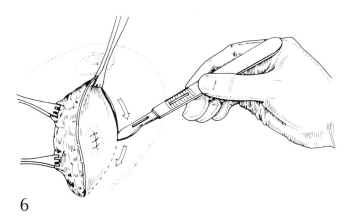

6

6

After the tumour is cleared inferiorly, the lower skin incision is completed and again the scalpel is immediately beveled laterally to ensure a clear margin of normal breast tissue. The dissection down to the pectoralis fascia is repeated as with the superior flap.

7

The remaining attachments of the lesions are divided.

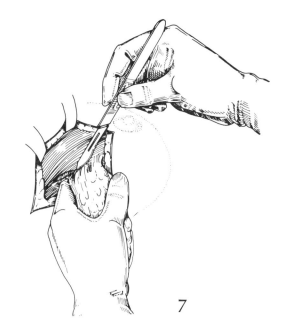

7

8

For lesions located in the upper outer quadrant, the lateral border of the incision may extend to the tip of the axillary hairline, thus permitting an in-continuity standard axillary dissection.

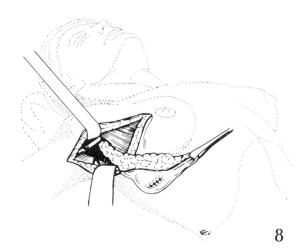

8

LONG THORACIC NERVE

THORACODORSAL NERVE
INTERCOSTOBRACHIAL NERVE

9

9

This technique removes all axillary tissue below the axillary vein and the thoracodorsal and long thoracic nerves are preserved.

10

Breast and subcutaneous tissue are reapproximated in layered fashion. Vacuum drainage minimizes accumulation of serous fluid.

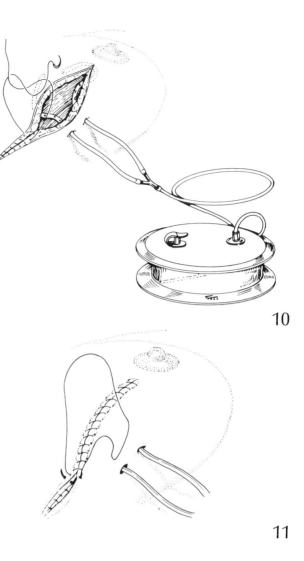

10

11

The use of continuous fine nylon or a subcuticular suture technique minimizes scarring.

11

Postoperative care

Full motion of the arm and shoulder and active exercises designed to return the patient to full activity are encouraged postoperatively. The suction catheters are left in place for about 4 or 5 days postoperatively, until daily suction drainage is less than 30–50 ml/day. The suction catheter is then removed and the patient is discharged from the hospital, usually on the fifth postoperative day.

Radiation therapy, if used postoperatively, can be started approximately 2–3 weeks postoperatively. Antitumour chemotherapy is given only for selected patients who have axillary lymph node metastases.

Results

From 1955 through 1972, 173 patients with carcinoma of the breast underwent partial mastectomy at the Cleveland Clinic[2]. This represents approximately 20 per cent of our total experience with various operative procedures for the treatment of breast cancer. In our earliest experience, a high percentage of patients who had partial mastectomy were elderly, had other diseases or refused mastectomy. In our more recent experience, the patients were younger with small, apparently early breast cancers.

Table 1 gives the 5- and 10-year survival results and incidence of recurrent disease for our patients who underwent partial mastectomy. *Table 2* gives the survival results for all patients treated for breast cancer at the Cleveland Clinic. A series of 106 patients, all of whom had invasive cancers, were matched for age of the patient, size of the

Table 1 Results of partial mastectomy: Cleveland Clinic 1955–1972

Stage	No. of patients	%
Clinical Stage I	144	83
Clinical Stage II	29	17
Radiation postoperatively	32	18
5-year survival	132/173	76
Lost to follow-up	3/173	2
10-year survival	28/63	44
Lost to follow-up	2/63	3
Died of other disease	14/63	22
Local recurrence	21/173	12
New cancer, same breast	6/173	3
New cancer, opposite breast	6/173	3

Table 2 Results of all operations for breast cancer: Cleveland Clinic 1955–1972, 1132 patients

	Survival (%)	
	5 years	10 years
All stages	58	44
Stage I	74	57
Stage II	54	29
Stages I and II	68	48
Stages III and IV	19	8

Table 3 Matched comparison of partial v. total mastectomy: Cleveland Clinic, 53 patients – 53 patients

	Partial mastectomy	Total mastectomy
Stage I/Stage II	32/21	32/21
Size of tumour (average)	2 cm	2 cm
Average age	57 yr	57 yr
5-year survival	41/53 77%	37/53 70%
Local recurrence	3/53 6%	4/53 8%
Died of other disease	3/53 6%	3/53 6%

tumour and involvement of axillary lymph nodes (*Table 3*). There appears to be no disadvantage to partial mastectomy when compared with complete mastectomy in this matched pair study.

Several clinical studies have been and are being reported from hospital centres throughout the world in order to study and define the role of partial mastectomy. Among the more important reports are those of Porritt[3] from London; Wise, Mason and Ackerman[4] from St Helier's Hospital, Surrey, England; the Guy's Hospital trial reported by Atkins *et al.*[5] and Hayward[6]; the report of Greening, Montgomery and Growing[7] from the Royal Marsden Hospital, London; the Milan trial reported by Veronesi[8] and Veronesi *et al.*[9]; the studies of Peters[10] at St Margarethe's Hospital, Toronto; the studies of Mustakallio[11] in Finland; the reports of Cope *et al.*[12] from Boston; and the studies of Montague *et al.*[13] in Texas. Additionally, the National Surgical Adjuvant Breast Project (NSABP protocol B-06) has now undertaken a prospective, randomized study in the United States comparing the results of partial mastectomy with and without radiation with the results of modified radical mastectomy. These studies confirm that, at present, for patients with small or potentially favourable breast cancer, there is no difference in long-term survival between patients who have had partial mastectomy with or without postoperative radiation and patients who have had modified radical or radical mastectomy.

References

1. Hermann, R. E., Esselstyn, C. B., Crile, G. Conservative surgical treatment of potentially curable breast cancer. In: Gallager, H. S., Leis, H. P., Snydermann, R. K., Urban, J. A., eds. The breast, Chapter 17, pp. 219–231. St Louis: C. V. Mosby Co., 1978

2. Crile, G., Cooperman, A., Esselstyn, C, B., Hermann, R. E. Results of partial mastectomy in 173 patients followed for from five to ten years. Surgery, Gynecology and Obstetrics 1980; 150: 563–566

3. Porritt, A. Early carcinoma of the breast. British Journal of Surgery 1964; 51: 214–216

4. Wise, L., Mason, A. Y., Ackerman, I. V. Local excision and irradiation: an alternative method for the treatment of early mammary cancer. Annals of Surgery 1971; 174: 392–401

5. Atkins, H., Hayward, J. L., Klugman, D. J., Wayte, A. B. Treatment of early breast cancer: a report after ten years of a clinical trial. British Medical Journal 1972; 2: 423–429

6. Hayward, J. L. The Guy's trial of treatments of 'early' breast cancer. World Journal of Surgery 1977; 1: 314–316

7. Greening, W. P., Montgomery, A. C. V., Gowing, N. F. C. Report on pilot study of treatment of breast cancer by quadrantic excision with axillary dissection and no other therapy. Journal of the Royal Society of Medicine 1978; 71: 261–264

8. Veronesi, U. Conservative treatment of breast cancer: a trial in progress at the Cancer Institute of Milan. World Journal of Surgery 1977; 1: 324–326

9. Veronesi, U., Banfi, A., Sacozzi, R., Salvadori, B., Zucali, R., Uslenghi, C. et al. Conservative treatment of breast cancer. A trial in progress at the Cancer Institute of Milan. Cancer 1977; 39: 2822–2826

10. Peters, V. M. Cutting the Gordian knot in early breast cancer. Annals of the Royal College of Surgeons of Canada 1975; 186–187

11. Mustakallio, S. Conservative treatment of breast carcinoma. Review of 25 years follow-up. Clinical Radiology 1972; 23: 110–116

12. Cope, O., Wang, C. A., Chu, A., Wang, C. C., Schulz, M., Castleman, B. et al. Limited surgical excision as the basis of a comprehensive therapy for cancer of the breast. American Journal of Surgery 1976; 31: 400–408

13. Montague, E. D., Gutierrez, A. E., Barker, J. L., Tapley, N. DuV., Fletcher, G. H. Conservation surgery and irradiation for the treatment of favourable breast cancer. Cancer 1979; 43: 1058–1061

Illustrations by Michael Courtney

Restorative prosthetic mammaplasty (non-mutilating mastectomy) in mastectomy for carcinoma and benign lesions

George T. Watts ChM, FRCS
Consultant Surgeon, United Birmingham Hospitals

Introduction

This procedure has been designed as an alternative to conventional forms of mastectomy as a means whereby the patient's figure may be maintained in a similar or improved form to that which precedes resection of the breast. It can be used in almost all cases of benign diseases of the breast where mastectomy is needed and in a proportion of those with malignancy. Excision and reconstruction may be in either one or two stages when reconstruction is carried out months or even years after the original resection of tissue. The objective is basically cosmetic: reconstruction must always be subordinated to that of adequate treatment of the breast lesion. Therefore,

selection of cases is extremely important and where doubt exists the operation should be carried out in two stages. This will allow both patient and surgeon to determine whether it is necessary or desirable. Cosmetic effects are not quite so satisfactory when reconstruction is carried out as a secondary operation, but from the technical point of view, delay is slightly simpler and safer and is, therefore, a more suitable course to follow for the inexperienced surgeon. The psychological impact of retaining the breast is great in most patients and the surgeon will find that he is pressed to carry out this procedure by patients once they know it is available.

Preoperative

Selection of cases

Though reconstruction is obviously most suited for the younger patient, it can be carried out at all ages and age alone should not be regarded as a contraindication. As the operation takes longer, however, age may be a factor which prevents use of an implant reconstruction. Similarly, the patient's general condition is a factor which must be weighed; local tissue and nutrition are also important. If there is doubt, operation should be held over as a second-stage procedure. Where time permits, of course, it may be possible first to improve the patient's general and local health, thus allowing a primary procedure to be carried out with safety.

In malignancy, choice of the operation should not normally be allowed to prejudice the patient's chance of survival. Nevertheless, some patients, knowing the diagnosis, elect to have an operation which does not destroy their femininity, rather than one which might in theory give longer survival, but at a price which they regard as intolerable. Therefore, the ideal patient in malignant disease is one in whom a small lesion, localized entirely to the breast tissue, can be removed with the confidence that there is a reasonable chance of total extirpation of malignant tissue. The operation should not be refused to a patient with advanced, even disseminated disease, for in these patients the outcome is determined but the psychological advantages may be very great indeed.

Fat patients should, in general, not be offered the operation until their weight has been reduced; in the obese patient with malignant disease the prosthesis can be inserted as a secondary procedure when the weight has been lowered by dieting. In the fat patient the skin and subcutaneous tissues tend to be stretched and thin and such tissues do not heal satisfactorily. In addition, the prosthesis needed is larger and therefore produces greater tension and pressure on the skin flaps with liability to complications. A further problem is that at a later stage the patient may wish to lose weight; the prosthesis will then remain constant in size and an asymmetry will result of most undesirable form. A similar problem may present when patients change their shape for other reasons (e.g. pregnancy). This is not a contraindication to the operation, but the patient should be warned that asymmetry may result and that subsequent corrective procedures may be required to match the breasts.

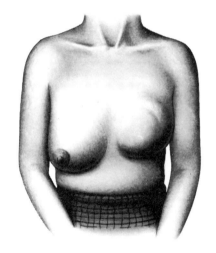

1a

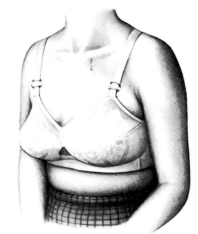

1b

1a & b

Skin tension

The most important single consideration in success for this procedure is the absence of skin tension along suture lines. Therefore, if it is necessary as part of the operation to remove skin, it will be necessary to insert a smaller prosthesis than the size of the breast tissue removed and for the patient to accept a breast which is smaller than her original one, or the other breast. Though it is possible as a second-stage procedure to replace the prosthesis and insert a larger one when the tissues have stretched, in general this is not a wise policy and the patient should be warned that it may be necessary, to achieve symmetry, to reduce the size of the remaining breast. Alternatively, the patient may be asked to accept asymmetry of the breasts and the necessity of wearing a partial external prosthesis. For the majority of patients the most important consideration of mastectomy is alteration in the decolletage of their clothing. Therefore, if it is possible to reconstruct the upper part of the breast, the patient may be able to wear normal clothing, though some padding is still necessary. If there is a liberal amount of skin available in the remaining breast, a flap of this may be swung across as an intermediate procedure to augment the skin supply available where the mastectomy has been carried out. With a pedicle, such skin survives well; grafted skin, if full thickness, may also be used, but then it is not wise to insert prostheses underneath unless part of the skin is attached to an undisturbed base.

2

Site of lesion and incision

Almost any incision site may be chosen in these patients, but it should not include or skirt the areola. From the point of view of cosmetic appearance and satisfactory healing, the inframammary incision is by far the best. However, this is not always suitable in cases where carcinoma is present. The most unsatisfactory site for incisions is the upper inner quadrant of the breast (as shown in the illustration). The reason for this is the poor blood supply of the skin in this area. In these cases, especially when excision of skin is concerned, great caution should be employed when considering the insertion of a prosthesis. The worst site of all for an incision is a vertical one extending upwards from the nipple in the midline, or one extending from the nipple towards the sternoclavicular joint.

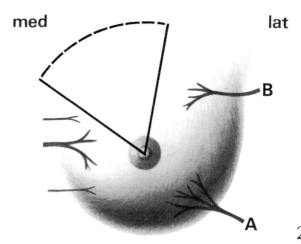

2

The most important blood supply is at A. A lesser vessel but one which is often quite large may be present at B. On the inner side, blood supply to the skin and breast is variable in amount and distribution. Rarely are more than two significant branches to the skin present and usually the lower the vessel the greater the size. Incisions in the quadrant shown are those most likely to give trouble in healing due to ischaemia.

Preoperative preparation

3

The normal routine investigation of all patients undergoing straightforward operation should be carried out. No special procedure is required. Before admission to hospital, the patient should be provided with a soft cotton broad-strapped brassiere to be worn in the postoperative period. The straps should be detachable for easy application; the main fastening should be, by preference, between the breasts in front. There should be no stiff quilting or wires; ideally, a soft supporting sponge insert may be used, but this is not essential. Some types of maternity nursing brassiere are satisfactory. A 'plunge type' brassiere will certainly do, but if this pattern is used it should have greater depth than usual. The cross-over type of brassiere, popular to give deformed shapes to women in fashion, is totally unsuitable. These have rigid edges which press on the breast and by confining it in a rigid way, interfere with the nutrition of the skin flaps postoperatively. The brassiere should not be tightly fitting in order to allow for dressings and supporting wool which will be inserted in the immediate postoperative period. The girth measurement of the chest should be the patient's normal size.

Attempts should be made to choose an appropriate size of prosthesis before the operation; usually after experience with a small number of cases it is possible to do this without recourse to other aids. Sizing cups are available and a set of unsterile prostheses may also be a help with comparison with the size of breast preoperatively. In the operating theatre, further assistance can be obtained by having a pair of scales available; the weight of the breast tissue can then be measured after its removal. A prosth-

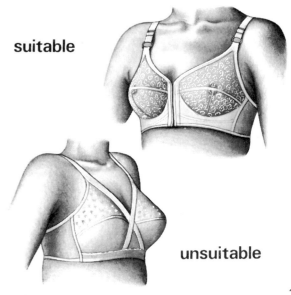

3

esis of about two-thirds of the capacity of the breast tissue is usually ideal. However, a range of prostheses should be available at the time of operation, both in case of mishap and in case of unsuitability of size.

Blood transfusion should not be necessary. In carrying out this procedure precise haemostasis is necessary and, therefore, blood loss should be minimal. Pre-existing anaemia should, of course, be treated appropriately before the patient is taken to surgery.

The operation

4a, b & c

Position of patient

The patient should be placed symmetrically on the table with both arms abducted on arm boards. Routine skin preparation is carried out on both sides. It is important to paint beneath the patient's arm and shoulder on both sides. To do this the patient is lifted from the table and before lowering back, a towel is inserted under the shoulder. The arm is then tied down to the arm board and the skin prepared and towelled, leaving both breasts bare. Sutures are preferable to towel clips as they cause less damage to the skin. They should be accurately placed on both sides to give complete symmetry in site. It will be found that a suture at the lower border of the axilla is an advantage, as well as the one at the uppermost part. A further towel is now applied to cover the normal breast; this may be fixed by towel clips which are attached to the drapes only.

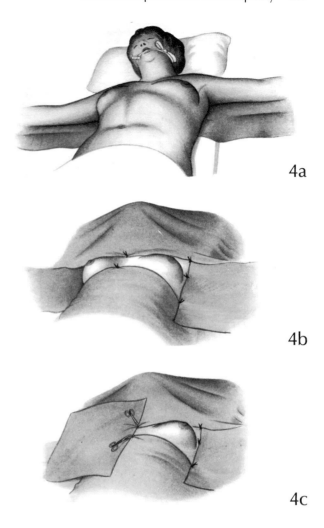

4a

4b

4c

5

Choice of incision

Whenever possible the incision of choice is the inframammary (a). This may be made more extensive than the axillary (b), medial (c), polar (d) or lateral (e) incisions with least likelihood of prejudicing the blood supply to the skin flaps. The marginal incision (f) also gives little trouble. When using such a marginal incision along the outer border of the breast, great caution must be exercised to avoid damage to the main blood supply. The lateral incision gives good access, but carries more hazard to nutrition of the skin. The medial and polar incisions should be avoided whenever possible.

The amount of skin to be excised will depend on the lesion. When no involvement of the skin is recognizable it is not necessary to remove skin overlying the tumour. If there is doubt, a frozen section of the tissue just beneath the skin can be carried out in the operating theatre for verification that involvement is absent. The conventional excision of the skin advocated by older surgeons has been found not to be necessary if the surgeon stays strictly in the correct plane of dissection.

The nipple does not need to be removed unless the lesion lies in the tissues immediately underlying it. Lymphatic drainage is away from the nipple in all directions

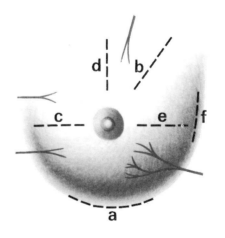

5

and therefore, unless a lesion actually starts at the nipple, involvement is rare. It is essential to avoid invasion of the nipple and areola by the incision if they are to be preserved. Ideally, an incision will stop short of the areola by at least 6–7 mm.

Technique of incision

6

The site of incision should be marked on the skin by a ball point pencil or some similar marker. The skin must be held under tension and pressure, the surgeon and his assistant pressing on the skin and drawing it apart with fingers spaced evenly along the wound. It will be noted that the surgeon does not touch the skin. This is a vital point in the whole of the operation. It is impossible to sterilize skin by any known means and therefore contact with the skin implies infection of the surgeon's or his assistant's gloves. Any instruments or swabs which have been in contact with the skin are discarded as soon as they have been used. Throughout this operation asepsis of the highest order is mandatory. When making the incision a flatter blade than that normally employed is an advantage. We prefer the Gillette A type of blade.

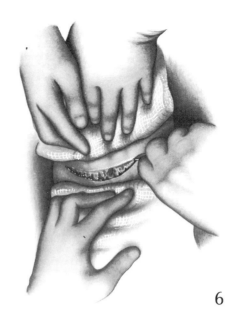

6

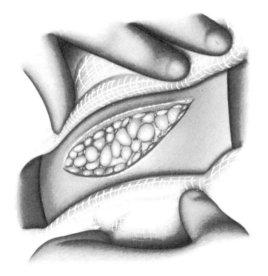

7

7

The knife is pressed on the skin in the usual fashion; as the skin is pierced, the pressure and tension applied by the surgeon and his assistants cause the skin to split apart, revealing the plane of separation between breast and subcutaneous tissues. This is easily recognized by the difference in size of the fat lobules, these being larger in the breast, and also by the presence of a plexus of veins covering the breast tissue.

Dissection

8a, b & c

Blunt and sharp dissection is carried out in this plane; pledgets of gauze on forceps (a) and blunt scissor dissection by the Hilton method (b) are both satisfactory, but with experience by far the best method is found to be dissection using a knife held flat to the tissues (c). The knife wipes across the surface of the breast, whilst the skin and subcutaneous tissues are lifted upwards, rather as though the breast were being spread with a coating of substance on the knife. Dissection proceeds in the same way as with conventional mastectomy to the margins of the breast.

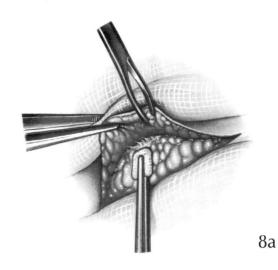

8a

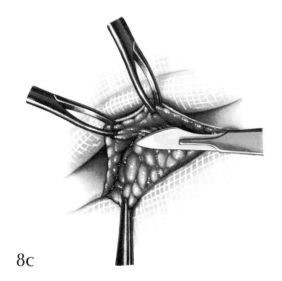

8c

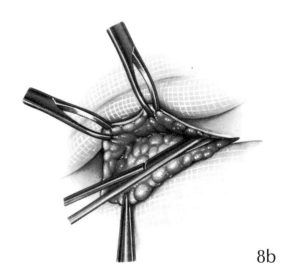

8b

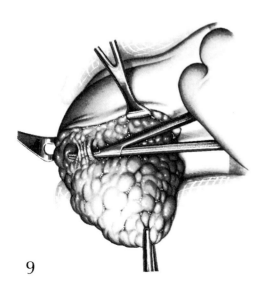

9

9

At the nipple, the dissection proceeds as close as possible to the ducts. To divide these it is found helpful to pass a curved artery forceps or similar instrument round behind the ducts and then to divide them with a scalpel held in the same plane as the general dissection.

10

In separating the breast from the underlying tissues, it will be found that it is an advantage to dissect to the edge of the breast at one point and then separate the breast from the pectoral muscles by blunt dissection. To do this, a pair of blunt sponge-holding forceps is passed behind the breast in the plane between breast and muscle. This is an easy manoeuvre unless fixation of the breast to the underlying tissues has occurred. After the instrument has been passed to the extremes of the breast, it is serially opened and then withdrawn.

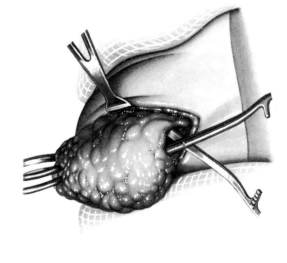

10

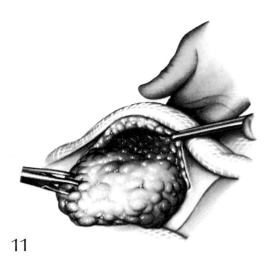

11

11

Once this has been done, it is often much easier to separate the breast from the rest of its integument by turning the skin and subcutaneous tissues inside-out rather in the fashion of removal of a surgical glove, or skinning a rabbit for the pot.

12

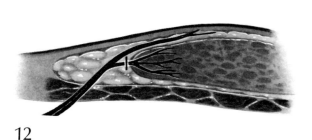

12

As the periphery of the breast is reached, it is possible to isolate the blood vessels supplying the breast and skin. It will be found that usually the blood vessels divide before entering the breast and therefore it is possible to separate the branch entering the breast tissue from that supplying the skin. Thus, the blood supply to the skin can be preserved, while the branch entering the breast can be severed. On the medial side of the breast these branches are small enough to be sealed by diathermy. However, it is much preferable to ligate the vessels with fine silk, as this produces less risk of causing thrombosis in the branches to the skin. On the lateral and inferior side, the main trunks are much larger and it is rarely wise to do anything other than ligate these vessels. Our preference lies with silk, but fine thread is sometimes more suitable.

Mastectomy is completed by dissection of the axilla or any other procedures found necessary. It differs here in no way from normal procedures. At the end of this phase, it will often be noted that the nipple is pale or cyanosed. This is without significance.

Insertion of prosthesis

13

Before insertion of the prosthesis it is essential to see that complete haemostasis has been achieved. This is best done by first inserting a large dry, clean pack. After several minutes this is withdrawn and points where haemorrhage is occurring are noted and the bleeding is arrested. The whole cavity should then be inspected carefully using a large retractor. Absolute haemostasis is essential. The skin area is then completely isolated, using large soft packs. The surgeon should then don a second pair of gloves over his first as an extra precaution and wash off all glove powder with *sterile* Cetavlon solution.

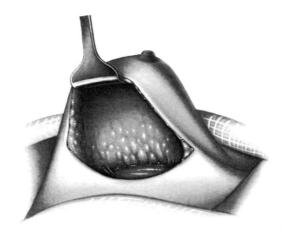

13

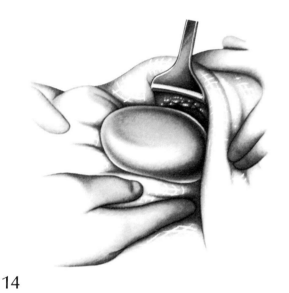

14

14

The prosthesis is brought to the wound in a towel and inserted, if possible, without contact between the surgeon's gloves and the patient's skin. It should not be handled by any of the assistants *en route*. Insertion, as far as possible, is carried out direct from the carrying towel to the wound. Adjustment can usually be made by handling the prosthesis with a pack. Only rarely should the surgeon need direct contact between his gloves and the prosthesis. The second pair of gloves provides protection in these circumstances. A sterile Teflon spatula may be of help. It will be found that contact with the tissues and blood makes it possible to manoeuvre the prosthesis more easily once in position. Minor adjustment can be carried out after closure of the wound, but the basic position should be established at the time of insertion.

15

After insertion of the prosthesis, skin tension should be checked. Unless the skin edges can be apposed easily and without any measurable degree of tension, the prosthesis is too large.

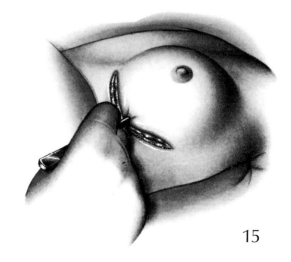

15

16

The prosthesis may be of various types, but in general the round, thin-walled patchless type is suitable for almost all cases. In a few instances a tear-drop type of prosthesis of the same basic pattern can be substituted. If such a prosthesis is used, the patchless type is preferable. Very rarely it is necessary to use a more shaped prosthesis, such as the Cronin pattern. These are normally only necessary when a fairly rigid shape of very large form is required. In no circumstances should sutures be inserted into the patches, nor should any attempt be made to anchor the other types of prosthesis in any way.

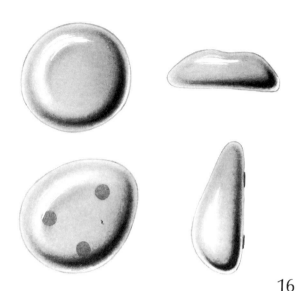

16

17

17

Next, the choice of prosthesis should be checked by a comparison with the normal breast. To do this, the extra drape previously applied is removed and the skin edges held together, as when testing for tension. It may be necessary to exert pressure on the remaining normal breast to push it into a reasonable shape, such as it assumes when wearing clothing. The best view obtainable is that from the anaesthetist's end of the operating table, but where possible, matching from all angles should be satisfactory.

If all is satisfactory, the wound may now be closed. This is done in two layers. The first in the capsule of the breast is of continuous 2/0 plain catgut. As the end of the closure is approached, the air in the cavity should be expelled by gentle pressure from all directions. The skin is then closed separately by the suture method of choice; the author's preference is for a subcuticular suture. It is important in all layers that the prosthesis is not perforated – though this is not disastrous, it is obviously undesirable.

18

Dressings are now applied. Support for the breast is best provided by adhesive foam dressing. Curved recesses are cut in the region of the nipple on both sides and the foam is applied over a thin layer of dressing or gauze or other preferred material. The patient's brassiere is now applied and fastened. It will be found that a pad of cotton wool inserted between the breast and the outer side of the brassiere is an advantage for the first 24–48 h. This should not be large (about the size of the palm of the hand) or particularly thick. However, it will prevent pressure on the breast from the brassiere and provide comfort for the patient. After this period, removal of the wool will relieve the patient of the discomfort caused by swelling and irritation.

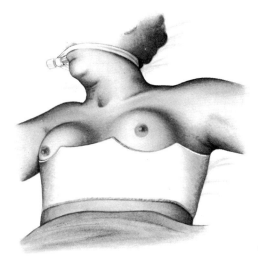

18

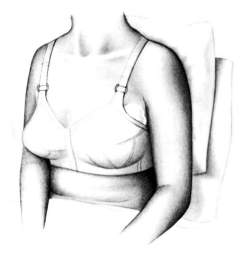

19

19

The patient is now transferred to the bed in the sitting position and minor adjustments to the prosthesis may be made if required.

Note the cotton wool pad on the axillary side. This is removed after 24 h.

Postoperative care and complications

The patient requires no special postoperative care. However, movement of the arm should be somewhat restricted for the first 2 weeks and the upper arm should not be raised above the horizontal during this period. Afterwards, full activity of the shoulder can be allowed and activities generally increased if healing has occurred naturally and soundly. The original dressing and the brassiere must be retained undisturbed for the first 2 weeks. After this they should be removed by the surgeon with care to ensure that any adhesive is pulled away along the line of the wounds and not across them.

The patient is told to wear a brassiere day and night for the first 2 months postoperatively, even when activity has been increased. After this, the brassiere may be gradually abandoned and the patient's normal habits in terms of clothing adopted once more.

Gentle frequent handling of the breast can be carried out after 2 weeks and helps keep the new breast soft and supple.

Complications

Skin necrosis

This is the most important complication. It is rare in lower incisions, though occasionally a form of pseudonecrosis may be noted where the skin becomes scaly and dry close to the edge of the incision. This is easily differentiated from true necrosis as the skin is dry and a gentle rub with a spirit swab removes the horny dried layer of skin. In true necrosis, the skin becomes wet and lifeless. When this occurs it should be excised promptly; it must be excised in all layers until sound tissue is reached and reapposition must also be obtained at all layers. Approximation of the skin by strapping only is not satisfactory as this will lead to a thin scar over the prosthesis and may give rise to trouble even years later.

In avoiding necrosis, the most important factor is preservation of blood supply; avoidance of tension is also important. It is vital in dissecting the flaps to maintain the correct plane. The danger is greatest during the later stages of dissection, especially if the integuments have been turned inside out, as it is then possible to stray from the correct plane into the subcutaneous tissues. The presence of bleeding is a useful warning that this is occurring. Normally, as dissection proceeds, bleeding should be almost non-existent.

Sepsis

Sepsis should be a rare phenomenon if true aseptic measures have been carried out meticulously as outlined above. Antibiotics should not be used, especially locally, as these may lead to excessive formation of fluid with an unsatisfactory final result from the formation of a rather rigid capsule round the prosthesis. Drainage is not necessary and should not be used as it provides a portal of entry for infection and a drain may also prevent close approximation of the surrounding tissues to the prosthesis.

Should sepsis unfortunately occur, panic should be avoided. Drainage of the cavity from below to give adequate dependent drainage is often sufficient to solve the problem, the track of the incision closing spontaneously when all the pus has been discharged. As the prosthesis has a smooth surface, it will not be contaminated by absorbent foreign bodies (for this reason prostheses with porous surfaces are most unsuitable and dangerous).

Some confusion exists about the method of sterilizing prostheses because manufacturers' advice differs. In addition to the precautions mentioned above, care should also be taken before the prostheses are sterilized. They should not be handled by bare hands, nor should they be allowed to become greasy or to remain in contact with infected surfaces. Reliance on manufacturers' claims of sterility is unwise. Prostheses should be handled with clean, preferably fresh sterile gloves; where necessary, they should be washed with simple soap and water in a sterile solution. They should not be cleaned with antiseptics. Occasionally, a tacky surface appears on prostheses that have been sterilized more than once; this can be eliminated by gentle washing with a dilute sodium bicarbonate solution.

The actual sterilization is best accomplished by heat. Precaution should be exercised when vacuum sterilization is used. This may produce vacuoles in the prosthesis. Though these have an unpleasant appearance, they do not appear to have any disadvantageous effects. It is most important that sterilization should not be effected as recommended by some authorities, with chemical methods. Some chemical adsorbs on the prosthesis and may cause great irritation at a later stage. As the prosthesis is impermeable, a short sterilization period is satisfactory.

Fluid collection

This is less of a problem than with conventional mastectomy. If adequate support of the breast has been attained as described, it is very rare for any fluid of note to collect. We have rarely found it necessary (3 cases in 140 patients) to aspirate fluid which formed. Should this be necessary, great care must be taken to avoid damage to the prosthesis by milking the fluid away from it. Drainage tends to increase the tendency to fluid formation, rather than prevent it. Excessive fluid formation has the drawback that the capsule formed round the prosthesis tends to be somewhat more rigid than normal and hence the re-formed breast will be more rigid than normal. Collection of fluid by haemorrhage should not occur, though it has been reported by some surgeons. In this event, immediate exploration would be necessary.

Formation of a rigid capsule

This is a rare complication and paradoxically occurs following over-zealous restriction of the patient's arm movements in the postoperative period. It can be dealt with simply by removal of the prosthesis, incision of the capsule at the point where it is adherent or restricting and reinsertion of the prosthesis. Fairly rapid mobilization of the arm can be allowed, as when prostheses are inserted for augmentation of the breasts in cosmetic surgery.

Change of shape

This normally occurs after some overall change in the patient's configuration, e.g. increased obesity, but in our experience it is most common following pregnancy. In these instances it is usually preferable to operate on the sound breast to augment or reduce it as necessary. In cases where gross changes have occurred, ir may be advisable to excise the whole of the remaining breast tissue and replace it with a matching prosthesis. Some surgeons advocate this procedure in cases of cancer of the breast.

Late changes

In our experience these are minimal except in cases of carcinoma. Here recurrence may constitute a problem. Where the recurrence is a small localized lesion, it may be excised and the wound sutured without difficulty as long as all layers are closed as in the primary operation. It is possible, without hazard, to excise the tissues right down to the surface of the prosthesis. Where more widespread dissemination occurs, it is possible to irradiate the breast or to give antimitotic drugs alone or in combination. No adverse effects on the prosthesis or its surrounding capsule have been noted and from the point of view of irradiation dosage, the presence of the prosthesis can be ignored. It is our personal experience that the recurrence rate locally following insertion of a prosthesis appears to be less than with simple mastectomy, though no explanation for this can be offered.

A late change which has also been noted is the stretching of the tissues with age. It has been found that the prostheses change shape slightly with age in the same way and at the same rate as a normal breast; therefore, it is not necessary for patients to modify their habits in terms of wearing brassieres. Those who prefer to abandon this garment can do so without fear that it would jeopardize their figure any more than would normally occur.

Further reading

Watts, G. T., Caruso, F., Waterhouse, J. A. Mastectomy with primary reconstruction. Lancet 1980; 2: 967–969

Illustrations by Kate Crowle

Chest wall coverage after radical surgery

Bryan C. Mendelson   FRCS(Ed.), FRACS
Lecturer in Surgery, Monash University Department of Surgery,
Alfred Hospital, Melbourne

Introduction

The surgical problem of chest wall coverage following radical surgery has been greatly simplified following the introduction of several new flaps.

Their characteristics of safety and large size provide the means for immediate coverage of virtually any conceivable defect. Irrespective of the indication for radical surgery, be it palliative mastectomy for an extensive primary carcinoma, wide resection of locally recurrent breast carcinoma, excision of radionecrosis or excision of chest wall tumours, the same flaps are utilized for chest wall coverage.

In general the latissimus dorsi musculocutaneous flap is the preferred flap, because of its versatility, proximity to most defects and minimal donor deformity. The transverse thoracoabdominal flap is indicated for an anterior or lateral defect if the latissimus dorsi flap is contraindicated because of damage to its vascular pedicle. A contralateral pectoralis major flap may be preferred for a midline or parasternal defect. The greater omentum is nearly always available failing the availability of the above three flaps and can be transposed to cover virtually any anterior chest wall defect, pedicled on either of its gastroepiploic vessels. It is the need for a laparotomy which relegates this flap to that of last resort.

THE LATISSIMUS DORSI FLAP

Historical

The latissimus dorsi flap was frequently used in the early years of radical mastectomy, before the wider acceptance of Halsted's method. In 1896 Tansini[1], Professor of Surgery in Pavia, advised that to minimize local recurrences, the principle of removing all the mammary skin rather than thinning the breast flaps should be used. The resultant defect was closed with a posterior transposition flap based superiorly. By 1906 his anatomical studies[2] had solved the problem of skin necrosis by recognizing that the underlying latissimus muscle provides much of the skin circulation and must be included with the skin flap.

Tansini's method, radical mastectomy with excision of all breast skin and wound closure utilizing the latissimus dorsi flap, was reportedly popular in Europe between 1910 and 1920. Hutchins[3] of Baltimore subsequently used the muscle alone as a superiorly based flap, transposed during radical mastectomy as padding between the chest wall and the skin flaps.

Interest in the flap thereafter lapsed, presumably because of failure of surgeons at that time to appreciate the principles on which the flap is based. In the last decade understanding of the blood supply of flaps in general has improved; the safety and versatility of the newly discovered arterialized (axial) flaps liberated flap surgery from many of the limitations inherent with traditional flaps based on a random circulation. While axial skin flaps exist in only a few areas of the body (e.g. deltopectoral, transverse thoracoabdominal), inclusion of the underlying muscle, as a compound musculocutaneous flap, permits skin flaps in certain areas of the body which do not have an axial circulation to utilize the axial circulation of the underlying muscle.

The latissimus dorsi musculocutaneous flap is probably the largest, safest and most versatile of all these flaps. It was rediscovered and its potential only then appreciated, because of an understanding of the scientific basis of flap design.

Principles

The latissimus dorsi flap is a musculocutaneous flap based on an axial circulation. The skin over the latissimus receives its circulation via multiple short muscle perforator vessels which exit from the muscle and course perpendicularly to the dermis. Because the skin circulation is dependent on the integrity of the muscle circulation, the skin flap can be completely severed from the surrounding skin with no impairment of its circulation. The skin is then transposed as part of the muscle flap.

The dominant axial blood supply to the latissimus dorsi, and therefore indirectly the overlying skin, is the thoracodorsal artery. The secondary circulation via multiple posterior intercostal perforating vessels is expendable with no loss of muscle viability. Apart from some small branches to the serratus anterior and mid axillary skin, the thoracodorsal artery carries its predominant and terminal flow to the ramifications within the latissimus muscle. The vascular pedicle provides no restriction to flap mobility, as it enters the muscle in the mid axilla near the rotation point of the muscle flap, and it can be further lengthened to 10 cm by ligation of the small side branches. The muscle itself can be severed of all its attachments yet maintain complete viability provided the thoracodorsal vascular axis remains intact. Normally the humeral insertion of the muscle is left attached, and part or all of the muscle used, which may include the aponeurotic part extending distally to the iliac crest and paravertebral region.

During surgery, care must be taken to protect the thoracodorsal vascular pedicle and to avoid shearing the skin from the muscle during handling of the flap. As integrity of the thoracodorsal vascular axis is the basis for the flap's remarkable safety, there is a potential risk in the patient who has had an axillary node dissection. If the flap is being used at the same operative procedure one can easily confirm the integrity of the thoracodorsal artery. If the axillary dissection was antecedent, the presence of a contractile muscle is a suggestion of vessel integrity. The nerve and artery are in such proximity that preservation of the nerve implies in all probability preservation of the artery.

If the muscle is not contractile, an alternative flap should be considered. However, the latissimus dorsi flap can still be attempted, but with an inherently increased risk. It has been demonstrated experimentally and confirmed clinically that collateral circulation may nourish the flap, coming either axially from the branch of the thoracodorsal artery passing into serratus anterior, or from the random circulation entering from around the tendinous insertion of the muscle. If operating in such a situation one should preliminarily dissect in the axilla to identify the vessel and thereafter strictly minimize further axillary dissection.

The operation

In practice the flap may be used in two basic ways,
according to the manner in which the skin component is
obtained.

1 & 2

TRADITIONAL – TRANSPOSITION FLAP

The skin component is marked tangential to the outer
edge of the chest wall defect. The anterior border of the
flap is parallel to the free lateral border of the latissimus
and should be no more than 5 cm anterior to it. The base
of the flap is superior. As transposition of the flap tends to
be restricted by skin tension from the medial end of its
base, i.e. the pivot point of the flap, it is important to
design the flap of sufficient length to reach easily the
upper and inner end of the defect.

The muscle beneath the flap is left attached to the skin
and elevated by transecting the muscle beneath the lower
end and posterior border of the skin flap, being cautious
to preserve the large vascular branch within 2 cm of the
axillary border of the muscle.

Though this flap may be adequate for limited defects it
is less effective than the island flap.

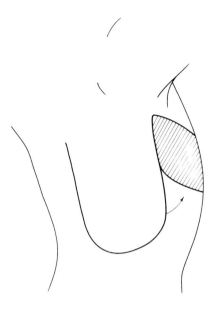

1

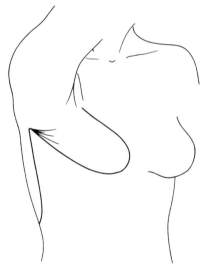

2

LATISSIMUS DORSI ISLAND FLAP

This method takes full advantage of the flap's potential without increased risk and is recommended.

3

The skin is completely incised as an island, remaining attached only to the underlying muscle. The pedicle therefore consists only of the superolateral muscle, thereby avoiding unnecessary bulk in the medial axilla. The potential difficulties associated with traditional transposition flaps, i.e. tension across the base from the pivot point and problems getting the flap to fit, are completely eliminated because of the independence of the skin island from the surrounding skin. The resultant change of the pivot point to the axilla allows remarkable mobility of the flap with ease of fit.

   In practice three sets of markings are outlined on the skin.

(a) The borders of the latissimus muscle, i.e. the posterior axillary fold extending to the iliac crest and the upper horizontal border at the level of the angle of the scapula.
(b) The planned skin island. This is outlined to fit the dimensions of the chest defect exactly. It is usually orientated nearly transversely across the upper muscle, but with increased obliquity as a longer flap is designed (see inset). The distance from the axillary end of the skin flap to the muscle insertion should be somewhat longer than the distance from the muscle insertion to the axillary end of the anterior chest defect.
(c) The planned borders of the muscle excision, usually several centimetres on the inferior and medial aspects of the skin flap, and including the full width of the muscle in the pedicle region.

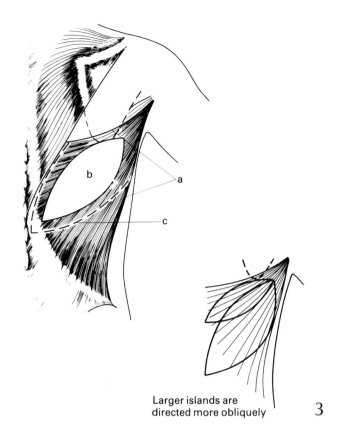

Larger islands are directed more obliquely

3

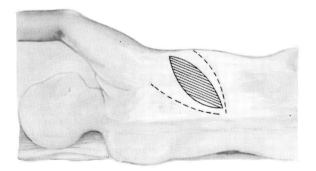

4

4

Position of patient

The patient is ideally placed in the true lateral position. The upper arm is placed on an overhead arm board, so that satisfactory exposure of the axilla and anterior chest can be obtained in addition to the back.

   The sterile draping includes the entire upper arm to allow repositioning during the procedure.

5

The incision

The entire skin flap is incised down to the fascia over the latissimus dorsi. As a precaution against inadvertent shearing of the skin from the muscle, several temporary tacking sutures may be placed between the dermis and the muscle fascia. To define the fringe of muscle beyond the skin island, the surrounding skin and subcutaneous tissue are dissected off the muscle fascia to the planned borders of the muscle incisions. Over the muscle pedicle this dissection continues up towards the axilla, as this manoeuvre frees the pedicle for later rotation. The upper edge of the muscle is located and freed up into the axilla. On dissecting this border lateral to the scapula, the ill defined cleavage plane between the latissimus dorsi and the outer border of teres major, is located by inferolateral retraction of the latissimus and then more easily opened by medial to lateral dissection.

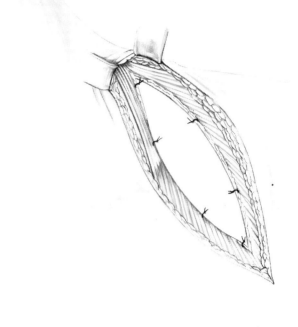

5

6

Muscle elevation

The tissue plane beneath the latissimus is entered by dissection around the free lateral border of the muscle, commencing low near the level of planned muscle transection. Blunt dissection medially in the relatively avascular plane between serratus anterior and the deep surface of latissimus allows bidigital control of the muscle with minimization of haemorrhage during its transection. Continuing medially beyond the oblique lower border of serratus, the latissimus is elevated off the periosteum of the lower ribs to where the muscle becomes aponeurotic. The posterior perforating branches of the intercostal vessels encountered here are the only major vessels requiring ligation throughout the entire dissection.

The muscle transection continues superiorly to where the free upper border of the muscle is encountered. At the same time the flap is being elevated by medial to lateral dissection, with increasing care to protect the axial vessels on the undersurface of the muscle as the axilla is approached. It should be verified that the superior border and outer surface are sufficiently released. Axillary dissection on the deep aspect may be deferred until exposure from the front is achieved.

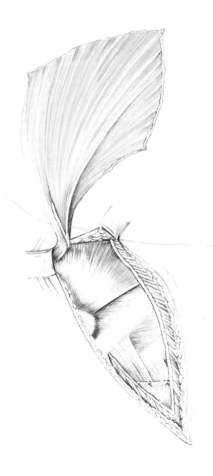

6

7

Dissection from anterior

Axillary dissection continues from the front by elevation of the skin flap adjacent to the previous radical extirpation. By continuing dissection over the external surface and tendon of latissimus dorsi, this wound now communicates with the posterior operative field. With the muscle gently retracted laterally, dissection is performed on its deep aspect with care to protect the thoracodorsal vascular pedicle, and proceeds proximally only to the extent required for satisfactory rotation of the flap. Not infrequently it is necessary to isolate and transect the branch of the thoracodorsal artery which passes medially into serratus anterior when it is responsible for tethering the rotation point of the flap to a low level (*see inset*). Rarely is dissection proximal to this level required.

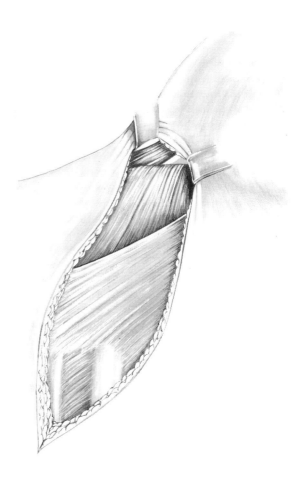

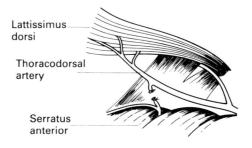

Lattissimus dorsi

Thoracodorsal artery

Serratus anterior

7

8 & 9

Tunnelling the flap

With the pedicle of the flap now mobilized and the axillary skin bridge sufficiently yet not excessively freed, the flap is tunnelled beneath the intact axillary skin bridge into the anterior defect. Particular care is required during this manoeuvre to avoid shearing the skin and subcutaneous fat from the muscle. The flap now rests in the axilla and over the anterior chest defect while attention is given to the posterior closure. Any temporary vascular spasm of the vessels supplying the flap will now have a chance to subside.

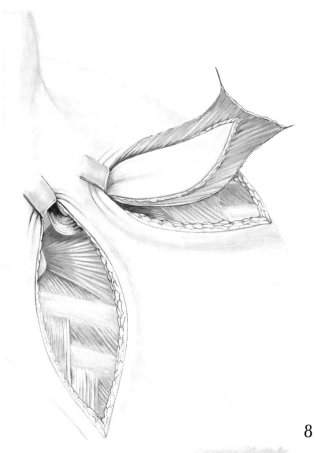

8

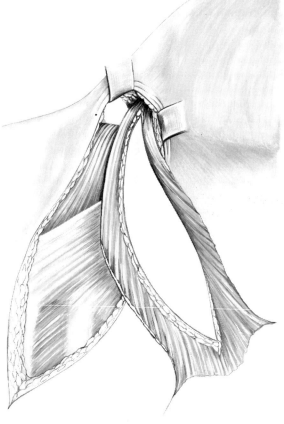

9

10

Closure of posterior defect

The posterior closure is often under tension and may be aided by adduction of the arm and shoulder. Failing this, wide undermining is required, and at times skin grafting of the tightest part of the closure is necessary.

A closed suction drain in the operative area is brought out through a laterally placed stab incision. The final layer of the closure utilizes a running subcuticular suture, as the patient will be lying on this incision postoperatively.

11

Insetting of flap

The flap is now inset into the defect over the anterior chest. This final step is most conveniently performed with the patient repositioned supine (and redraped) but can be somewhat awkwardly performed with the patient still in the lateral position. The muscle edges are first sutured in position to either the underlying chest wall or the undersurface of the skin flaps elevated during mastectomy. Care is required near the axillary end of the flap to avoid the axial vessels.

A second closed suction drain is placed beneath the flap, then the final skin closure performed.

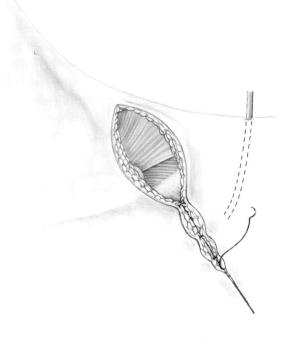

10

Postoperative care

Postoperatively, the arm is positioned away from the side to avoid possible compression of the muscle pedicle. Shoulder movement is minimized for several days to allow early adherence of the skin flaps and prevent serum collection. When wound drainage has become minimal, usually about 5 days, complete restoration of shoulder function is encouraged.

Results

Despite the sacrifice to function of a large muscle, there is negligible, if any, weakness of shoulder movement in everyday activity. Such weakness can be detected only on gymnastic-like manoeuvres.

The flap has a remarkable safety record, with only a few instances of minor skin edge necrosis in several hundred reported cases. Major flap necrosis is exceedingly rare and presumably reflects gross breach of proper technique.

The most troublesome complication, serous fluid collection under the skin flaps of the donor area of the back, can be minimized by proper use of drain tubes, early minimization of shoulder activity and the judicious use of elasticized pressure dressings commencing several days after surgery.

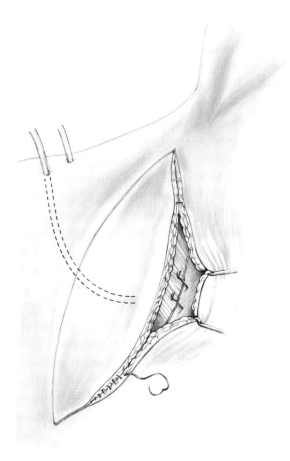

11

THE TRANSVERSE THORACOABDOMINAL FLAP

12 & 13

The axial vessels emerging from the rectus sheath 2–4 cm from the linea alba provide the vascular basis for this flap, as they course laterally in the subcutaneous layer adjacent to the deep fascia. The flap is designed transversely across the lower ribs, with its upper limit at the xiphoid. A mastectomy incision across the flap is a contraindication to its use.

The flap can safely extend to the anterior axillary line and usually the mid axillary line, but the need for a longer flap mandates a preliminary delay procedure. The width of the flap is according to need. Usually direct closure of the donor site is possible by advancement of the lower skin edge, aided if necessary by extensive undermining to release the subcutaneous fibrous attachments to the iliac crest. A skin graft is rarely needed. On elevation of the flap, inclusion of the underlying deep fascia enhances viability, while cautious dissection medially over the rectus sheath is essential.

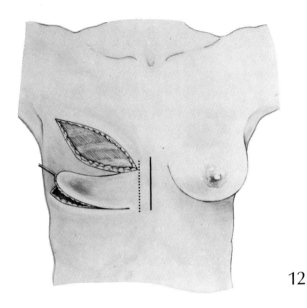

12

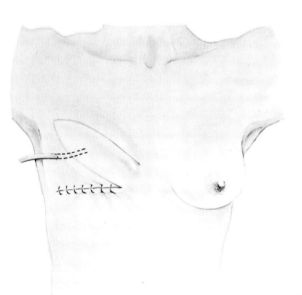

13

TRANSPOSITION OF THE GREATER OMENTUM

14 & 15

The greater omentum maintains viability from either of its axial vessels, the left and right gastroepiploic arteries. When transposed extra-abdominally it provides a satisfactory coverage for virtually any anterior chest wall defect, and provides an ideal vascularized bed for the final coverage provided by a split-thickness skin graft. At operation the omentum is meticulously dissected off the transverse mesocolon; the entire series of short gastric vessels is then ligated, close to the greater curvature of the stomach, so preserving the gastroepiploic arcade. According to the region of the chest being covered and after digitally confirming the patency of the intended axial vessel, the omentum is liberated from the opposite end.

A tunnel of adequate dimensions is created, passing obliquely through the musculature over the subcostal margin, and continued subcutaneously to the lower edge of the defect of the chest wall. The omentum is passed through the tunnel, then spread out over the defect, where it is tacked into position without tension and immediately covered with a skin graft.

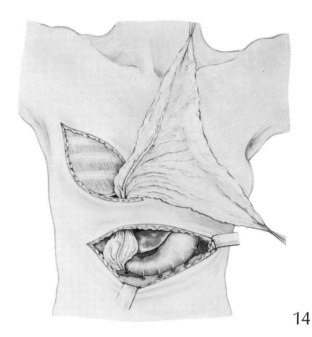

14

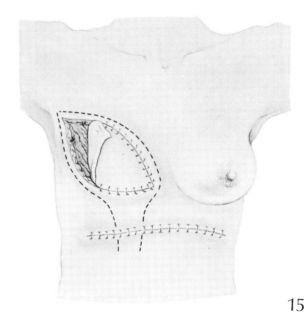

15

References

1. Tansini, I. Nuovo processo per l'amputazione della mammella per cancro. Riforma Medica 1896; 12: 3

2. Tansini, I. Sopra il mio Nuovo Processo di amputazione della mamella. Riforma Medica (Palermo, Napoli) 1906; 15: 757A

3. Hutchins, E. H. A method for the prevention of elephantiasis chirurgica. Surgery, Gynaecology and Obstetrics 1939; 69: 795–804

Further reading

Arnold, P. G., Pairolero, P. C. Use of pectoralis major muscle flaps to repair defects of anterior chest wall. Plastic and Reconstructive Surgery 1979; 63: 205–213

Bostwick, J., Nahai, F., Wallace, J. G., Vasconez, L. O. Sixty latissimus dorsi flaps. Plastic and Reconstructive Surgery 1979; 63: 31–41

Davis, W. M., McCraw, J. B., Carraway, J. H. Use of a direct, transverse, thoracoabdominal flap to close difficult wounds of the thorax and upper extremity. Plastic and Reconstructive Surgery 1977; 60: 526–533

Jurkiewicz, M. J., Arnold, P. G. The omentum: an account of its use in the reconstruction of the chest wall. Annals of Surgery 1977; 185: 548–554

Maxwell, G. P. Iginio Tansini and the origin of the latissimus dorsi musculocutaneous flap. Plastic and Reconstructive Surgery 1980; 65: 686–692

Maxwell, G. P., McGibbon, B. M., Hoopes, J. E. Vascular considerations in use of a latissimus dorsi myocutaneous flap after mastectomy with axillary dissection. Plastic and Reconstructive Surgery 1979; 64: 771–780

Mendelson, B. C. The latissimus dorsi flap for breast reconstruction. Australian and New Zealand Journal of Surgery 1980; 50: 200–204

Mendelson, B. C., Masson, J. K. Treatment of chronic radiation injury over the shoulder with a latissimus dorsi myocutaneous flap. Plastic and Reconstructive Surgery 1977; 60: 681–691

Olivari, N. The latissimus flap. British Journal of Plastic Surgery 1976; 29: 126–128

Olivari, N. Use of thirty latissimus dorsi flaps. Plastic and Reconstructive Surgery 1979; 64: 654–661

Purpura, F. Tansini method for cure of cancer of the breast. Lancet 1908; 1: 634–637

Breast reconstruction after modified-radical and radical mastectomy

Ernest D. Cronin MD, FACS
Plastic Surgery Section,
St Joseph Hospital, Houston, Texas

Thomas D. Cronin MD, FACS
Clinical Professor of Plastic Surgery,
Baylor College of Medicine, Houston, Texas

Introduction

After a woman has had a mastectomy, aimed at curing her of cancer, she may suffer a devastating emotional shock because she feels mutilated by the loss of a breast. The physician would both like to cure his patient and restore her to her original condition, so far as it is possible.

Several factors have made breast reconstruction feasible and easier in many cases.

1. The early discovery of lesions, because of periodic self-examination by women and the use of screening procedures such as mammography or xeromammography, allows surgery of a less radical nature to be done, thereby making simpler reconstructive techniques possible.
2. The realization by general surgeons that in most cases of breast cancer, the pectoralis major muscle may be preserved without altering the survival rate, simplifies reconstruction.
3. The development of the Silastic gel implantable breast prosthesis by Cronin and Gerow[1] has greatly simplified the construction of a breast mound.
4. The development of new skin and musculocutaneous flaps has facilitated breast reconstruction.

Preoperative

Indications

A strongly motivated patient is mandatory. There must also be reasonable assurance that the surgeon has accomplished complete local eradication of the tumour.

Contraindications

Reconstruction is not performed after mastectomy for inflammatory carcinoma, very large aggressive tumours, or extensive axillary metastasis. In essence, we would not wish to attempt reconstruction on any patient likely to have a local recurrence.

Timing

In favourable cases, reconstruction of the breast is delayed for a few months after the mastectomy to allow the tissues to soften and return to normal. Also, psychologically, the woman is more likely to appreciate a reconstructed breast (which will be less than perfect) if she has had an opportunity to compare it with the flat, scarred chest. If the patient receives postoperative irradiation, the reconstruction is delayed for one year. In patients with aggressive tumours and an increased likelihood of local recurrence, a delay of 3 years might be considered.

The operations

Three techniques will be considered. If the surgeon has done a modified radical mastectomy with a transverse or oblique incision, and has left reasonably thick skin flaps, the surgeon may be able to insert a Silastic gel prosthesis either under the skin flaps alone, or preferably under the pectoralis major muscle, which provides better cover and minimizes the tendency to fibrous capsule formation. In cases of radical mastectomy, or in cases of modified-radical mastectomy where the skin flaps are very thin and closely adherent to the chest wall, additional skin coverage is added by use of the thoracoepigastric flap or the latissimus dorsi musculocutaneous flap.

WITHOUT ADDITIONAL SKIN FLAP

1

When there is adequate loose and thick flap coverage after modified-radical mastectomy, a breast reconstruction may be accomplished without the use of flaps. The horizontal scar is most favourable as this allows for some undermining and advancement of the skin from below as in a reverse abdominoplasty. The old horizontal scar is either excised, or incised, and then minimal undermining between the subcutaneous tissue and the pectoralis major muscle is performed.

2

The pectoralis major is then split parallel to its fibres for 6 or 7 cm. A plane of dissection is developed between the pectoralis major muscle and the pectoralis minor. A fibreoptic headlight and long retractors to facilitate the dissection under direct vision are used. Superiorly, the dissection is in the loose plane between the pectoralis major and the chest wall. Laterally, the pectoralis major is also separated from the pectoralis minor, which is left attached to the chest wall. The pocket is extended almost to the clavicle, taking care to avoid the thoracoacromial vessels. Medially, the dissection continues to the origin of the pectoralis major muscle, and in the medial and inferior portion of the pocket a portion of the origin may be cut, if necessary, to accommodate the proper-sized implant. Inferiorly and laterally the pocket is usually continued under the serratus anterior and external oblique until the corresponding inframammary line is reached. Laterally, the pectoralis minor muscle is separated from under the surface of the pectoralis major muscle so that the cavity is extended to the midaxillary line. The electrosurgical knife may facilitate this dissection. It is important to dissect inferiorly so that with an implant in place, the inframammary fold is at the same level as the opposite breast.

Placing the patient in a sitting position by flexing the operating table will enable a better evaluation to be made of the size, shape and position of the reconstructed breast with relation to the other breast. After the pocket has been completed and meticulous haemostasis has been obtained the space is irrigated copiously with saline. A percutaneous plastic catheter is placed into the pocket for instillation of Kenalog (triamcinolone acetonide) 40 mg + bacitracin 50 000 units in 30 ml volume after wound closure. This is agitated to create a foam before instillation.

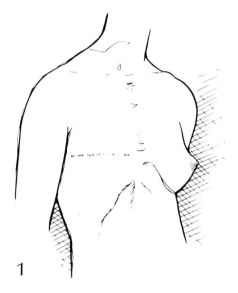

1

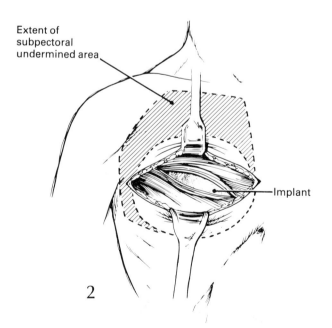

Extent of
subpectoral
undermined area

Implant

2

3

The selected implant is then inserted and the wound closed. Occasionally, suction drainage may be used; if so, the Kenalog and bacitracin solution is instilled after removal of the drain at 24 or 48 h. First, the pectoralis muscle is closed with interrupted absorbable sutures. Then the subcutaneous layer is closed with absorbable sutures and the skin is closed with a subcuticular 3/0 monofilament suture. Occasionally, when the muscle is loose but the skin seems inadequate, a split-thickness skin graft may be placed directly on the muscle to prevent a tight closure. This will blend best if there is little subcutaneous tissue on the skin flaps. Nipple-areola reconstruction is usually delayed 2 or 3 months.

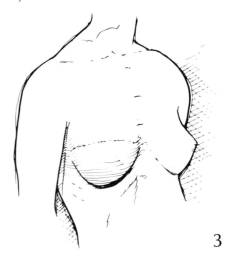

3

THORACOEPIGASTRIC FLAP

4

When a patient presents after a modified-radical mastectomy with tight and thin or scarred skin flaps, the use of the thoracoepigastric flap may be the answer for additional skin coverage. It is best suited for modified cases with oblique or vertical scars. This flap is based on perforating vessels from the superior epigastric artery, specifically a large lateral branch. The flap can be transposed in one stage if it extends only to the midaxillary line. It is usually about 10 cm in width. When a longer flap is needed, multiple delays may be necessary. In the first delay, the flap is elevated as in the illustration, leaving a central bridge undisturbed. The second delay procedure consists of incision and elevation of the bridge area only, 1 or 2 weeks later.

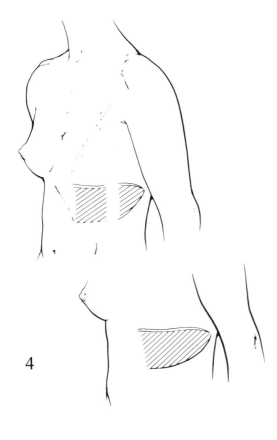

4

5

At the third procedure, the entire flap may be elevated and transferred. The flap is elevated beneath the fascia and transposed after opening or excising the old scar. Minimal undermining of the skin flaps is done.

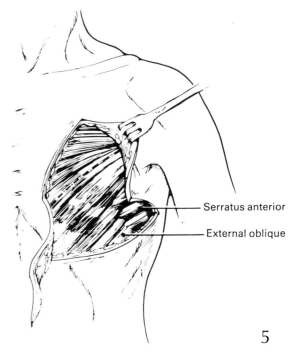

Serratus anterior

External oblique

5

6

The pectoralis major muscle is then split parallel to its fibres and the dissection plane is developed beneath it and over the pectoralis minor muscle. Inferiorly and laterally, the dissection continues beneath the external oblique and serratus anterior to ensure adequate coverage of the implant and adequate extent of the pocket. After haemostasis is obtained, the cavity is irrigated with saline. A percutaneous plastic catheter, for later instillation of Kenalog 40 mg + bacitracin 50 000 units, is inserted. The muscle is then closed with 3/0 absorbable simple interrupted sutures.

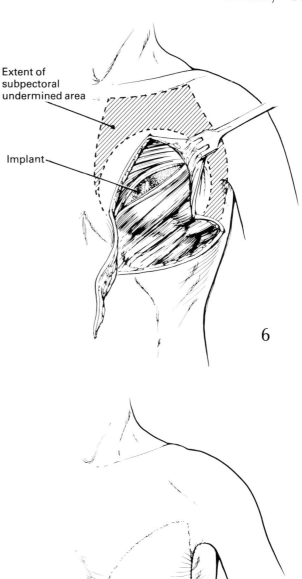

6

7

The thoracoepigastric flap is rotated and sutured in place with 3/0 absorbable suture in the subcutaneous layer and 3/0 monofilament suture in the subcuticular layer. The donor area may be closed primarily by undermining inferiorly toward the iliac crest. Flexing the table will facilitate the closure. The nipple-areola complex is reconstructed 2 or 3 months later to allow for changes in the breast contour with healing.

7

LATISSIMUS DORSI MUSCULOCUTANEOUS FLAP
(see also chapter on 'Chest wall coverage after radical surgery' pp. 306–315)

8

The latissimus dorsi musculocutaneous flap is the most versatile flap available and in radical mastectomy cases is now used almost exclusively. It is able to replace a broad expanse of muscle over the anterior chest, as well as provide additional skin. A patent thoracodorsal artery is assumed to be present if function of the latissimus muscle can be demonstrated.

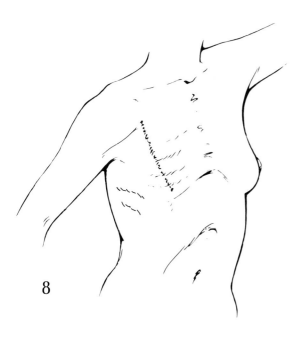

8

9

When the skin portion is to fall in an oblique fashion on the anterior chest, the design of the flap on the back is as shown. The skin island is outlined in an oblique manner so that it overlies the latissimus dorsi muscle from which it obtains its blood supply. The latissimus dorsi is a broad, thin, fan-shaped muscle arising from the lower six thoracic lumbar and sacral vertebrae and the posterior crest of the ilium. The insertion is on the intertubercular groove of the humerus. The muscle's function is to extend, adduct and rotate the arm medially. However, patients hardly notice any functional change with the use of this flap as the teres major takes over. There is a dominant vascular pedicle arising on the undersurface of the muscle about 10 cm from its insertion. The thoracodorsal vessel is accompanied by the thoracodorsal nerve and two venae comitantes. The skin is supplied by small musculocutaneous vessels. First the skin island is incised. This may be as large as 10 by 20 cm and still allow for primary closure of the donor site. Care must be taken not to shear the skin and subcutaneous tissue from the muscle.

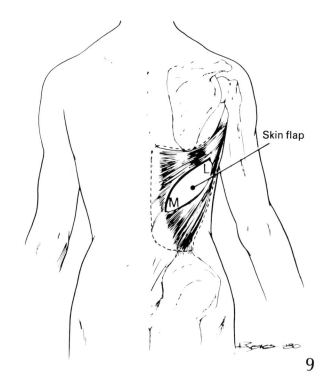

Skin flap

9

10

Next, the dissection plane is developed between the subcutaneous tissue and the muscle, peripherally, around the island to outline the muscle totally. The upper edge is found at about the level of the inferior edge of the scapula. The anterior border of the muscle is also delineated. Next, a dissection plane is developed beneath the muscle. Some care must be taken so as to separate the serratus anterior muscles which tend to interdigitate with the latissimus. When most of the undermining is done, the muscle is incised near the origin medially and inferiorly.

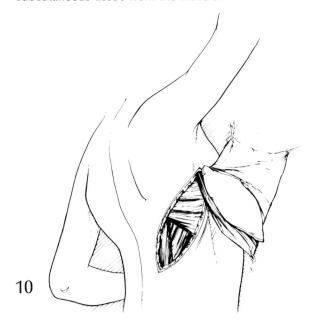

10

11

The muscle is then elevated and dissection superiorly beneath the muscle is completed, taking care not to damage the thoracodorsal neurovascular bundle superiorly.

Next, a tunnel is developed from the posterior wound subcutaneously to join with the anterior wound which is usually placed in the old scar. The tunnel is made as superiorly as possible. Then, the skin and muscle flap is tunnelled through and brought out onto the anterior chest and the posterior wound is closed primarily. This is facilitated by flexing the table. At completion of this closure, the patient is moved from the lateral decubitus position to the supine position.

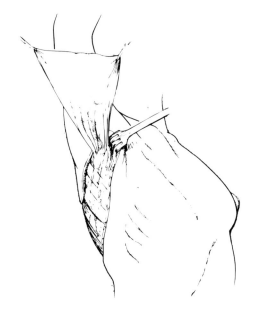

11

12

The pocket on the anterior chest is then completed. A wide subcutaneous or possibly subpectoral pocket if the pectoral muscle is still present is made, and the latissimus is rotated to the anterior position.

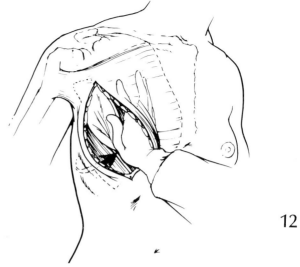

12

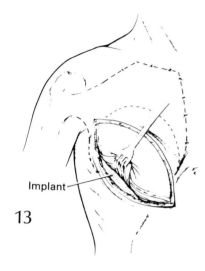

Implant

13

13

Following this, the muscle is spread out widely on the anterior chest and secured with permanent sutures on the edge of the pocket.

14

The implant is then inserted beneath the musculocutaneous flap and muscle and skin closure completed. This flap allows for an adequate amount of skin coverage and also muscle to help fill in when the ribs are showing prominently.

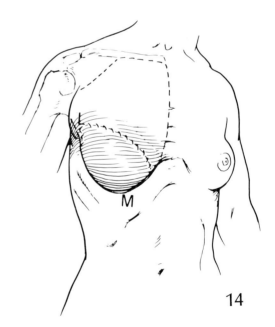

14

15

The nipple-areola reconstruction is usually delayed for a few months.

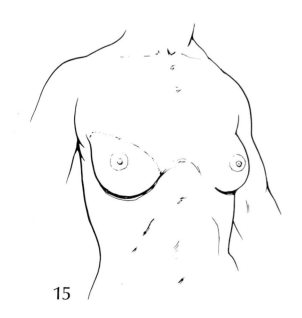

15

NIPPLE-AREOLA RECONSTRUCTION

The nipple-areola is usually reconstructed a few months after the breast reconstruction because changes in the contour of the reconstructed breast and the greater mobility in the opposite breast make it difficult to locate the nipple-areola in a symmetrical position primarily. There are two nipple-sharing techniques which are used if the donor nipple is large enough (0.70 times the donor diameter equals the new nipple diameter).

16a–d

The conjoined spiral method

This method utilizes full-thickness nipple-areola grafts. A pattern is made as shown in (*a*). The nipple is bisected and then split in a curvilinear fashion to meet the edge of the areola 180 degrees away (*b*). Each graft is then coiled and sutured to form a new nipple-areola complex (*c*). This is placed on a dermal bed after removal of a split-thickness layer of skin (*d*).

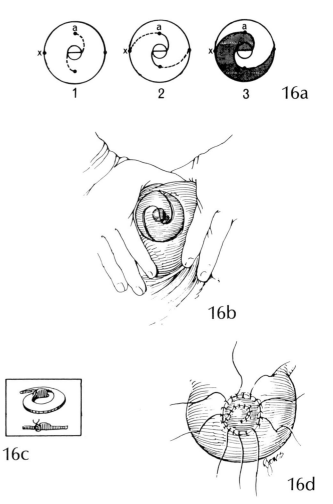

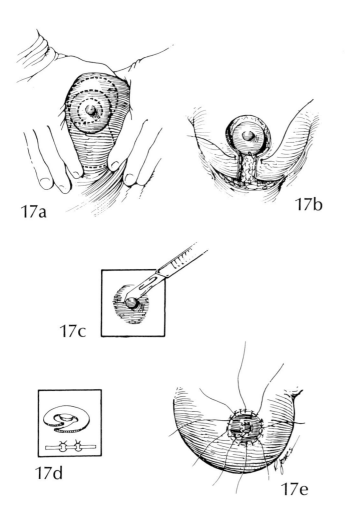

17a–e

The concentric circle method

The concentric circle method uses the excess areola at the periphery of the large areola obtained during reduction mammaplasty or mastopexy on the opposite breast (*a* and *b*).

The areola is used in conjunction with either a composite nipple graft, obtained by taking the top 3 or 4 mm of the opposite nipple, or with a labial graft (*c* and *d*).

The new nipple-areola constructed with the grafts is placed on a dermal bed and a bolster dressing is tied over it (*e*).

18a, b & c

Another satisfactory method for nipple-areola reconstruction utilizes a full-thickness skin graft from the upper, inner thigh area (*a*). The donor site is closed primarily. A nipple donor is taken from the opposite breast by removal of the top 3 or 4mm of the nipple (*b*). Then the full-thickness skin graft together with the composite nipple graft is placed on a dermal bed for reconstruction of the nipple-areola complex (*c*).

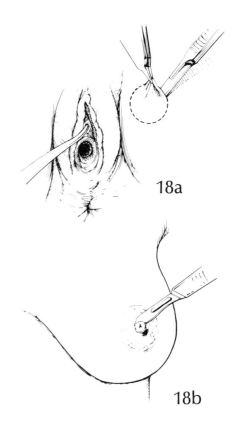

18a

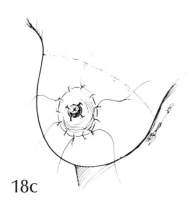

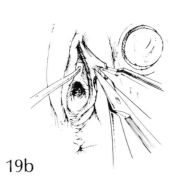

18c

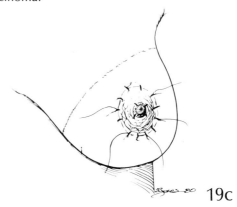

18b

19a, b & c

A fourth method utilizes the same upper inner thigh full-thickness skin graft, together with a portion of full-thickness labium minus to be used as the nipple graft (*a* and *b*). The areola and nipple grafts are then placed on a dermal bed and a tie-over bolster is usually used (*c*).

Labial grafts are usually too darkly pigmented for use as the areola. A small portion of ear lobe may be used for nipple graft. Banking of the nipple-areola complex in the abdominal wall or thigh at the time of the mastectomy has been used but it carries a small risk of transferring carcinoma.

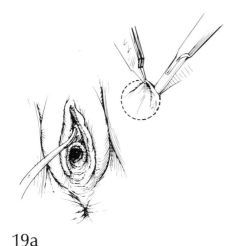

19a

19b

19c

THE OPPOSITE BREAST

Following reconstruction of one breast, consideration must be given to the opposite breast. It may be that no treatment at all is indicated, or possibly procedures such as subcutaneous mastectomy, simple mastectomy, reduction mammaplasty, augmentation mammaplasty or mastopexy may be done.

Conclusions

Facilitation of reconstruction

The general surgeon can facilitate breast reconstruction by preserving the pectoralis major muscle, preserving as much skin as possible and avoiding excessive thinning of skin flaps. In addition, the surgeon should spare the thoracodorsal neurovascular bundle to the latissimus dorsi muscle, and use a horizontal incision or an oblique incision which does not extend far beneath the inframammary crease. Wide retention sutures should be avoided. Care must be taken in selecting candidates for reconstruction and early reconstruction should be avoided when local recurrence is likely.

Problems in breast reconstruction

The main difficulties that exist in breast reconstruction are attaining symmetry of the breasts and nipples, securing adequate projection of the breast mound, obtaining a well-defined inframammary crease, correcting the infraclavicular hollow, recreating the anterior axillary fold and selection of suitable skin for nipple-areola. However, reasonably aesthetic results varying from excellent to fair may be expected in most cases.

Reference

1. Cronin, T. D., Gerow, P. J. Augmentation mammaplasty; a new 'natural feel' prosthesis. Translations of the Third International Congress of Plastic Surgery. Amsterdam; Excerpta Medica, 1963

Further reading

Biggs, T. M., Cronin, T. D. Breast reconstruction following mastectomy. In: Murphy, Gerald P., ed. International advances in surgical oncology, Vol. III, pp. 29–40. New York: Alan R. Liss, 1980

Bostwick, J. Breast reconstruction: a comprehensive approach. Clinics in Plastic Surgery 1979; 6: 143–162

Bostwick, J., Scheflan, M. The latissimus dorsi musculocutaneous flap: a one stage breast reconstruction. Clinics in Plastic Surgery 1980; 7: 71–78

Bostwick, J., Vasconez, L. O., Jurkiewicz, M. J. Breast reconstruction after a radical mastectomy. Plastic and Reconstructive Surgery 1978; 61: 682–693

Bostwick, J., Nahai, F., Wallace, J. G., Vasconez, L. O. Sixty latissimus dorsi flaps. Plastic and Reconstructive Surgery 1979; 63: 31–41

Brent, B., Bostwick, J. Nipple-areola reconstruction with auricular tissues. Plastic and Reconstructive Surgery 1977; 60: 353–361

Cronin, T. D., Cronin, E. D. Reconstruction of the breast following mastectomy for malignancy. In: Marchant, D. J., Nyirjesy, I., eds. Breast disease, pp. 279–285. New York: Grune and Stratton, 1979

Cronin, T. D., Cronin, E. D. Reconstruction of the breast without additional skin or muscle flaps. Clinics in Plastic Surgery 1979; 6: 47–55

Cronin, T. D., Upton, J., McDonough, J. M. Reconstruction of the breast after mastectomy. Plastic and Reconstructive Surgery 1977; 59: 1–14

Maxwell, G. P., McGibbon, B. M., Hoopes, J. E. Vascular considerations in the use of a latissimus dorsi myocutaneous flap after a mastectomy with axillary dissection. Plastic and Reconstructive Surgery 1979; 64: 771–780

McGraw, J. B., Bostwick, J., Horton, C. E. Methods of soft tissue coverage for the mastectomy defect. Clinics in Plastic Surgery 1979; 6: 57

McGraw, J. B., Dibbell, D. G., Carroway, J. H. Clinical definition of independent myocutaneous vascular territories. Plastic and Reconstructive Surgery 1977; 60: 341

Vasconez, L. O., Johnson-Giebink, R., Hall, E. J. Breast reconstruction. Clinics in Plastic Surgery 1980; 7: 79–88

Augmentation mammaplasty

Ernest D. Cronin MD, FACS
Plastic Surgery Section,
St. Joseph Hospital, Houston, Texas

Russell C. Romero DDS, MD
Resident, Plastic Surgery Section,
St. Joseph Hospital, Houston, Texas

Thomas D. Cronin MD, FACS
Clinical Professor of Plastic Surgery,
Baylor College of Medicine, Houston, Texas

Introduction

The modern era of augmentation of the female breast began in 1963, with the introduction of the Silastic gel prosthesis[1]. This soon replaced other less satisfactory methods such as dermal fat grafts, pedicle flaps, implants of plastic sponge or other synthetics, and the dangerous injection of silicone fluid. Since that time, modification in both the implant and technique of operation has occurred. We prefer silicone-gel-filled low-profile-round or round implants. These are seamless, contain no fixation patches and come in numerous sizes. The implants we use most frequently are 200 ml, 235 ml, and 270 ml low-profile-round implants.

Preoperative

Indications

The indications for augmentation mammaplasty are hypoplasia, aplasia, atrophy, asymmetry of the breasts and mild ptosis (if the patient has more than mild ptosis, augmentation will only accentuate the problem). There are no specific age limitations for augmentation mammaplasty, but adequate time should be allowed after puberty for natural development of the breast to be complete.

Patient evaluation

The desire for augmentation mammaplasty must be that of the patient herself and not of others if an optimal result is to be obtained. The physician should determine whether the breasts have always been small or whether there have been changes after pregnancy. Previous biopsies, infections or family history for breast cancer should be taken into consideration.

Physical examination

The breasts should be examined for masses. Xeromammography should be considered if there are any lumps, or if the patient is over 40 years of age.

Asymmetry of the breasts, even if it is minor, should be noted. Often one breast is somewhat larger, and sometimes one nipple may be at a slightly different level from the other. Any discrepancies should be measured preoperatively and pointed out to the patient. The relationship of the breast to the patient's body-build, height and weight must be correlated. Preoperative and postoperative photographs are strongly recommended.

Preoperative discussion

The motivation, desires and expectations of the patient should be elicited; there should then be a thorough discussion of the entire procedure, including placement of incisions and possible complications.

Although the final decision about implant size is usually made by the surgeon at the operating table, the patient's desires and her individual physical characteristics must be expressly kept in mind.

325

Preoperative preparation

The procedure may be performed on an inpatient or outpatient basis, under either general or local anaesthesia; general anaesthesia is preferred.

1

The patient is taken into the surgical suite for preoperative measurements, which are most accurately done in the sitting position. The proposed incision is 5 or 6 cm long. It is placed in the inframammary crease or about 5 cm below the inferior edge of the areola. The innermost extent of the incision is in vertical alignment with the medial edge of the areola. The relative position of the two incisions is checked by measuring the distance from the midline and from the inferior edge of the areola.

The patient is then placed in the supine position for induction of anaesthesia. The hands are placed over the lower abdomen, with the elbows padded and away from the sides. The entire chest, neck and upper abdomen are prepared as for any major operation. The operative field is then blocked off with four sterile adhesive plastic drapes; paper or cloth drapes are used to complete isolation of the area. Before the procedure, the surgical gloves are wiped with alcohol and then with saline, to rid them of powder.

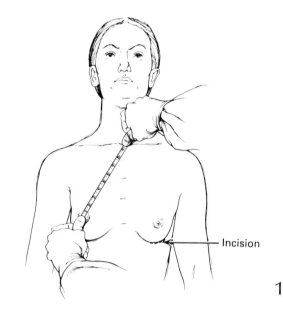

Incision

1

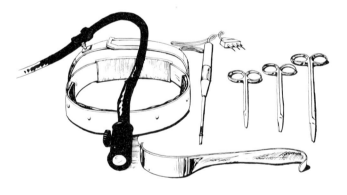

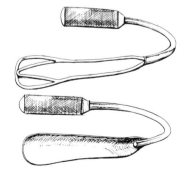

2

2

Instruments

In addition to the usual surgical instruments, the following items are needed: fibreoptic headlight, electrosurgical knife, insulated extender, Metzenbaum scissors up to 28 cm in length, special long retractors (e.g. Biggs retractors, Paget instruments, 2838 Warwick TFWY, Kansas City, MO 64108; or Cronin retractors, Royal Surgical Instruments, PO Box 12662, Houston, TX 77017) and a smooth-surface Deaver retractor.

The operation

3

The incision is made through the skin; then, bevelling slightly superiorly, it is carried down to the fascia overlying the superficial musculature. The dissection is then continued upward superficial to the pectoral fascia and may be performed with either the electrosurgical knife or a scalpel and Metzenbaum scissors of increasing length. If scissors are used, a spreading action with minimal cutting diminishes bleeding. Haemostasis is maintained at all times with the electrocautery. Initially, a sharp rake retractor is used, exerting slight tension at the junction of the breast and muscle fascia. The plane of dissection leaves a layer of fascia on the pectoralis major muscle.

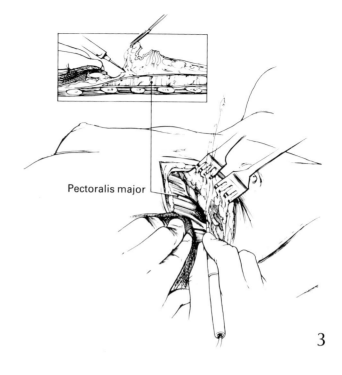

Pectoralis major

3

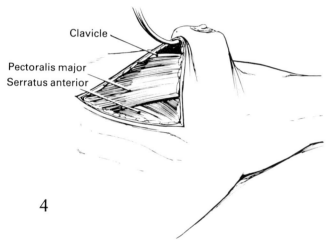

Clavicle

Pectoralis major
Serratus anterior

4

4

A large pocket is then created in this plane between the breast and muscle fascia. As the dissection progresses, special long retractors are used to maintain exposure, and extension devices are used on the electrosurgical instrument so that a large pocket can be created. A fibreoptic headlight gives a good view and is essential.

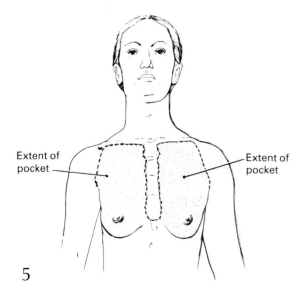

Extent of
pocket

Extent of
pocket

5

Extent of dissection

5

The dissection extends medially to the sternal border, with care being taken to isolate and not cut the perforating branches of the internal mammary vessels. Superiorly the pocket extends to the clavicle. Laterally the entire edge of the pectoralis major muscle is freed, and the dissection extends to the mid-axillary line[2].

6

The illustration shows the internal mammary artery which sends perforating branches through the costal interspaces and through the pectoralis major muscle in the medial aspect of the dissection. Also depicted are the fourth intercostal nerve and its lateral cutaneous branch, which carries sensory innervation to the nipple. In the lateral aspect of the dissection, it is desirable to identify and preserve this branch, which comes through the serratus anterior just lateral to the pectoralis major muscle and enters the undersurface of the breast[3,4].

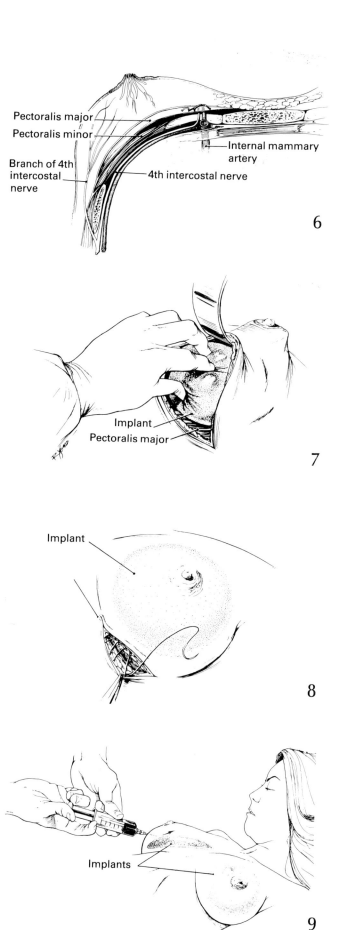

7

Sponges are kept out of the wound to minimize possible foreign-body contamination. When creation of the space is completed, a Deaver retractor is placed in the wound, and trial implants are used to determine the correct size for the prosthesis. The patient may be raised to a sitting position for better evaluation, if desired. Because the implants are not fixed, the spaces created must be symmetrical.

After selection of the prosthesis, the cavity is copiously irrigated with saline to remove all tissue, debris and clotted blood; haemostasis is again checked; and an 18 gauge Intracath Teflon catheter is percutaneously introduced into the pocket. The new implant is immersed in saline before being touched by the surgeon. It is then inserted into the space, with care being taken to minimize contamination.

8

The wound is then closed in layers using 3/0 absorbable suture for deep layer closure, 4/0 absorbable suture at the subcutaneous dermal level and 3/0 monofilament suture for intradermal closure. The subcuticular suture is removed in 10 days. The most commonly used absorbable sutures are Vicryl and Dexon.

9

A solution of 30 ml saline containing bacitracin 50 000 u, oxacillin 125 mg and triamcinolone acetonide 40 mg (Kenalog) is foamed by vigorous aspiration into and expulsion from a syringe, then instilled into the cavity through the plastic catheter. Foaming the solution increases the volume that can be instilled and allows better distribution[5].

Subpectoral implantation

Occasionally a patient with little or no breast development and thin subcutaneous tissue may benefit from subpectoral implantation, to give more coverage for the prosthesis.

10a, b & c

In this case, after the submammary incision is made, the dissection is carried beneath the free edge of the pectoralis major muscle when its inferior and lateral border is reached. Much of the dissection is in the loose areolar plane beneath the pectoralis major muscle and can be performed bluntly. This dissection is superficial to the pectoralis minor muscle. The inferior and medial costal origins of the pectoralis major muscle may be cut if necessary for proper relaxation of the muscle and positioning of the implant.

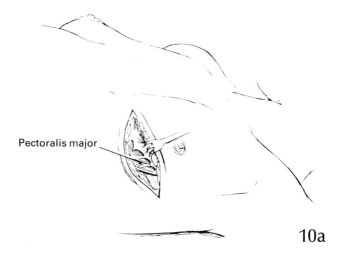

Pectoralis major

10a

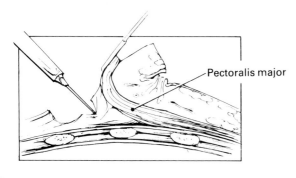

Pectoralis major

10c

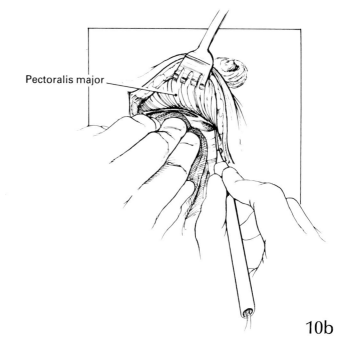

Pectoralis major

10b

11a, b & c

These sagittal views show the relative position of the breast tissue and pectoralis major muscle preoperatively (a) and the prosthesis in a retromammary augmentation (b) and in a subpectoral augmentation (c).

Dressing

The skin closure may be reinforced with Steri-strip tapes; 10 × 10 cm (4 × 4 inch) gauze pads are then placed over the incisions and the nipples. Adhesive-type microfoam tape is placed across the chest in a supportive fashion.

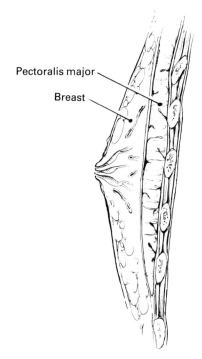

Pectoralis major

Breast

11a

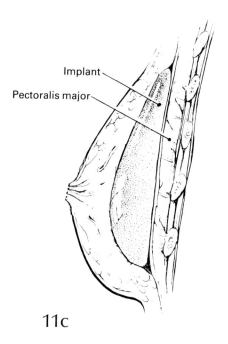

Implant

Pectoralis major

11c

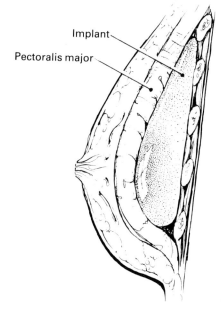

Implant

Pectoralis major

11b

Postoperative care

Whether augmentation of the breast is performed on an inpatient or outpatient basis, the patient should always be seen on the first postoperative day to check for haematoma formation. If a haematoma is recognized, the patient is taken back to the operating room for its evacuation and a careful search for the bleeding point.

12

On the first or second postoperative day, manipulation of the implant within the pocket is begun. The purpose is to move the implant to the extent of the large pocket that has been created, in order to maintain a bursa-like potential space. Using her opposite hand, the patient cups the inferior half of the breast and pushes inward against the ribs, in order to displace the implant superiorly to the full extent of the space. In addition, she will push the implant superomedially and superolaterally.

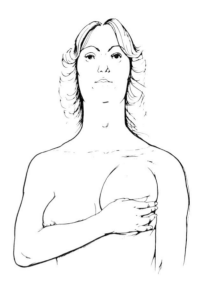

12

During the postoperative period, frequent manipulation of the implants by the patient is encouraged. After the first week, a regular regimen of twice-daily manipulations is then maintained for life.

The patient is allowed to resume most normal activities the day following surgery. Vigorous activity such as tennis or jogging is forbidden for 4–6 weeks.

Complications

Complications most commonly encountered in augmentation mammaplasty are haematoma, infection, hypertrophic scarring, spherical fibrous capsular contracture and alteration of sensation to the nipple-areola complex.

Infection, a serious complication, usually requires the removal of the implant for several months.

The fibrous capsule is the pseudomembranous lining which develops at the interface between the prosthesis and surrounding tissues. This capsule may contract, the result being a firm or distorted-appearing breast. There are varying theories about the cause of fibrous capsular contractures.

In our experience, certain measures will diminish the likelihood of fibrous capsular contractures: creation of a large pocket relative to the size of the implant, instillation of antibiotic and steroid solution into the operative space, administration of systemic antibiotics immediately before and for a short time after the operative procedure, and faithful and regular manipulation of the implant by the patient in the early postoperative course and forever afterward.

References

1. Cronin, T. D., Gerow, E. J. Augmentation mammoplasty: a new 'natural feel' prosthesis. Transactions of the International Congress of Plastic Surgery, pp. 41–49. Amsterdam: Excerpta Medica Foundation, 1964

2. Biggs, T. M., Cukier, J., Worthing, L. F. Augmentation mammaplasty: a review of eighteen years. Presented at the American Society of Plastic and Reconstructive Surgeons Annual Meeting, Sept. 28 – Oct. 3, 1980, New Orleans, La.

3. Farina, M. A., Newby, B. G., Alani, H. M. Innervation of the nipple-areola complex. Plastic and Reconstructive Surgery 1980; 66: 497–501

4. Courtiss, E. H., Goldwyn, R. M. Breast sensation before and after plastic surgery. Plastic and Reconstructive Surgery 1976; 58: 1–13

5. Dubin, D. B. The etiology, pathophysiology, predictability, and early detection of spherical scar contracture of the breast: a detailed protocol for prevention of spherical scar contracture of the breast. Presented at the American Society for Aesthetic Plastic Surgery Annual Meeting, May 18–22, 1980, Orlando, Florida

Thyroid needle aspiration and biopsy

Eugene D. Furth MD
Chairman, Department of Medicine, School of Medicine,
East Carolina University, Greenville, North Carolina

Introduction

Nodules of the thyroid are common and usually benign. Identification of the rare malignant lesion should begin with various non-invasive means, including a careful history of previous childhood X-ray treatment to the head and neck, evaluation of the rapidity of development of the nodule, with or without adjacent nodes, clinical impression on palpation, and appraisal of the degree of function by either radioiodine or technetium scanning and ultrasonography, in order to differentiate between solid and cystic lesions. One can then proceed if necessary to needle aspiration and biopsy, which is the most direct and reliable method for diagnosis of thyroid malignancy and other thyroid disorders, short of open thyroid biopsy.

General considerations

A detailed historical review and summary of fine needle aspiration, cutting needle biopsy and aspiration needle biopsy has recently appeared[1, 2]. Needle biopsy is technically simple. Cutting needle biopsy is usually limited to nodules of at least 2 cm or larger, while aspiration needle biopsy is employed for cysts and the smaller nodules, provided they are not extremely hard.

Needle aspiration and biopsy should be performed only if a competent trained histopathologist is available for interpretation of tissue. A member of the department of pathology should be available during the procedure to process aspirated material.

Materials and methods

Materials at hand before the procedure is begun should include one or two disposable 10 or 20 ml syringes; 22, 25, or 27 gauge needles 3.8 cm (1.5 inches) in length for fine needle aspiration; 16 gauge needles for needle aspiration biopsy; and Tru-Cut cutting needles (Baxter–Travenol Laboratories, Michigan) or Silverman needles for cutting needle biopsy. Single-handed aspiration can be facilitated by use of a Cameco syringe pistol (Precision Dynamics Corporation, California). Alcohol preparation sponges, sterile gauze pads, glass slides with frosted end, Papanicolaou's stain for fine needle aspiration, Bouin's solution for fixation, and paper towels and/or filter paper and appropriate specimen jars for tissue should be at the bedside.

Fine needle aspiration

1 & 2

The needle biopsies are usually performed on an out-patient basis. The patient is placed in a recumbent position with a pillow under the shoulders to hyperextend the neck. The skin is cleansed with an alcohol swab. Lignocaine may be used to infiltrate the tissue if multiple punctures or cutting needle biopsy are anticipated, but aspiration of cysts does not usually require anaesthesia. A 25 gauge needle is attached to a 10 ml Luer–Lok disposable syringe mounted in the Cameco pistol holder. A right-handed person fixes the nodule with the left hand. The needle is then inserted directly into the nodule.

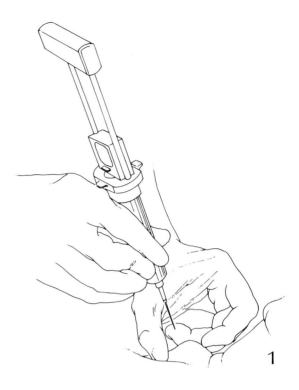

1

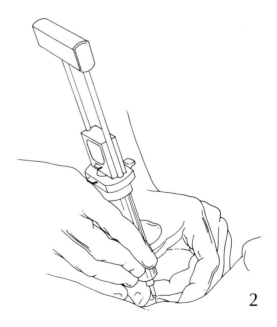

2

3

The barrel of the syringe is withdrawn and then allowed to return to the initial position. No material should enter the barrel of the syringe unless fluid is being aspirated, in which case the liquid may be dark brown or yellowish brown, suggesting degeneration or old blood. Should difficulty be encountered in aspirating the cystic material, which may be gelatinous, a 20 gauge needle may be used instead.

Before removal, the syringe and the needle may be rotated 360° with suction, to use the bevel as a cutting edge. Clots in the syringe during aspiration of cysts may be prevented by drawing up to 1 ml of citrate solution or heparin before aspiration. Cystic fluid can be poured out onto paper towel or filter paper for identification of tissue, which may then be fixed as described below.

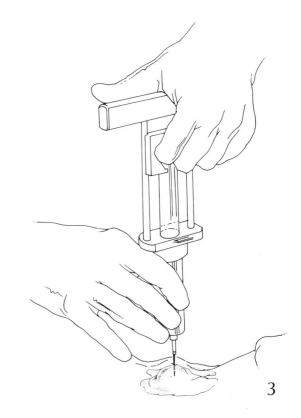

3

4

After aspiration has been completed, the needle is withdrawn from the nodule and detached from the syringe. A few millilitres of air are taken into the syringe, the needle is reattached and air is blown through the needle over a glass slide.

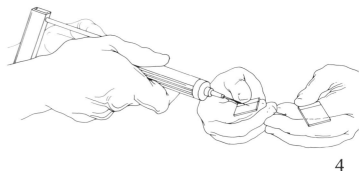

4

The material is then examined for quantity or quality. Four to six aspirates should be taken from different parts of the nodule. Cystic fluid should be saved for centrifugation and cytopathology. Some investigators recommend spraying the smear of cyst fluid with a fixative such as hairspray to prevent drying. An alternative is to place the liquid material directly on a slide to which fixative has been previously added. The material should then be stained by the Papanicolaou technique for the usual cytological criteria of benign versus malignant cells. It may be desirable to have the patient wait while the tissue is being examined, in order to ascertain whether an adequate sample has been taken.

Cutting needle biopsy

Cutting needle biopsy may be performed with either a Tru-Cut needle or a Vim–Silverman needle. The patient is positioned in a manner similar to that for fine needle biopsy. The skin is anaesthetized with xylocaine and nicked with a scalpel blade in order to facilitate insertion of the needle. The needle should be inserted in a direction parallel to the long axis of the neck in order to avoid damage to major vessels or nerves. It is essential that the Tru-Cut needle be inserted through the skin and the thyroid capsule prior to extension and return of the cutting obturator (see chapter on 'Operations for benign breast disease', pp. 239–253, for illustrations).

Complications

Small haematomas and recurrent laryngeal nerve damage from cutting needle biopsies have been reported. Recurrence of cysts following therapeutic aspiration may necessitate reaspiration. Cutting needle biopsy and aspiration needle biopsy should be employed with extreme caution for nodules at the thoracic inlet, since haemorrhage and airway obstruction may occur. Seeding of the needle track with tumour is exceedingly rare. It may be extremely difficult to make the differential diagnosis between well differentiated follicular carcinoma and follicular adenoma, but this is also true of fixed tissue removed at surgery.

Results

Most histopathologists will interpret tissue as 'cancer probable', 'cancer possible' or 'tissue benign'. Follicular carcinoma may be confused with follicular adenoma, and Hashimoto's thyroiditis may be confused with lymphoma of the thyroid. Fine needle aspiration, cutting needle biopsy or aspiration needle biopsy has a 90 per cent accuracy when interpreted as 'cancer probable'. Approximately 20 per cent of fine needle aspirations interpreted as 'cancer possible' and 10 per cent of cutting needle biopsies categorized as 'cancer possible' prove to be malignant. When tissue has been interpreted as 'benign', diagnosis is 95 per cent accurate.

References

1. Lowhagen, T., Willem, J. F., Lundell, G., Sundblad, R., Granberg, P. O. Aspiration biopsy, cytology and diagnosis of thyroid cancer. World Journal of Surgery 1981; 5: 61–73

2. Hamburger, J. I., Miller, J. M., Kini, S. Clinical-pathological evaluation of thyroid nodules. Handbook and atlas. Limited edition, private publication, 440 Prudential Town Center, Suite 275, Southfield, MI 48075.

Illustrations by Carol J. Pienta

Thyroglossal duct cyst

Walter J. Pories MD, FACS
Professor and Chairman, Department of Surgery, School of Medicine,
East Carolina University, Greenville, North Carolina

1

Presentation

The most common cause of a midline cervical lesion is a thyroglossal duct remnant. The usual presentation is that of a soft rubbery mass, 2–5 cm in diameter, in or just beside the midline near the hyoid bone. Although most are diagnosed during childhood, they are encountered in all ages and have been reported in the elderly. Frequently the lesions are inflamed and there is a history of previous flare-ups or even previous drainage procedures.

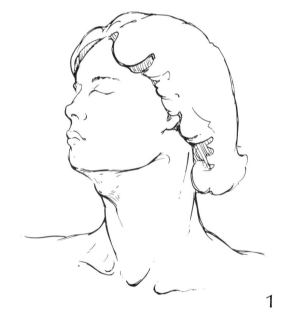

1

336

2

Position of thyroid tissue

Thyroid tissue demonstrates more variation in position and in form than any other gland. It has been identified in humans from the foramen caecum of the tongue to the heart and diaphragm.

Thyroid tissue begins to form during the fourth week of embryonic life as a ventral diverticulum in an epithelial thickening of the ventral pharyngeal wall – the tuberculum impar. This new tissue grows caudally in the loose sub-pharyngeal plane of mesoderm through tissue where the body of the hyoid bone will develop. It is this intimate developmental relationship to the hyoid bone which explains the necessity for excising the centre of the hyoid bone to avoid recurrence. Thyroid remnants may occur at any level along the descending thyroglossal tract, even if normal thyroid is present. Indeed, such rests may represent the entire functioning thyroid when there is failure of the thyroid to migrate to its normal position.

The duct usually fibroses and becomes obliterated, but remnants may persist anywhere along its course as simple cysts or fistulas, especially in the area of the hyoid bone. The amount of thyroid tissue in such cysts or fistulas is usually negligible.

Thyroglossal duct cysts should be removed surgically because of their propensity for recurrent infection, their unattractive appearance and their occasional tendency to become malignant. Although most such cancers are papillary adenocarcinomas, squamous carcinoma has also been reported[1].

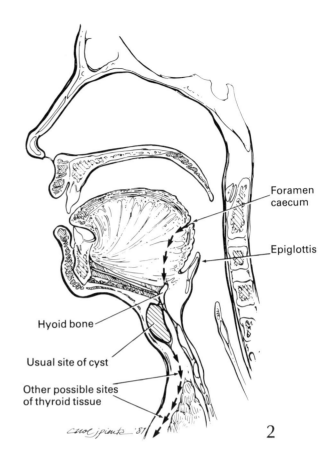

Foramen caecum

Epiglottis

Hyoid bone

Usual site of cyst

Other possible sites of thyroid tissue

2

Preoperative

Preoperative study does not need to be extensive but should include a bimanual oral examination and a thyroid radionucleide scan to determine the location of all thyroid tissues before proceeding with excision of the cyst and tract. Infection can usually be avoided by administering cephazolin 1g intravenously 2h before surgery, at the beginning of the operation and every 6h for 24–36h after operation.

Nasotracheal anaesthesia is preferred but orotracheal intubation is acceptable. The mouth should be draped into the surgical field in order to allow intraoral manipulation of the posterior tongue during the procedure.

If a sinus is present, it is occasionally useful to inject the tract with a dilute solution of methylene blue.

The operation

The incision

3 & 4

The incision is made transversely directly over the cyst in the infrahyoid region. The platysma muscle is divided and reflected, the cyst is exposed and gently dissected from the surrounding tissues. Usually an identifiable cleavage plane guides the dissection over most of the cyst's surface. The dissection is pursued toward the base of the cyst and along the tract until the hyoid bone is encountered. This excision is directed superiorly and posteriorly in a sagittal plane at an angle of approximately 45° to the long axis of the body.

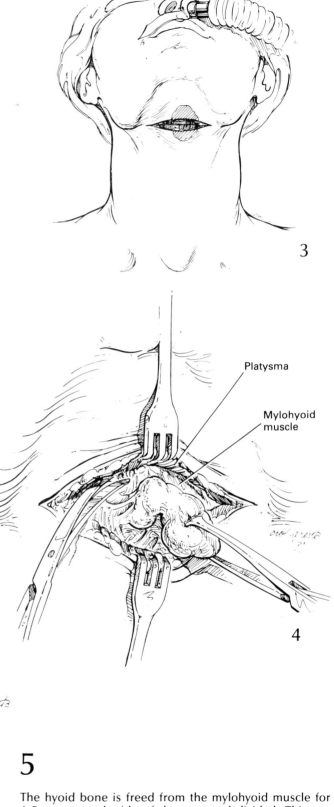

3

Platysma

Mylohyoid muscle

4

5

5

The hyoid bone is freed from the mylohyoid muscle for 4–5 mm on each side of the tract and divided. This can usually be done with stout scissors, but a small bone cutter may be needed in adults.

6

The dissection is then pursued further along the tract, continuing the excision through the mylohyoid raphe and the geniohyoid and genioglossus muscles, avoiding the fibrous scarred tissues of the tract. This produces a core of tissue 5–10 mm in diameter. Care must be taken not to pull too hard on the specimen; the tract is easily torn apart.

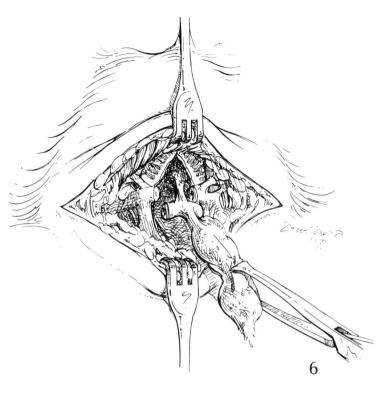

6

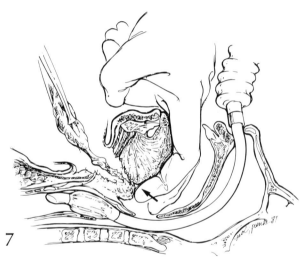

7

7

The dissection is aided considerably by a finger inside the mouth which elevates the foramen caecum and defines the base of the tract. The specimen is then divided just below the oral mucosa; if the mouth is entered during the excision, the mucosa should be closed with one or two sutures of absorbable material.

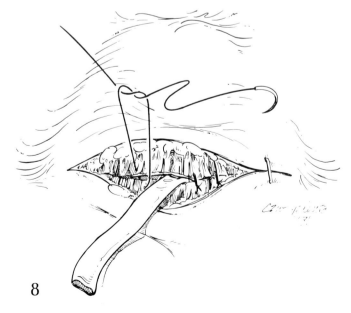

8

8

Closure

The hyoid bone does not need to be repaired. A small rubber drain should be left in the site of the tract and cyst; it can be brought out through the wound.

Closure should be loose, particularly in cases with a history of infection. Generally a few absorbable sutures in the platysma suffice. Skin may be closed with sutures or staples.

Postoperative care

The postoperative period is usually benign. Patients may be fed the day after surgery and usually go home on the following day. The drain can be removed 24h after surgery and the skin sutures or staples may come out at 72h.

Results

Results have been excellent if the central portion of the hyoid bone is excised. Deane and Telander[2] reported a 4 per cent recurrence rate in 277 cases, with a minimum of one year follow-up, but only 2 of these 11 patients had neither infection nor a previous attempt at excision. In their total list of 338 patients, 8 patients experienced major complications and 2 of these died. Their minor and major complications are shown in *Table 1*.

Table 1 Complications of surgery for thyroglossal duct remnants in 338 patients[2]

Complications	No. of patients
Major	
Haematoma with respiratory obstruction	3
Respiratory obstruction without haematoma	2
Postoperative bleeding requiring transfusion	1
Postoperative hepatic necrosis	1
Moderate to severe pneumonitis	1
	8
Minor	
Wound haematoma	12
Wound infection	9
Poor cosmetic result requiring scar revision	3
Wound granuloma	1
Parotitis	1
Temporary paresis of marginal branch of VIIth nerve	1
	27

References

1. Benveniste, G. L., Hunter, R., Cook, M. G. Squamous carcinoma of thyroglossal duct remnants: a case report and review of the literature. Australian and New Zealand Journal of Surgery 1980; 50: 53–55

2. Deane, S. A., Telander, R. L. Surgery for thyroglossal duct and branchial cleft anomalies. American Journal of Surgery 1978; 136: 348–353

Illustrations by Carol J. Pienta

Thyroidectomy: subtotal lobectomy and lobectomy

T. S. Reeve CBE, FACS, FRACS
Professor and Chairman, Department of Surgery,
The University of Sydney, Royal North Shore Hospital,
St Leonards, New South Wales

Preoperative

Indications

The indications for thyroidectomy are both absolute and relative.

Absolute

Compression of the trachea.
Suspicion of malignancy.

Relative

Thyrotoxicosis not responsive to drug therapy.
Thyrotoxicosis in the young, under 45 years of age.
Cosmetic reasons.

Choice of operation

Total thyroidectomy, total thyroid lobectomy, subtotal thyroid lobectomy and bilateral subtotal thyroidectomy are the common operations performed on the thyroid gland. Local lymph node excision or modified radical cervical lymph node dissection may be added to total or near-total thyroidectomy for malignancy to complete local therapy of the disease.

Total thyroidectomy is usually reserved for treatment of thyroid malignancy. In some cases of thyrotoxicosis with severe exophthalmos total thyroidectomy (removal of target organ) may be indicated. In some patients with nodular goitre no normal tissue is present on gross review of the gland and total gland excision is practised if the surgeon is comfortable with this approach. Many surgeons leave a small rim of thyroid tissue to protect the parathyroid glands.

Single thyroid nodules are best treated by total thyroid lobectomy. Subtotal lobectomy is usually reserved for thyroiditis or to preserve the segment of thyroid in the tracheo-oesophageal gutter which frequently appears to be normal, in spite of otherwise generalized thyroid abnormality. Total lobectomy of the involved lobe is suggested as the form of biopsy in the management of single thyroid nodules. If the lesion proves malignant the surgeon can remove the remaining thyroid lobe without imposing any risk on the vital structures remaining in the bed of the original lobe.

Bilateral subtotal thyroidectomy is performed for thyrotoxicosis, 3–4 g of tissue being left on each side. It is also performed for multinodular goitre, when varying amounts of tissue may be left. The thyroid isthmus should always be removed when excisional thyroid surgery is performed, thus allowing easy access to the trachea in case of airway occlusion during the 24 h after surgery. In addition, a remnant of thyroid isthmus may enlarge after thyroidectomy and produce an unsightly and disturbing pretracheal lump.

Evaluation and preparation for surgery

All the following prerequisites should be met before progressing to thyroidectomy.

1. The function of the thyroid gland should be assessed clinically and by laboratory tests. This is essential if operation on patients with unexpected hypo- or hyperthyroidism is to be avoided.

   On presentation a full history and thorough total body physical examination should be carried out. When a morphological or functional disorder of the thyroid is either diagnosed or suspected after this review, further evaluation is necessary for optimal decision-making. Special note of thyroid nodules and enlarged cervical lymph nodes should be made.

   Thyroid function should be normal (euthyroid) before any surgery is undertaken, and a number of investigations may be done to verify euthyroidism. The choice varies with individual centres.

   (a) *In vivo.* Radioiodine uptake: if the radioiodine (^{131}I) uptake is elevated attempts to suppress it with thyroid hormone can be undertaken; suppression of uptake confirms euthyroidism and failure to suppress confirms the diagnosis of thyrotoxicosis. With improved *in vitro* tests this investigation is less frequently performed but may prove useful in confirming the appropriate diagnosis in difficult cases.

   (b) *In vitro.* A number of tests are available: serum triiodothyronine (T3) measured by radioimmunoassay provides accurate values and it is to be remembered that some patients may have only this hormone elevated. Serum thyroxine (T4) and serum levels of thyroid-stimulating hormone (TSH) are readily measurable. Where possible all three tests should be done to provide a basis on which to make a full assessment of thyroid function. A single test is insufficient to give a definite answer.

2. The distribution of function in the thyroid can be assessed by scanning patients who have thyroid disease with isotopes: ^{131}I and ^{99m}Tc and the more frequently used. 'Cold' areas on the scan should alert the observer to the risk of malignancy.

   Ultrasound scans can also be useful in this area of investigation. They can differentiate cystic from solid lesions. Low reflectance solid areas are said to be more common in malignant disease.

3. Fine needle aspiration cytology is now being used quite widely to screen thyroid nodules (*see* chapter on 'Thyroid needle aspiration and biopsy', pp. 332–335). This technique requires that both cytologist and surgeon acquaint themselves with the limits of its accuracy and relate it to both the clinical findings and laboratory data. When fully assessed it may become a standard investigation.

4. Examination and recording of the function of the larynx by indirect laryngoscopy should be carried out by an experienced observer before thyroidectomy and repeated after operation.

   Paresis of a vocal cord may not always lead to clinically noticeable voice changes. Medicolegal problems may be avoided if the cord function is clarified before surgery.

5. Careful evaluation of the cardiovascular and respiratory systems should precede surgery. An electrocardiogram may be necessary. Auricular fibrillation, when present, should be controlled by digitalis, and cardioversion considered after surgery. Chest X-rays that include the thoracic inlet should be performed in goitrous patients. Where intrathoracic extension is suspected a lordotic view of the thoracic inlet gives a good view of the trachea (by air contrast) and any impingement on its lumen. The extent of any mediastinal intrusion may be judged on this form of X-ray.

6. Parathyroid function should be carefully monitored before and after thyroidectomy. This is best done by measuring the serum calcium concentration in venous blood collected without stasis.

Final preoperative evaluation in hospital

A full discussion regarding the surgery itself should involve both surgeon and anaesthetist and a final assessment assuring euthyroidism should be made. If the patient has been thyrotoxic the surgeon should ensure that controlling drugs are maintained and the leucocyte count is normal at the time of surgery, and he should liaise with the endocrinologist as appropriate. Attention to clinical details cannot be overstressed.

A frank discussion the night before surgery outlining the course of events for the patient is most useful.

The operation

1

Position of the patient

Patients must be positioned carefully for thyroidectomy. As for other operative procedures, optimal positioning of the patient facilitates the operation. A small sandbag or cloth roll, 9 × 35 cm (3.5 × 14 inches), is placed under the shoulders across the midscapulae. This manoeuvre gives adequate cervical elevation and extension and ensures that symmetry of the neck and shoulders is maintained throughout the operation.

Care must be taken not to overextend the neck, as this may result in postoperative cervical pain and discomfort. Patients with a previous history of neck difficulties should have preoperative cervical spine X-rays, and some will then be precluded from having their neck extended during thyroidectomy. Excessive extension may provoke postoperative headache.

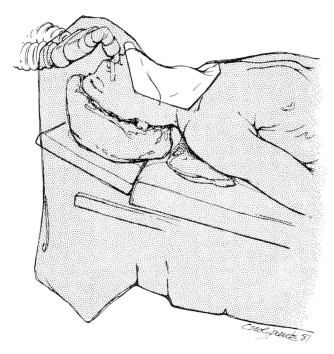

1

2

The incision

When the patient has been appropriately positioned, the site for the operative incision is marked.

The incision is approximately 2 cm (one finger's breadth) above and parallel to the clavicle and its line is marked by blue ink. It is customary to draw longitudinal lines down the midline and along the anterior jugular veins. These lines are useful both in providing guidance as to the width of incision and when closing in helping align the wound to ensure accurate skin apposition and to prevent distortion. The area under the line marked for incision is infiltrated subcutaneously with 30 ml of 1:30 ornithine-vasopressin (POR–8; Roche) before the operative site is prepared.

The width of the incision is determined by need. If the surgeon knows that he is operating upon a patient with a 2 cm single thyroid nodule situated centrally in the lobe, there should be little difficulty in making a decision; the incision will not be as wide as that made for a large multinodular gland in which retrosternal extension has been demonstrated and in which retropharyngeal extension is suspected. In general, for smaller glands the incision extends from 3 cm lateral to the anterior border of the sternomastoid to a similar position on the opposite side and approximately 1–2 cm wider bilaterally in larger glands.

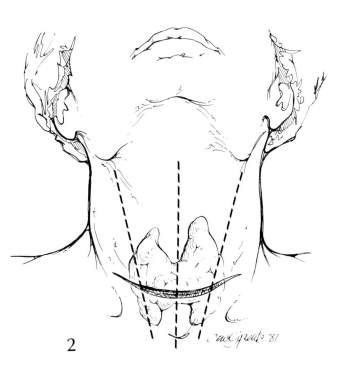

2

3

The incision is carried down through platysma; upper and lower flaps are mobilized. The upper flap is raised to the level of the superior border of cricoid cartilage superiorly and the lower to the level of the clavicle inferiorly. This degree of skin elevation allows for better mobility of the thyroid gland.

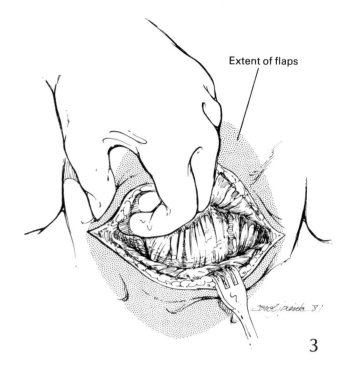

Extent of flaps

3

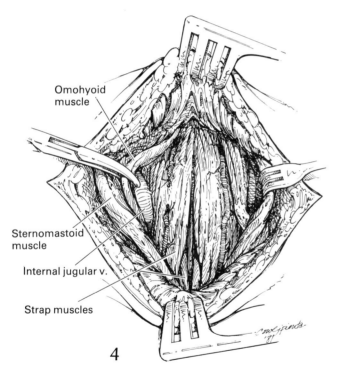

Omohyoid muscle

Sternomastoid muscle

Internal jugular v.

Strap muscles

4

4

The sternomastoid muscles are then mobilized, an incision is made along their anterior border and the muscles are separated from the strap muscles. The omohyoid is isolated and its tendon grasped with a haemostat. This tendon is an accurate anatomical landmark, directly overlying the internal jugular vein, and identifies the position of the vein for the surgeon as he divides the strap muscles, thus helping to prevent venous injury. Before the strap muscles are divided, the veins coursing over them should be doubly clamped, divided and ligated.

(Although a self-retaining retractor is illustrated, the author prefers when possible to provide exposure with hand-held instruments.)

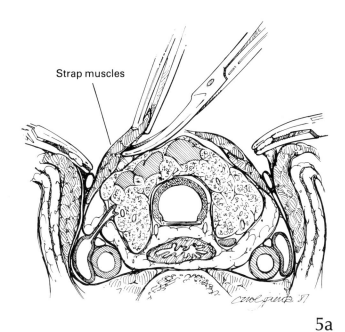

Strap muscles

5a

5a & b

The strap muscles are then divided. Initially, a small incision is made through the fascia overlying the thyroid isthmus in the midline. When the gland is reached the muscle is lifted with dissecting forceps, and the dissecting scissors (14 cm (5⅝ inches) curved Mayos) are gently advanced deep to the strap muscles while lying on the thyroid surface in the direction of the omohyoid tendon.

When appropriately cleared from the thyroid gland the muscles are divided over the scissors at the level of the second and third tracheal rings by coagulation diathermy.

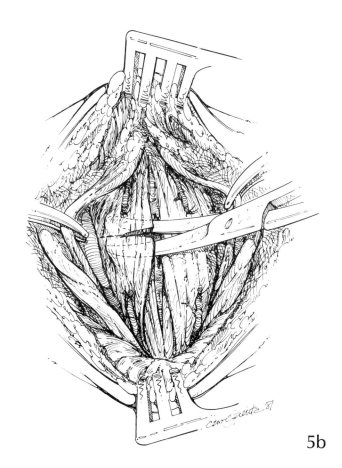

5b

6

The muscles of both sides are divided, and careful inspection of each lobe precedes palpation. The muscles are not separated along the midline for two reasons. First, this manoeuvre offers a poorer view of thyroid tissue and can cause abnormalities to be overlooked. Second, there is a longer healing line which may adhere to the trachea and lead to a tethered wound. The strap muscles are retracted cephalad and the sternomastoid is retracted laterally, so allowing access to the upper pole of the thyroid gland.

The gland is grasped with a heavy haemostat (Dunhill) (largely hidden under the operator's fingers) and drawn caudad. This manoeuvre allows for more ready separation of muscle and gland at the upper pole and if carefully utilized it minimizes bleeding.

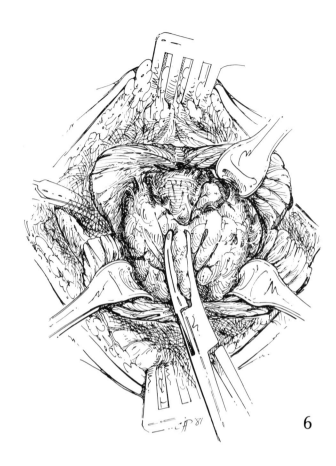

6

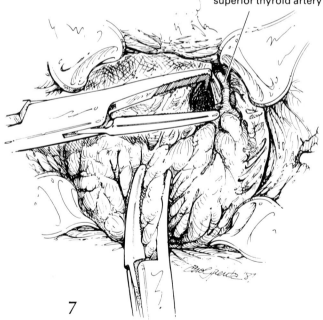

Marginal branch of superior thyroid artery

7

7

A fine pointed right-angle clamp (Dietrich) is then taken and its points insinuated through the pretracheal fascia at a site where the fascia seems to thin and provide a natural 'window'. This lies about 1 cm from the tracheo-isthmal-lobar junction. When the fascia has been penetrated, a Lahey's swab can readily clear the thyroid from the cricothyroid muscle surface, leaving two glistening surfaces, one over the cricothyroid and one over the upper pole of the thyroid gland. Small parasitic vessels between the gland and muscle can sometimes make this area difficult to dissect. Great care must be taken because damage to the external laryngeal nerve or to the cricothyroid muscle during this phase of dissection can be harmful to the voice. The cricothyroid muscle is tensed by the external laryngeal nerve, and damage to the nerve may produce a flat voice; the ability of a young mother to raise her voice and warn her child may be considerably impaired, as may the voices of singers, teachers and others who are heavily voice-dependent in their daily round.

External laryngeal nerve

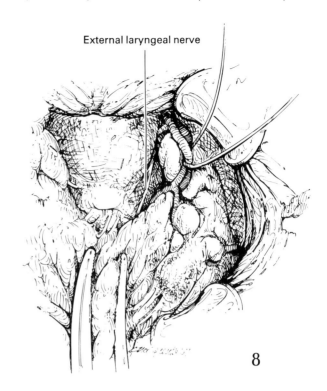

8

8

The marginal branch of the superior thyroid artery and accompanying vessels are then ligated and divided on the gland capsule, so avoiding the external laryngeal nerve. This nerve is well defined and is most unlikely to be damaged if individual vessel dissection is followed at the upper pole. Once the apex of the upper pole has been freed the dissection is not carried back any further than 1 cm from the cricoid-tracheal junction. Beyond this point the recurrent laryngeal nerve can be distorted and ligated inadvertently with upper pole vessels; its further dissection should be left until later. Mass dissection of the superior thyroid vessels above the apex of the upper pole may also inadvertently include the external laryngeal nerve and lead to its transection. This error is caused by distortion when the gland is drawn caudad. When the upper pole is mobilized the lobe is rotated towards the opposite side.

Parathyroid gland

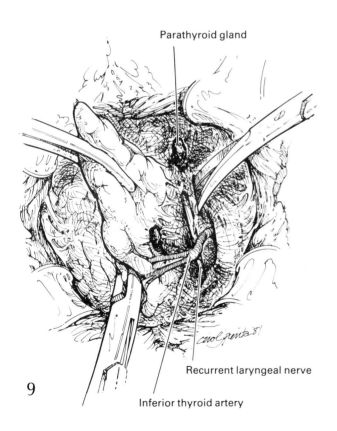

Recurrent laryngeal nerve

9

Inferior thyroid artery

9

The inferior thyroid artery is next identified and the areolar tissue overlying the trachea and oesophagus is gently split longitudinally (not transversely) by scissor dissection to expose the recurrent laryngeal nerve. Although some tissue is teased apart none is formally divided until the recurrent laryngeal nerve has been clearly demonstrated. The nerve can frequently be felt as a tight cord by fingernail palpation, usually in the region of the tracheo-oesophageal groove. The nerve should be checked along its course from the anterior mediastinum to the larynx. The recurrent laryngeal nerve is a distinct structure, and attention to its location during dissection is frequently attracted by the vasa nervorum which runs as a distinct 'thin red line' along the nerve; superiorly, the nerve may terminate in one branch or a virtual delta of nerve branches.

The parathyroid glands should be protected during surgery; the classic sites are inspected and, if observed, the glands carefully avoided. If it is difficult to avoid either the excision of or damage to a parathyroid gland, it should be freed from its site while still attached to its blood supply and dissected back until there is a clear length of artery allowing the surgeon to place the gland out of harm's way (clearly noted in this dissection). While not always possible, this manoeuvre improves with practice and may be helped by magnification. Up until this point there is essentially no difference between the approach to the thyroid for total lobectomy or subtotal lobectomy.

SUBTOTAL LOBECTOMY

In planning a subtotal thyroid lobectomy a decision must be made to leave tissue on the ipsilateral side. The residual amount is usually in the range of 3–5 g. Therefore it is useful to develop a working knowledge of remnant size in relation to weight. When the upper pole has been fully mobilized and the recurrent laryngeal nerve identified, the lower pole of the thyroid is mobilized. In subtotal lobectomy malignancy is not expected and the surgeon can 'hug' the gland, ligating and dividing individual vessels on the gland capsule. This usually allows full protection of the inferior parathyroid glandule. The recurrent laryngeal nerve, which is a constant reference point, is sighted until it turns back into the larynx, either as a single fibre or multiple fibres.

   The upper parathyroid is identified at this point and the isthmus cleared from the trachea by dissecting on its deep surface with a large haemostat. This allows a distinctive level to work towards when sectioning from the lateral to the medial surface of the gland.

10

A line of curved mosquito haemostats is carefully placed along the capsule, first biting into gland substance from superior to inferior poles, and the tissue held by the clamps is then incised with curved scissors. (This method used to be the prime treatment for thyroid adenomas but is no longer routine practice. Total thyroid lobectomy is now the standard procedure for treating single thyroid nodules).

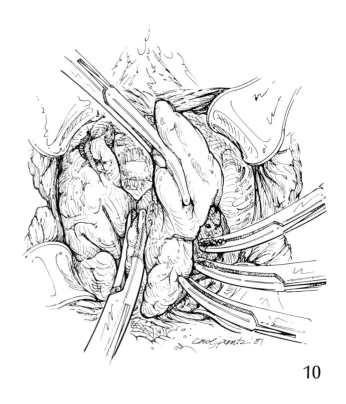

10

11

This process is repeated, progressing across the gland but not impinging on it at an angle of more than 180° to the anterior trachea. To do so may mean injury to the recurrent nerve at its high point. The nerve should be checked once or twice during this procedure, particularly if the lobe is large.

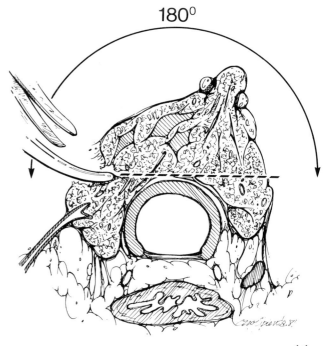

11

12

When the transection is completed the clamped vessels are ligated and haemostasis should be secured. The size of the remnant is judged by eye and is designed to meet individual need, e.g. thyroid tissue 2.75 × 1 × 1 cm weighs 2.1 g. Measurement of gland tissue *in situ* can give considerable assistance in leaving remnants of appropriate size.

Ligation of the inferior thyroid artery as a routine measure is not necessary. In fact, ligation is avoided as it is likely to interfere with blood supply to the parathyroid glands.

We have now reached the end point of bilateral subtotal thyroidectomy. The remnant of the left is approximately 5 × 2 × 1.5 cm and approximately 8 g in weight and that of the right is 3 × 1 × 2 cm, weighing 2.5 g. There is more tissue remaining than would follow a resection of thyroid for Graves disease, when approximately 5–8 g is left, though some authors recommend 10 g. Remnant size depends on size of gland, severity of disease and sometimes technical factors, particularly the site of parathyroid glands which must be carefully protected.

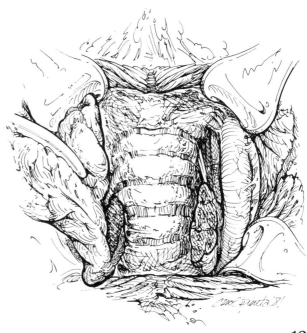

12

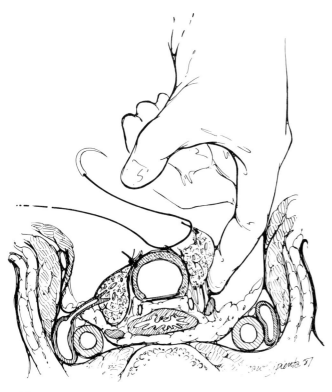

13

13

Should bleeding from the cut surface of the gland persist and securing of the bleeding points by haemostat be considered a risky manoeuvre, a useful alternative is to suture through the thyroid capsule and tracheal fascia. A finger is then insinuated deep to the lobar remnant which is gently elevated, the suture tied snugly in this elevated situation and the gland allowed to fall back into its normal position. This puts extra tension on the capsule and is usually sufficient to control remnant bleeding. Several such sutures may be necessary.

TOTAL LOBECTOMY

The mobilization of the lobe – upper pole, lower pole and inferior thyroid artery – and location of the recurrent laryngeal nerve proceed as already described. The remainder of this operation is really a dissection of the recurrent laryngeal nerve and, where appropriate, preservation of the parathyroid glands.

14

Dissection of the recurrent laryngeal nerve is an exercise in gentle dissection and patience, and if the procedure has been well conducted, the surgeon is rewarded by the complete exposure of the nerve from the base of the neck to the larynx with its single or, when present, multiple components intact. Fine instruments are ideal, and a magnifying loupe can be helpful at the upper end. Full visualization – the key factor in successful nerve exposure – cannot be compromised. The surrounds are dissected away from the nerve, being careful not to handle the nerve and not to be lured to the superior end before dissecting the lower end to save time; one should dissect from below.

The parathyroid glandules are protected with great care. Their anatomical location is not fixed: the superior gland is relatively constant, but the sites of the lower glands are less predictable. The clearest guide is to follow the branches of the inferior thyroid artery which can be skeletalized and leave the parathyroid attached to its blood supply. In the presence of malignancy this may not be the appropriate approach and the parathyroids may have to be taken with the thyroid lobe to achieve a complete clearance of malignant tissue.

15

If the parathyroid has to be excised it can be macerated and inserted into a bloodless muscle pocket in either sternomastoid muscle. Such tissue can, it appears, 'take' and produce parathormone.

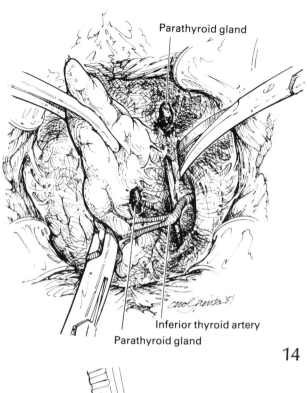

Parathyroid gland

Inferior thyroid artery
Parathyroid gland

14

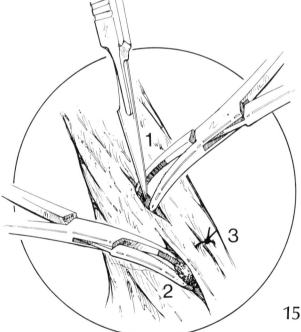

15

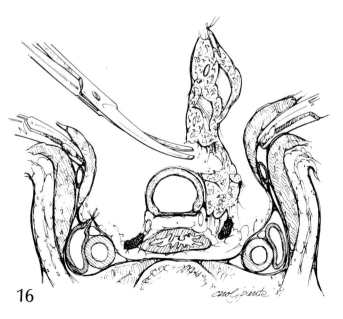

16

16

The left lobe has been rotated medially, and the recurrent laryngeal nerve has been exposed in the tracheo-oesophageal groove and is seen passing under the lower fibres of the cricothyroid to enter the larynx. The superior parathyroid remains *in situ*. The isthmus has been cleared from the trachea; the dissected lobe is sectioned along the line of junction of the isthmus and right thyroid lobe. This achieves total lobectomy. In young patients the upper lobe of the thymus may be noted, as in this illustration.

Wound closure

17

When haemostasis is secured the wound is closed in layers. The strap muscles are reapposed with 2/0 chromic catgut and care is taken to have fascia coapted to fascia in an attempt to avoid wound adhesion.

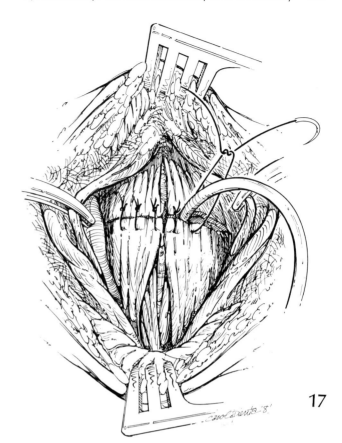

17

18, 19 & 20

The platysma is then reapproximated with 3/0 plain catgut and the skin wound with subcuticular 4/0 synthetic absorbable polyglycolic acid (Vicryl). One vacuum drainage tube is placed deep to muscle and a second subcutaneously. These are connected to a single drainage bottle. The wound is painted with povidone-iodine and left exposed.

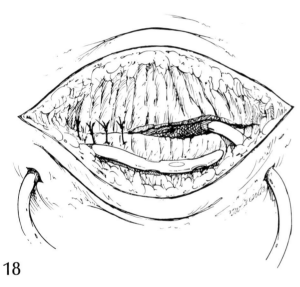

18

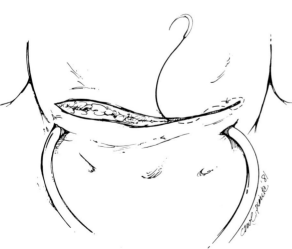

19

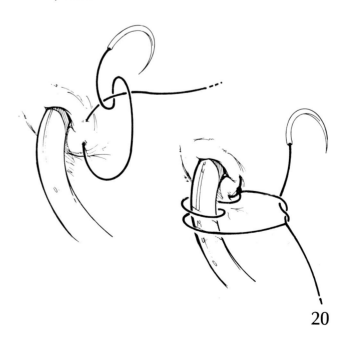

20

Postoperative care

The patient is nursed in a recovery facility until fully conscious. The absence of dressings allows nursing staff to have a clear and early view of any change in the neck. This allows for intervention in any early airway problem or haemorrhage. The anaesthetist should check vocal cord function after removal of the endotracheal tube. The respiratory and cardiovascular systems should be carefully monitored, the time for particular trouble being the night of the operative day. The drains are removed on the second postoperative day.

Due attention must be given to medication and, in particular, where blockade has been used to control thyrotoxicosis, it must be maintained for up to one week postoperatively. It will be remembered that blockade does not treat thyrotoxicosis; it simply protects the end organs from the effects of thyroid hormone.

Complications

There are two categories of complications: those occurring soon postoperatively, and those that are delayed.

Postoperative complications

Haemorrhage, causing tracheal obstruction

This occurs after approximately 1 per cent of thyroid operations. Early operation may obviate the need for tracheostomy.

Respiratory distress

1. From idiopathic laryngeal oedema
2. Secondary to
   (a) haemorrhage
   (b) bilateral recurrent laryngeal nerve palsy
   (c) traumatic laryngeal intubation
   (d) vocal cord oedema secondary to allergy to the endobronchial tube
   (e) collapsing trachea due to a large compressing goitre and subsequent tracheomalacia

Vocal cord paresis

This should be an uncommon complication of thyroidectomy if the recurrent laryngeal nerve is deliberately dissected throughout its whole length in the neck. Published series vary somewhat, but in my experience permanent recurrent laryngeal nerve palsy has been observed in approximately 0.3 per cent of patients on a University Surgical Unit and transient recurrent laryngeal nerve palsy in 2.8 per cent (1975). These results have been observed following pre- and postoperative laryngoscopy by an independent ear, nose and throat surgeon and the results have further improved in the last few years. Careful nerve dissection does not lead to vocal cord palsy.

Delayed complications

Hypocalcaemia

This may be present in two forms: transient or permanent. Care to protect the parathyroid glands during surgery leads to a low incidence of their damage.

The glands are supplied by easily damaged end-arteries and venous infarction may also be seen.

If serum calcium concentrations are carefully monitored before and after thyroidectomy, a fall the day after operation is almost universally observed (of about 0.25 mmol). This recovers in all but the permanent cases within a few days. The permanent rate is now under 1 per cent but at last report (1975) was 1.2 per cent and the transient rate was 2.1 per cent. These patients require close long-term follow-up.

Further reading

Barraclough, B. H., Reeve, T. S. Postoperative complications of thyroidectomy: a comparison of two series at an interval of ten years. Australian and New Zealand Journal of Surgery 1975; 45: 21–29

Blackburn, G., Salmon, L. F. W. Cord movements after thyroidectomy. British Journal of Surgery 1961; 48: 371

Hunt, P. S., Poole, M., Reeve, T. S. A reappraisal of the surgical anatomy of the thyroid and parathyroid glands. British Journal of Surgery 1968; 55: 63–66

Reeve, T. S. Right subtotal thyroid lobectomy. Surgical techniques illustrated 1977; 2: 61

Reeve, T. S. Thyroidectomy – transoperative and postoperative problems. In: Hardy, J. D., ed. Rhoads textbook of surgery, 5th ed., p. 713. Philadelphia: J. B. Lippincott, 1977

Thompson, N. W., Olsen, W. R., Hoffman, G. L. The continuing development of a technique of thyroidectomy. Surgery 1973; 73: 913–927

Illustrations by Kevin Marks

Thyroid cancer

T. S. Reeve   CBE, FACS, FRACS
Professor and Chairman, Department of Surgery,
The University of Sydney, Royal North Shore Hospital,
St Leonards, New South Wales

A. G. Poole   FRACS, FACS
Visiting Surgeon, Royal North Shore Hospital,
St Leonards, New South Wales;
Clinical Tutor, Department of Surgery, The University of Sydney

Introduction[1]

Thyroid cancer accounts for about 1.5 per cent of all human malignancy and for about 0.5 per cent of all cancer deaths. All tumours except medullary ones arise from the follicular cell and may present in one of three pathological forms: papillary carcinoma, follicular carcinoma and anaplastic carcinoma. The first accounts for approximately 55 per cent of all thyroid malignancy and tends to remain localized for a long time, eventually spreading to lymph nodes and lungs. In people aged less than 40 years it carries a good prognosis when appropriately treated. Papillary carcinoma becomes more aggressive with advancing years, particularly after age 40.

Follicular carcinoma is found in about 25 per cent of all patients presenting with thyroid carcinoma. It may spread locally, but blood vessel invasion provides its most frequent metastatic route. Papillary and follicular carcinoma may present as a 'mixed' lesion in about 15 per cent of instances and this seems to follow the papillary pattern of behaviour.

Anaplastic thyroid malignancy is uncommon – representing approximately 3 per cent of thyroid cancer. It may be seen as small cells, giant cells or spindle cells. Local infiltration, respiratory obstruction and widespread metastases are the rule. Some 'anaplastic carcinomas' are probably lymphomas. Treatment with surgery and radioiodine are of little value. Chemotherapy is still on trial. Death within 18 months is the rule.

The current treatment for papillary and follicular carcinoma is total or near-total thyroidectomy, combined with local excision of isolated cervical nodes and modified neck dissection where nodal involvement is more extensive. After clearance of the thyroid gland and involved nodes, a scan dose of 5 mC: $(18.5 \times 10^{10}$ Bq) of ^{131}I should be administered. If residual thyroid function is present it should then be ablated with the same radionucleide and maintenance thyroxine administered. This allows for subsequent scans with ^{131}I to seek functioning metastases.

Suppression with thyroid hormone is said to help control thyroid carcinoma. A further aid to follow-up is the detection of radioimmune thyroglobulin because when this is raised in patients who have undergone thyroid ablation, recurrent carcinoma must be strongly suspected. Any metastases that can be excised should be so treated in order to reduce radiation dosage.

Medullary carcinoma arises from the thyroid C cell and should be treated similarly surgically. However, subsequent ^{131}I therapy has no role to play. Radiotherapy has been useful on occasions and the data on chemotherapy are as yet sketchy.

Survival rates after treatment of thyroid carcinoma at 5 years are as follows.

Papillary	92%
Follicular	85%
Anaplastic	0%
Medullary	65%

Neck dissection in thyroid cancer

The surgical treatment of thyroid cancer is still somewhat controversial, particularly as it applies to papillary carcinoma. There is however a slow but definite trend towards total thyroidectomy followed by ablative ^{131}I being the optimal therapy in this disease as it is in the follicular carcinoma.

When lymph nodes are present the surgeon must decide on his approach. Local lymph nodes, if involved, should be locally removed. When lymph nodes are very extensively involved more extensive surgery is necessary,

and modified radical neck dissection has become the standard approach. Preservation of the spinal accessory nerve, the sternomastoid muscle and the internal jugular vein still allows adequate neck clearance, optimal residual function and cosmesis.

The modified neck dissection may need to be done at the time of original thyroid surgery or later. The overall approach is similar. If the procedures are done simultaneously the thyroidectomy is performed first and neck dissection follows.

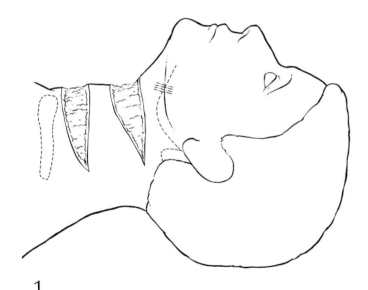

1

1

Skin incisions

Parallel incisions after McFee[2] are routinely used in modified neck dissection for carcinoma of the thyroid. The lower one is a continuation of the thyroidectomy incision. In those cases where upper neck dissection is planned, the incision should be at least 2 cm below the angle of the mandible to avoid the ramus mandibularis of the facial nerve. The submandibular gland is rarely involved in metastatic thyroid cancer and therefore the submandibular triangle is not routinely cleared. The approach from the upper incision gives good access to the hypoglossal nerve, the jugular foramen and the digastric triangle.

Elevation of skin flaps

2

Skin flaps are elevated in a subplatysmal plane to the lower border of the hyoid and mastoid bone, posteriorly to the anterior border of the trapezius and inferiorly to the clavicle. During the subsequent dissection careful retraction on skin flaps is mandatory to avoid bruising and subsequent damage to vascular supply. Langenbach or similar retractors are ideal.

The ramus mandibularis should not be at risk if the dissection proceeds in a subplatysmal plane to the level of the hyoid. If greater definition or more extensive surgery is planned the nerve should be identified.

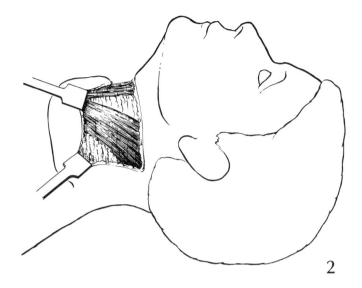

2

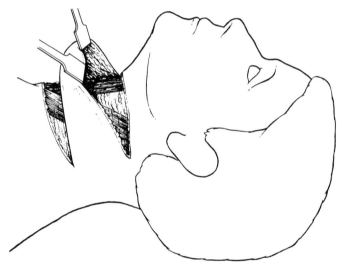

3

3

The central skin bridge is elevated and demonstrates that ample room is available beneath the flaps to allow for cervical structures to be identified and dissected.

Posterior triangle dissection

4

The contents of the posterior triangle are approached first[3]; and areolar tissue, fat and lymph nodes are dissected away from the anterior border of the trapezius posteriorly and the clavicle inferiorly. Care is exercised in this region as the spinal accessory nerve is very superficial.

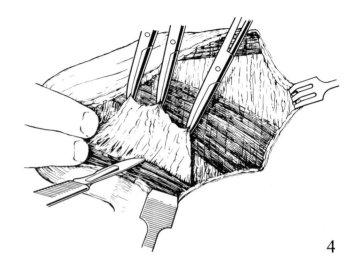

4

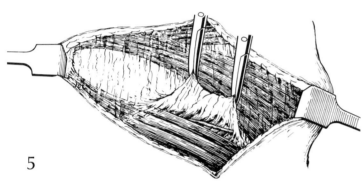

5

5

The nerve is located at the junction of the lower and middle third of the anterior border of the trapezius.

In the presence of thyroid malignancy the accessory nerve is preserved unless obviously involved with cancer.

This nerve may be difficult to locate, but meticulous dissection along the border of the trapezius should allow identification. It is almost always a significant structure.

6

The accessory nerve has been identified then dissected away from the contents of the posterior triangle until the nerve emerges from the posterior border of the sternomastoid. Once this has been done the nerve must be protected whilst the remainder of the posterior triangle contents is mobilized off the anterior border of the trapezius and the muscles of the posterior triangle, scalenus posterior, scalenus medius and the levator scapulae. It is best to avoid disturbing the fascia over these muscles as damage to motor branches of the cervical plexus will inevitably result. The transverse cervical artery may be removed with the block or can be left bare on the muscles low down in the posterior triangle free of any fatty tissue.

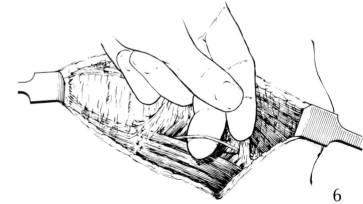

6

7

During the dissection in the posterior inferior angle (trapezius-clavicle angle) the inferior belly of the omo-hyoid is transected with a knife.

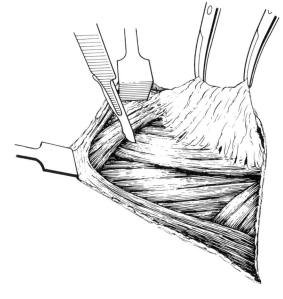

7

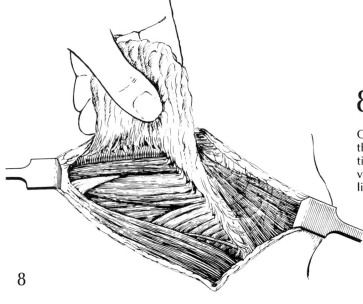

8

8

Once this has been performed the block is mobilized off the brachial plexus by gentle traction and scalpel dissection until the scalenus anterior and the internal jugular vein are exposed. The vein when retracted and elevated lies in a superoanterior plane to the carotid artery.

9

The phrenic nerve is seen and preserved as it courses downwards on the scalenus anterior within that muscle's fascia. At the upper end of the phrenic nerve, the lower trunk of the cervical plexus is transected, again preserving any muscular branches as well as the phrenic nerve.

The upper end or apex of the posterior triangle is approached through the superior incision, and the contents of the triangle are again divided at the anterior border of the trapezius up to the mastoid process. By gentle traction and elevation of the sternomastoid, the contents are carefully dissected from the levator scapulae and the splenius capitis.

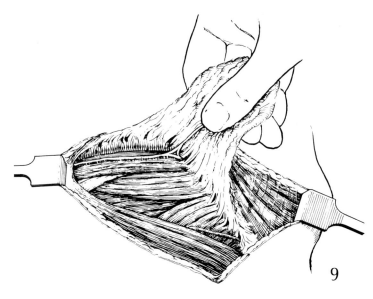

9

10

With the contents of the posterior triangle now replaced, the posterior border of the sternomastoid muscle is freed and the bare muscle elevated from the deeper structures over the whole length of the sternomastoid. In surgery for thyroid carcinoma the sternomastoid muscle is usually preserved.

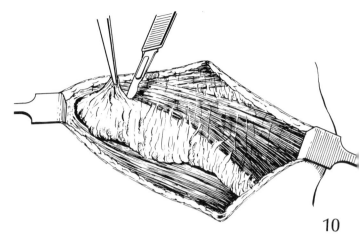

10

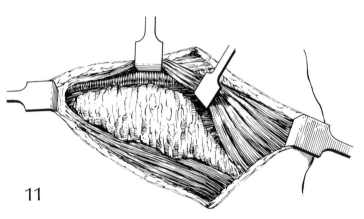

11

11

By dissecting to the anterior border of the sternomastoid inferiorly one can readily mobilize all of the muscle off the underlying structures – the internal jugular vein, the vagus nerve and the common carotid artery. These are too deeply placed medially to be visualized in this view, as they have been identified and dissected deep to the sternomastoid muscle.

12

Superiorly, as the sternomastoid is elevated and separated from the fatty tissue and lymph nodes, the accessory nerve comes into view anterior to the mastoid process at the level of the transverse process of the atlas which can be readily palpated and the nerve preserved.

   This manoeuvre is more difficult than in a standard neck dissection because the sternomastoid muscle remains *in situ*.

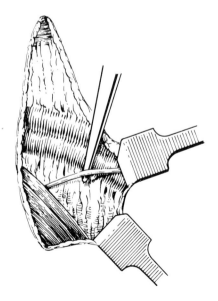

12

13

This nerve can then be separated from nodes and fibro-fatty tissue well up towards the base of skull. Dissection of the posterior belly of the digastric muscle and then elevation of this structure is mandatory in this part of the operation.

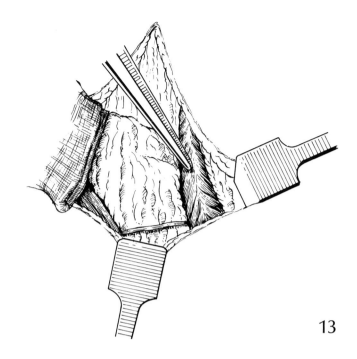

13

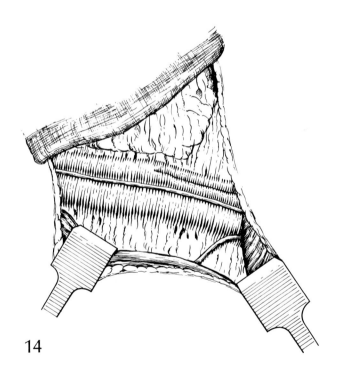

14

14

The upper end of the internal jugular vein is readily identified as the accessory nerve is in very close anterior and then lateral relation to it. The upper extent of the node dissection is now identified: anteriorly, it is the internal jugular vein; posteriorly, it is the fibrofatty tissue under the mastoid process level with the transverse process of the atlas. Division of this tissue which lies deep to the digastric is now performed, care being maintained as a large occipital artery can cause embarrassing haemorrhage if divided.

The next step is complete separation of the contents of the posterior triangle and deep cervical nodes off the upper end of scalenus anterior, medius and posterior and the levator scapulae, thus dividing further branches of the cervical plexus (sensory) to expose the carotid system and the vagus nerve.

15

The mass of tissue to be removed is thus mobilized off these structures, and in so doing superiorly the trunk of the hypoglossal nerve comes into view. This nerve is readily identified as the contents of the neck are mobilized off the upper end of the levator scapulae and following division of the upper trunks of the cervical plexus to expose the internal jugular vein and internal carotid more adequately. Furthermore the descendens hypoglossi can be easily seen as it descends down the internal jugular vein. The hypoglossal nerve may be seen near the tip of the hyoid bone anterior to the carotid system if approached from the front.

The contents of the neck are now mobilized inferiorly off the internal jugular vein, vagus and carotid vessels. It will be necessary to divide some veins (lingual, common facial and pharyngeal veins) to gain adequate exposure in this area. If the submandibular triangle is to be resected, it is conveniently done at this point. At the level of the hyoid bone the superior remnant of the superior thyroid artery and vein will be redivided, ligated and removed with the surrounding tissue which may include some lymph nodal structures as well as the superior attachment of the omohyoid.

In the lower one-half of the neck, the block is mobilized off the carotid, vagus and the internal jugular vein. Care must be exercised posterior to the lower end of the internal jugular vein – as the thoracic duct curves around to gain entry into the junction of that vein and the left subclavian.

Once this step has been completed the contents of the neck will be free; haemostasis is checked and any bleeding points identified and either ligated or coagulated with diathermy. Thoracic duct damage is noted by the pooling of opalescent fluid in the vicinity of the scalenus anterior in the supraclavicular fossa and care should then be taken to ligate the duct.

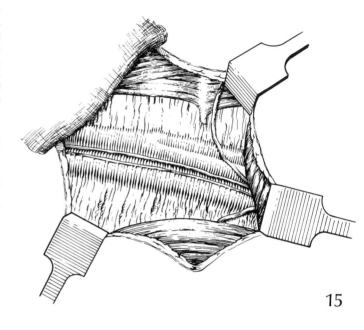

15

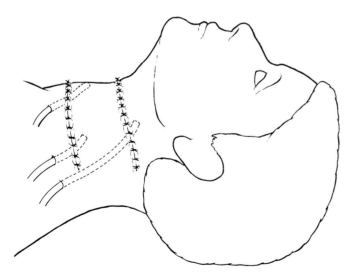

16

16

The wounds are then closed. Suction drains (Redivac) are used – at least two for the neck component of the surgery and at most two for the thyroid component. Skin may be closed by autoclips, subcuticular Vicryl or standard skin sutures. Vacuum drains are always used – any air leak through the skin incisions must be recognized and corrected prior to removal of the drapes.

Conclusion

Modified neck dissection is eminently suitable for the management of thyroid malignancy. It is in effect a functional dissection of the neck and the unfortunate sequelae of radical neck dissection are prevented.

References

1. Duncan, W., ed. Thyroid cancer. Berlin: Springer-Verlag, 1980

2. MacFee, W. F. Transverse incisions for neck dissection. Annals of Surgery 1960; 151: 279–284

3. Bakamjian, V. Y., Miller, S. H., Poole, A. G. A technique for radical dissection of the neck. Surgery, Gynecology and Obstetrics 1977; 144: 419–424

Illustrations by Carol J. Pienta

Total thyroidectomy

Walter J. Pories MD, FACS
Professor and Chairman, Department of Surgery, School of Medicine,
East Carolina University, Greenville, North Carolina

Introduction

Total thyroidectomy is not a common operation because there are few indications for the procedure. These include medullary carcinoma, multifocal papillary carcinoma, completion lobectomy after previous thyroid surgery and a few other unusual problems. The operation carries the considerable risks of hypoparathyroidism and damage to the laryngeal nerves. In addition, total thyroidectomy demands lifelong supplementation with thyroid medication to avoid the serious complications of myxoedema.

The operation

1

Position of patient

Patients requiring total thyroidectomy frequently present with large glands which may offer considerable problems of exposure. Access is usually obtained best by arching the neck with a rolled towel or sheet placed beneath the shoulders and by endotracheal anaesthesia in which the tubing is led out from beneath unsupported drapes or a low towel screen.

Blood loss from venous ooze can be reduced by the 'reverse Trendelenburg' position in which the head of the operative table is elevated. This does however increase the possibility of air emboli if a large vein is injured and thus requires special care.

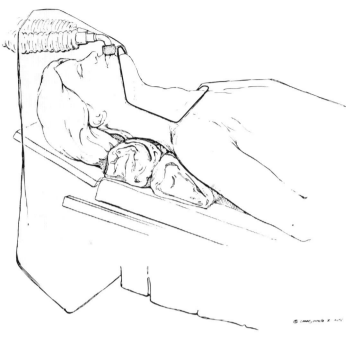

1

2

The incision

The best incision for exposure and a fine scar is a low transverse cut approximately 1–2 cm above the clavicle. Frequently, and especially in women, a transverse wrinkle line extending across the neck can be located; the use of such wrinkles produces an unusually fine scar. If such a line is not well defined, a depression left by a suture pressed briefly across the neck serves well as a guide to a straight horizontal incision.

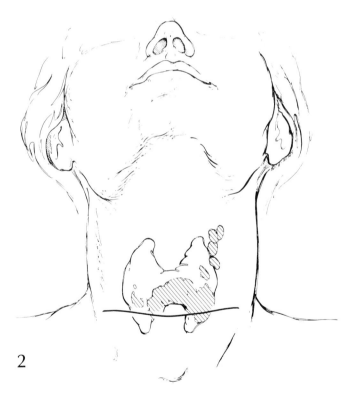

2

3

The incision is carried through the platysma muscle, a well defined layer. Cutaneous bleeding is controlled by gentle pressure on both sides of the incision. Most of the oozing will stop spontaneously and only a few vessels require ligature or cautery. Care must be taken not to injure the venous plexus directly under the platysma. If cutaneous oozing continues to be a problem after the superior or inferior flaps have been developed, it can generally be handled nicely by pressure from one or two self-retaining retractors.

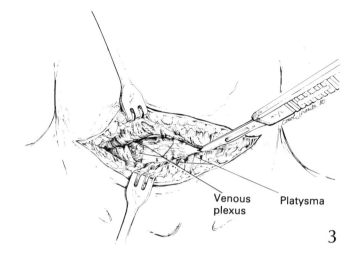

Venous plexus   Platysma

3

4

The superior and inferior flaps can be developed by sharp incision with a knife or a combination of blunt and sharp scissor dissection, but generally the fascial plane can be opened most easily by finger dissection. Gentle but firm traction pulling the flap from the underlying fascia on both sides of the midline will expose the operative field quickly with a minimum of bleeding. The remaining midline attachment can then be divided with scissors. Frequently the midline fascial band contains several large veins which require ligature.

After the flaps have been developed superiorly to the angle of the larynx and inferiorly to the sternal notch, they can be retracted with sutures to the drapes, with towel clips, or, as we prefer, with a Wheatlander retractor.

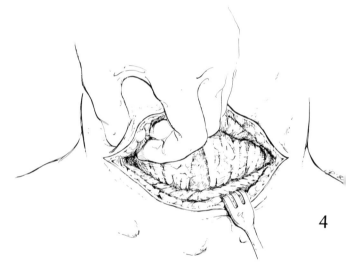

4

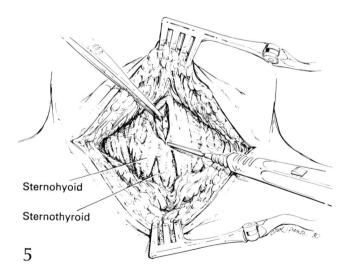

Sternohyoid

Sternothyroid

5

5

The strap muscles (sternohyoid and sternothyroid) are separated in the midline down to the thyroid gland. Because the large thyroid gland frequently distorts the tissues of the neck, the 'midline' may be deviated to either side; this 'bloodless' plane should be carefully identified and followed to avoid the veins encasing these muscles.

6

Although it is occasionally necessary to divide the strap muscles for better exposure, this step can usually be avoided by careful blunt separation of the muscles from the underlying thyroid structures. Often muscular fibres appear to invest the vessels of the superior pole of the thyroid; these can be swept away gently with the tip of the closed scissors to expose the vascular supply. The thin veil-like fascial layers overlying the thyroid should be thoroughly incised to the surface of the gland before exploration in order to minimize injury to the delicate veins within the fascial covers. Exploration should be thorough before proceeding with the excision of the gland.

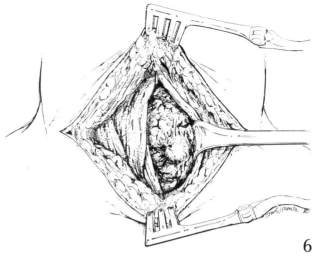

6

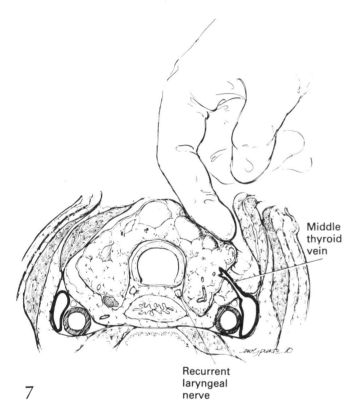

Middle thyroid vein

Recurrent laryngeal nerve

7

7

After the anterior surface of the thyroid has been thoroughly exposed, both lobes can be freed from their surrounding structures by gentle finger dissection. Special care must be given to the middle thyroid vein which surfaces early at about the middle of the gland.

If possible, veins should be divided first because this will allow rotation and better examination of the gland as well as identification of the recurrent laryngeal nerves.

The recurrent laryngeal nerve should be identified early in the thyroidectomy so it can be shielded from injury. It is easily found in the tracheo-oesophageal groove by gently spreading the tissues in a longitudinal axis. The nerve is a 1 mm glistening white structure, about the size of a wooden matchstick, running upward and forward from between the branches of the inferior thyroid to the base of the larynx.

8

The anatomy of the gland will generally determine the best approach to the division of the vasculature of the thyroid gland. Those vessels which are most easily exposed should be divided first. *Vessels should be carefully cleaned and divided as close to the gland as possible to avoid injury to the recurrent laryngeal or superior laryngeal nerves. Fine clamps should be used and a bloodless, clearly visualized field is mandatory. It is best to ligate with 4/0 suture or to clip each vessel immediately after it is divided; these arteries and veins are frequently friable and tear easily.*

The vessels of the superior poles are generally divided before those at the base of the gland because they are more easily exposed and because their early division facilitates mobilization of the thyroid gland. The superior thyroid arteries are often covered by fibres from the strap muscles. Division of these muscular fibres helps immeasurably in the exposure of the vessels. As shown in the illustration both the veins and arteries of the superior poles should be *doubly* ligated with 2/0 or 3/0 suture *before* division.

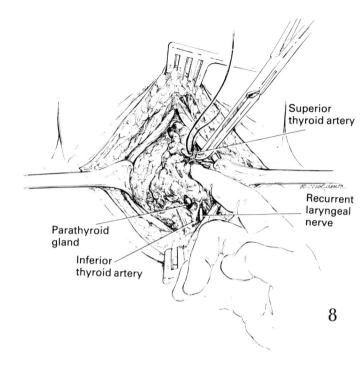

Superior thyroid artery

Recurrent laryngeal nerve

Parathyroid gland

Inferior thyroid artery

8

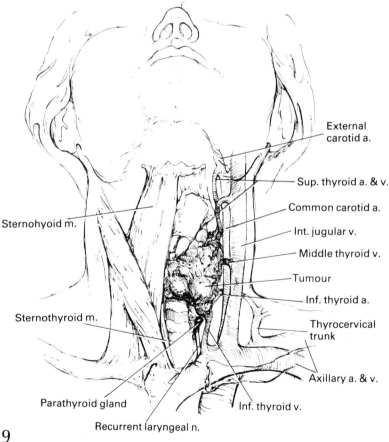

External carotid a.

Sup. thyroid a. & v.

Common carotid a.

Int. jugular v.

Middle thyroid v.

Tumour

Inf. thyroid a.

Thyrocervical trunk

Axillary a. & v.

Sternohyoid m.

Sternothyroid m.

Parathyroid gland

Recurrent laryngeal n.

Inf. thyroid v.

9

9

Injury to the superior thyroid artery can result in troublesome bleeding. Blind clamping must be avoided. The situation is best handled by pressure on the injured vessel and identification of the origin of the superior thyroid artery at the carotid bulb. The common carotid artery lies immediately behind the thyroid gland and lateral to the trachea. It can be traced upwards to its bifurcation and, because the superior thyroid artery is the first branch of the external carotid, the bleeding vessel can be readily ligated *in situ*.

The inferior thyroid arteries also require special care because they supply and frequently surround one or several of the parathyroid glands, and within their branches may be hidden the recurrent laryngeal nerve. Because of these anatomical relationships, it is safer to divide the inferior thyroid arteries by their branches *near* the thyroid gland than to ligate the main trunks.

10

After the major vessels of the lobe have been divided, the isthmus can usually be separated easily from the anterior surface of the trachea with sharp and blunt dissection. *Care must be taken not to injure the contralateral recurrent laryngeal nerve which can be tented up with the gland on traction.*

When the isthmus has been freed from the anterior trachea, the remaining lobe is removed in a similar manner to the first with division of the medial thyroid vein, identification of the laryngeal nerves and parathyroid glands, and double ligature and division of the superior and inferior thyroid vessels.

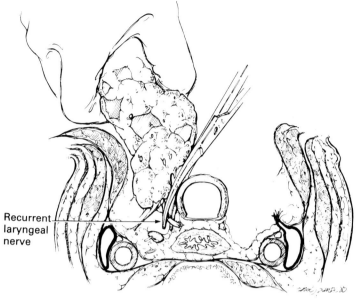

Recurrent laryngeal nerve

10

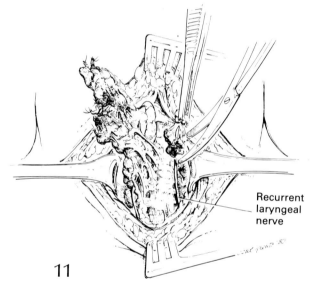

Recurrent laryngeal nerve

11

11

Node dissection

If the operation is performed for malignancy, the neck should be searched for involved nodes and, when possible, these should be removed *en bloc*. Usually, however, as in the case illustrated here, the nodes are anatomically separate from the thyroid and may have to be removed with a margin of normal surrounding tissues. A formal radical neck dissection is only rarely indicated for thyroid malignancies. These nodes should be examined by frozen section to guide the operative approach.

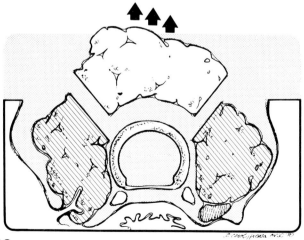

12

12

Morcellation of large thyroid glands

If the operation is performed for a benign lesion, such as a massive nodular goitre, or a large substernal gland, it may be helpful to morcellize the gland in order to make mobilization and safe identification of the various structures feasible. Morcellation can be done safely and cleanly by removing one or several wedges of tissue from the anterior surface of the gland overlying the trachea. As long as the excision is confined only to tissue anterior to the trachea, injury to an important structure is unlikely. When the central portion has been removed, both lobes can then be easily pulled out of their grooves.

Identification and management of the parathyroid glands

13

The four beige, soft parathyroid glands and their blood supply should be identified before resecting any thyroid tissue. At least two of these small glands should be preserved from injury. If this is not possible, or if the glands were removed inadvertently, two of the glands should be reimplanted. After identification by pathological examination of small portions of the glands, the tissue is wrapped in a sponge soaked with saline and chilled in a sterile metal basin in an ice bath covered with a sterile plastic sheet.

14

When the tissue has been confirmed to be parathyroid gland by pathological examination, it should be morcellized into 1–2 mm fragments and implanted into the anterior surface of the sternomastoid muscle. Implantation is easily accomplished in the following way: (1) a small slit is made into the muscle in the direction of its fibres, (2) the transplant is inserted into the pocket so that it is totally covered by muscle, and (3) the site is then closed and marked with a silk or other black non-absorbable suture.

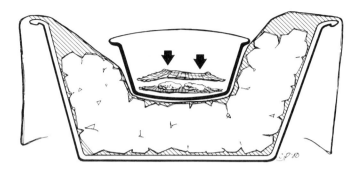

13

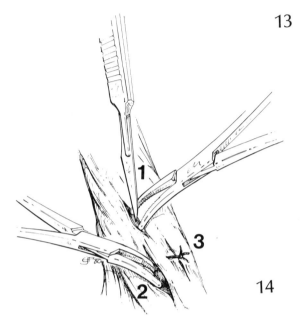

14

Closure

15

At the end of the procedure the field must be dry before the incision is closed. Small vessels can be controlled easily with the electrocautery, but voltage and placement must be precise to avoid damage to adjoining nerves.

The wound can be closed around a small Y-shaped drain through the centre of the wound or a small suction catheter which is placed through a separate stab wound.

16

The platysma is reapproximated with several sutures of 4/0 gauge and the skin is closed with carefully placed stitches of 4/0 polyethylene or nylon suture or skin staples. A small dressing consisting of a strip of paper tape or small absorbent bandage usually suffices.

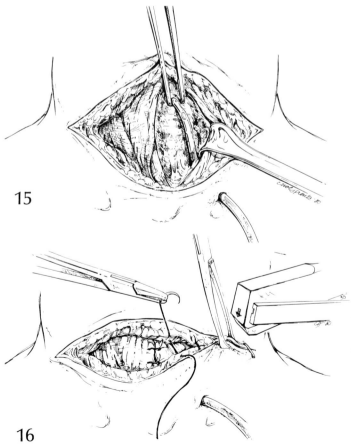

15

16

Postoperative management

During extubation *the vocal cords should be examined* to be certain these function well. If one cord is paralysed, an injury to the recurrent laryngeal nerve must be suspected. Although such paralyses are more likely to be caused by bruising of the nerve rather than transection, they can be the cause of serious respiratory complications during the postoperative period because of the loss of effective cough and glottal competence. Such patients require careful postoperative management and reassurance. If the nerve has not been transected, it will usually regain its function in 2–6 months.

If both vocal cords are paralysed, the patient will require endotracheal intubation during initial management. If function is not regained quickly, a tracheostomy will be required urgently.

Postoperative haemorrhage poses a particular danger because the trapped haematoma may compress the trachea. Some of the oozing can be avoided by gently compressing the neck during extubation so that any excessive straining does not, by increased venous pressure, reopen previously clotted veins. If the neck enlarges during the postoperative period, the patient's wound should be re-explored directly in the operating room, the haematoma removed and bleeding stopped. If this is done expeditiously there should be no delay in the patient's convalescence.

Hypocalcaemia should also be rare, but may occur. It is important to remember that serum calcium levels may not fall immediately. Early falls may be caused by migration of calcium ions into bone because of reduction of thyroid activity. Only if the values are normal at 72 h after operation can the surgeon be confident that parathyroid function is adequate. Measurement of serum calcium levels is therefore recommended on the second and third postoperative days.

Hypothyroidism is, of course, inevitable after total thyroidectomy. It can be handled by careful thyroid replacement. Patients and their families must be cautioned regarding the signs and symptoms of hypoparathyroidism, told to continue the medication daily and instructed that replacement will be required for the rest of the patient's life.

Wound care usually presents few problems. The drain can be removed in 24 h and alternate sutures or staples can be removed at 48 and 72 h. A strip of paper tape placed over the incision after the sutures are removed will tend to support the wound edges and may produce a finer scar. It also provides an aesthetic covering of the wound during the first few weeks after operation. Women patients are often gratified to learn that they can wear a strategically placed choker or string of pearls to hide the healing scar. It works well and seems to cause no wound problems.

Further reading

Attie, J. N., Moskowitz, G. W., Margouleff, D., Levy, L. M. Feasibility of total thyroidectomy in the treatment of thyroid carcinoma. American Journal of Surgery 1979; 138: 555–560

Edis, A. J. Prevention and management of complications associated with thyroid and parathyroid surgery. Surgical Clinics of North America 1979; 59: 83–92

Esmeraldo, R., Paloyan, E., Lawrence, A. M. Thyroidectomy, parathyroidectomy and modified neck dissection. Surgical Clinics of North America 1977; 57: 1365–1377

Foster, R. S. Morbidity and mortality after thyroidectomy. Surgery, Gynecology and Obstetrics 1978; 146: 423–429

Green, W. E. R., Shepperd, H. W. H., Stevenson, H. M., Wilson, W. Tracheal collapse after thyroidectomy. British Journal of Surgery 1979; 66: 554–557

Katz, A. D., Bronson, D. Total thyroidectomy. The indications and results of 630 cases. American Journal of Surgery 1978; 136: 450–454

Loré, J. M., Kim, D. J., Elias, S. Preservation of the laryngeal nerves during total thyroid lobectomy. Annals of Otolaryngology, Rhinology and Laryngology 1977; 86: 777–788

Retrosternal goitre

G. B. Ong MB BS, DSc, FRCS(Ed.), FRCS, FRACS, FRSE
Professor of Surgery, University of Hong Kong;
Head of the Department of Surgery, Queen Mary Hospital, Hong Kong

Introduction

Retrosternal goitres are usually extensions of thyroid enlargement originating from the lower poles of the right or left lobes. The retrosternal extension is in the anterior mediastinum and almost always above the aortic arch. However, occasionally, it may be in the posterior mediastinum and thus in the right side of the chest. This peculiarity is caused by the anatomical deviation of the aortic arch towards the left side of the mediastinum. The incidence is given as 25 per cent by Rietz and Werner[1], and 9.8 per cent by de Andrade[2].

In very few of these retrosternal goitres, an alternative source of blood supply may be acquired in the chest. However, in the vast majority the gland retains its blood supply from the thyroid vessels.

Most retrosternal goitres are benign, but malignant ones are also encountered. In 932 thyroidectomies, exci-sion of a retrosternal extension was done in 21 cases. Of these, 16 were benign and in 5 the operation was carried out for malignant goitres. In all except 2 malignant retros-ternal goitres, the gland was removed from the neck. The 2 malignant cases required median sternotomy.

Anaesthesia

The operation is carried out in each instance under general anaesthesia of nitrous oxide and oxygen with endotracheal intubation. As a rule, there should be no difficulty in inserting the endotracheal tube.

The operations

REMOVAL OF GLAND FROM NECK

1

The incision

A collar incision is made along the lowest crease of the neck. A low incision is desirable, as this allows extension downward for a median sternotomy. The platysma is cut along the line of skin incision, and the skin flaps are raised upward and downward. We have found it unnecessary to inject adrenaline to prevent excessive blood loss. This can be minimized if the flaps are raised with the diathermy knife.

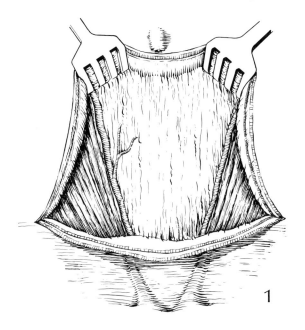

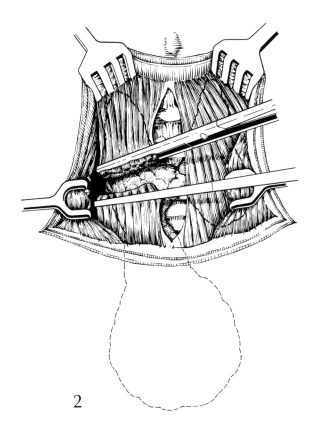

2

Division of strap muscles

After the skin flaps have been raised the anterior jugular veins may be divided and the two ends suture-ligated. The strap muscles are dissected clear of the investing fascia. The midline fascia between the two pairs of strap muscles is then divided longitudinally with scissors. The muscles are then divided between Kocher's forceps below the points where the ansae hypoglossi enter their lateral borders. By inserting the finger deep to the muscles the retrosternal extension of the thyroid can be confirmed.

3

Freeing the divided strap muscles and division of middle thyroid vein

By lifting the Kocher's forceps, the sternohyoid and then the sternothyroid muscles are peeled off the thyroid capsules. This can best be done with sharp dissection. Thus the thyroid gland is completely exposed. The middle thyroid vein, which may be absent, is exposed, ligated and divided.

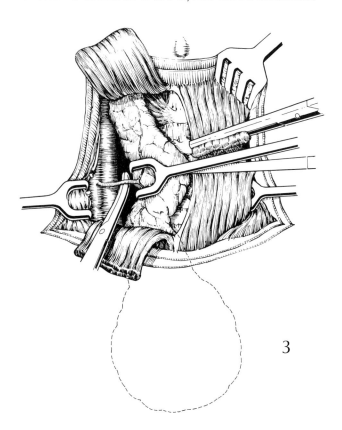

4

Exposure and division of superior thyroid vessels

Normally when the nodular goitre is not vascular, the strap muscles can be dissected to their origins without difficulty. However, some carcinomas of the thyroid gland may be very vascular, making exposure and ligation of the superior thyroid vessels difficult. The vessels are thin-walled and much blood may be lost, if the muscles are dissected off the thyroid capsule. In such cases it is best to leave the sternothyroid muscle intact and, at its upper insertion, split the fibres. This manoeuvre will allow exposure and division of the superior thyroid vessels with the minimum loss of blood.

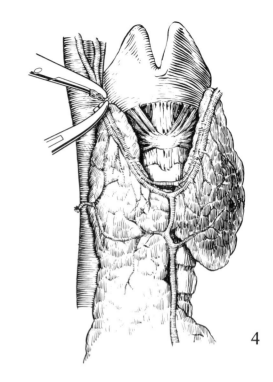

4

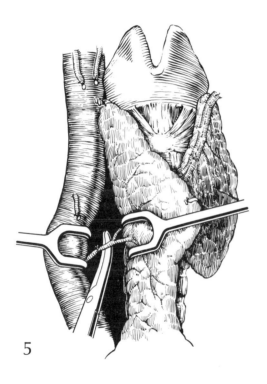

5

5

Isolation and division of inferior thyroid artery

With division of the superior thyroid artery, the glandular surface becomes less vascular. This allows the sternothyroid muscle to be stripped off the thyroid capsule. The carotid sheath can now be retracted laterally and the inferior thyroid artery ligated before it divides into branches.

6

Division of inferior thyroid veins

The inferior thyroid veins drain into the innominate vein and, when there is a retrosternal extension of the thyroid gland, are stretched and dip deep to the upper margin of the manubrium sterni. These veins may be large and are isolated with care and ligated and divided as low as possible.

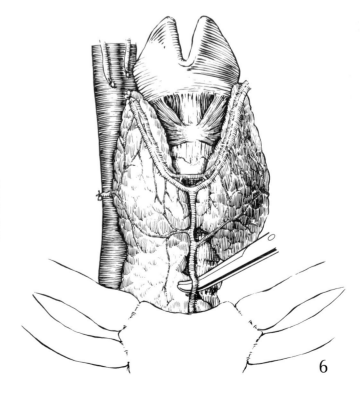

6

7

Delivery of retrosternal goitre

At this stage, the retrosternal extension may be freed from the cervical surface of the endothoracic fascia (Sibson's fascia). By insinuating the finger between the true capsule of the thyroid gland and the fascia, the retrosternal extension is freed and can be delivered into the neck. Delivery can be assisted by applying several tissue forceps (Babcock's) on the capsule and using gentle traction.

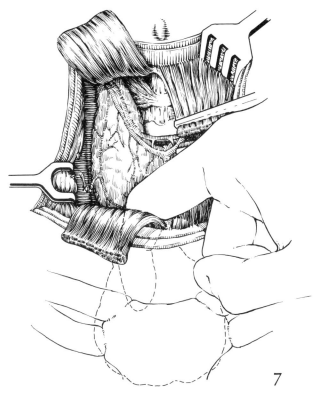

7

8

Intracapsular evacuation of retrosternal thyroid contents and delivery into the neck

Occasionally, the retrosternal goitre may be impacted behind the manubrium sterni. Delivery into the neck by traction then will not be possible. The capsule of the gland is incised and the thyroid contents are evacuated by scooping or, if they are fluid, removed by suction.

Thus the thyroid will be reduced in size and its delivery into the neck is eased.

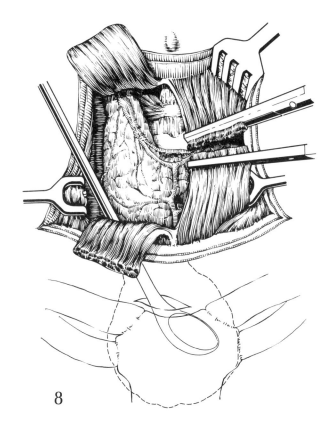

8

9

Identification of recurrent laryngeal nerve

After delivery of the retrosternal extension into the neck, the recurrent nerve needs to be identified. It is best to look for this in the tracheo-oesophageal groove. It may be displaced by the retrosternal goitre, but is much more constant in its location lower down in the neck than at the level of the thyroid gland. By tracing it upward any variation in its course and relation to the inferior thyroid artery and carotid sheath are detected and injury prevented.

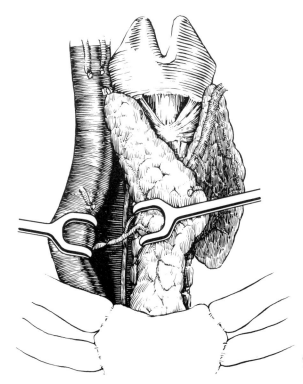

9

10 & 11

Resection of thyroid gland with its retrosternal extension

If the opposite lobe of the thyroid gland is normal, it is necessary to remove only the side of the gland containing the retrosternal extension as well as its isthmus. The isthmus is divided between clamps and the cut edge of the normal lobe is stitched. Bleeding from the posterior rim of the thyroid tissue is controlled by suture-ligatures and then the two edges are brought together with a series of interrupted chromic catgut sutures.

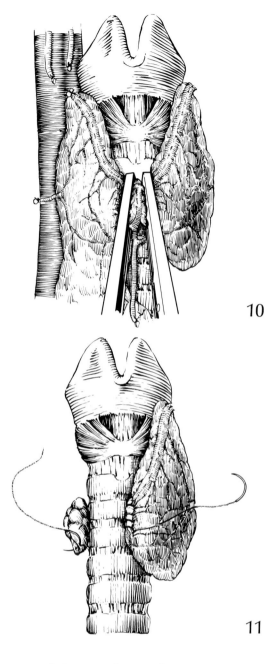

10

11

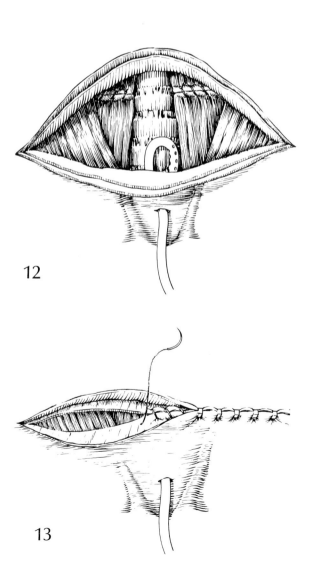

12

13

Drainage and closure of wound

12

After all bleeding points have been brought under control, a Redi-vac drain is inserted with its tip in the retrosternal space. Despite absolute haemostasis, drainage after thyroidectomy must be instituted; failure to do so will lead to accumulation of serum. Repeated tapping will lead to infection and thus causes delay in healing. The drain can usually be removed after 48 h. The strap muscles are brought together with catgut sutures.

13

The platysma is approximated by a continuous interlocking chromic catgut suture. The skin edges are then brought together by applying a series of skin clips.

MEDIAN STERNOTOMY FOR RETROSTERNAL GOITRE

Sectioning of the sternum for retrosternal goitre is, as we have indicated, a very rare operation. Almost all retrosternal goitres can be removed through a cervical approach. However, on rare occasions, when the thyroid gland has acquired a new blood supply (usually from the internal mammary or intercostal arteries), removal of the thyroid through the neck can be extremely dangerous. Bleeding from the newly acquired vessels may be difficult or impossible to control. A median sternotomy will permit ligation of these vessels before the thyroid is removed. Some cases of carcinoma of the thyroid with recognized extension in the mediastinum will also require a sternotomy. A complete instead of a partial sternotomy is performed. This allows clearance of the mediastinal lymphatics and the whole operation can be carried out with good exposure.

14

The incision

From about the middle of the cervical incision, a vertical limb extending from the neck to the upper part of the abdomen is made. Small vessels may be coagulated with diathermy.

Sectioning of sternum

15

The strap muscles are divided as near to the manubrium sterni as possible.

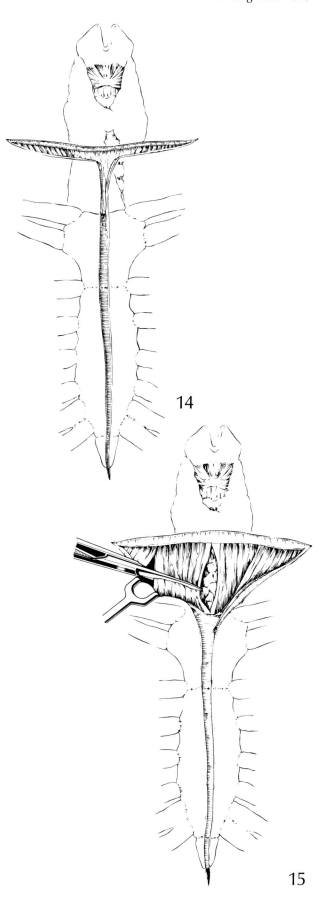

14

15

16

A finger is inserted into the anterior mediastinum, hugging closely the back of the sternum. This opens the anterior mediastinal space. A finger is also inserted into this space after division of the xiphisternum. Thus a finger inserted from the neck above meets in the mediastinum the other finger from the lower end of the sternum.

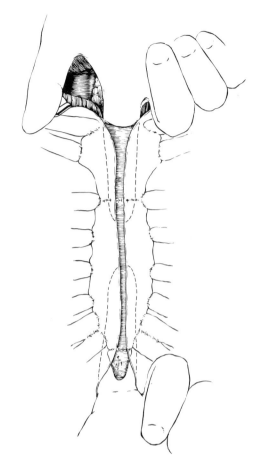

16

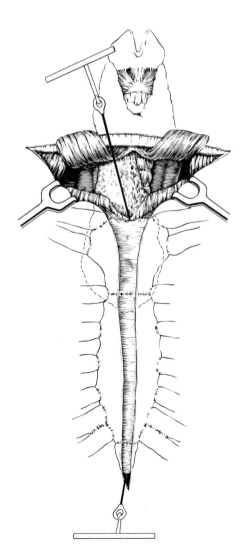

17

17

A Gigli saw with its guide is inserted and the sternum can now be split, taking care to avoid injury to the underlying heart and thyroid gland.

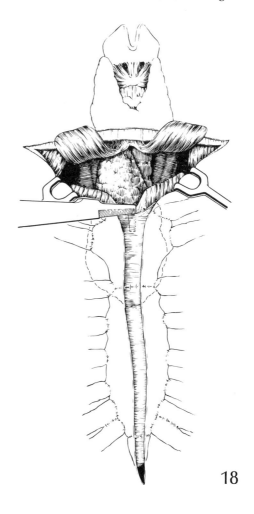

18

An alternative method of splitting the sternum is to employ the Lebsche chisel. This may be more convenient when, as a result of compression on the superior vena cava, there is extensive venous congestion. In using the Lebsche chisel it is wise not to exert pressure on the instrument, so that the guide may stay close to the back of the sternum. This will prevent the chisel from cutting the dilated veins.

Those experienced with the instrument will use a power-driven oscillating saw (*see* chapter on 'Thymectomy', pp. 387–396).

18

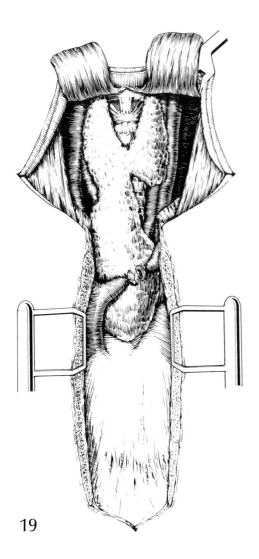

19

Dissection of mediastinal structures

When it is desirable to perform lymph node dissection, the left innominate vein is divided between forceps and transfixed. The remnants of the thymus need to be removed. The thyroid extension is dissected from the mediastinal tissues and is combined with a total thyroidectomy.

19

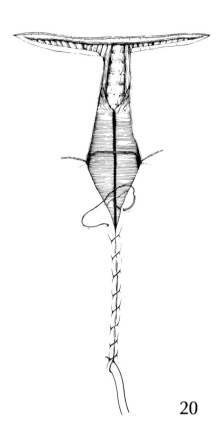

20

Closure and drainage of mediastinum

The edges of the sternum are brought together with three figure-of-eight stitches of braided stainless steel wire, applied at the lateral borders of the sternum. A drain is inserted in the anterior mediastinum and another in the pleural cavity. If both mediastinal pleura are torn, then both sides of the chest should be drained.

   The subcutaneous tissues over the sternum are brought together by a continuous suture of 0 chromic catgut. The strap muscles are reattached to the back of the manubrium sterni. A separate drain is inserted into the neck and the skin closed.

20

Postoperative care

Drains are removed within 24–48 h. The mediastinal drain is usually removed after 24 h. The chest drains, if necessary, may be kept in longer.

   Recurrent nerve palsy may occur and care must be taken to detect it early. Patients with recurrent nerve palsy will have difficulty in bringing up sputum and with physiotherapy may avoid the necessity of bronchial toilet or tracheostomy.

   Tetany caused by removal of parathyroids or interference with their blood supply will require intravenous calcium gluconate. Subsequently calciferol and calcium may be needed.

Results

Removal of retrosternal goitres gives excellent results. There have been no hospital mortalities in 21 such operations. In 2 cases, a median sternotomy was needed to remove extensive carcinoma of the thyroid. One was for a recurrent follicular carcinoma, while the other had medullary carcinoma of the thyroid with massive vascular lymph nodes in the mediastinum and retrosternal extension. Both have survived, one for more than 3 years and the other more than 5 years.

References

1. Rietz, K.-A., Werner, B. Intrathoracic goiter. Acta Chirurgica Scandinavica 1960; 119; 379–388

2. Andrade, M. A. de. A review of 128 cases of posterior mediastinal goiter. World Journal of Surgery 1977; 1: 789–797

Illustrations by Paul Darton

Parathyroid gland exploration

Euan Milroy MB BS, FRCS
Consultant Urologist, The Middlesex Hospital, London

Introduction

Parathyroid exploration is not an operation to be done occasionally. Although many of these operations are not particularly difficult and may be completed in a reasonably short time, the occasional extremely difficult case cannot be predicted in advance. The operations should only be undertaken by surgeons who are familiar with the surgery of the neck and who regularly carry out parathyroid explorations.

Hyperparathyroidism

The only indication for parathyroid surgery is to remove overactive parathyroid tissue in patients in whom it is causing hypercalcaemia, there being no satisfactory long-term drug therapy for hyperparathyroidism. Patients with hypercalcaemia may present in a great variety of ways. The stone, bone and gastrointestinal (peptic ulcers and pancreatitis) symptoms are well known, as are the less common psychological and psychiatric disturbances caused by hypercalcaemia. In a recent personal series of 200 patients with surgically proven hyperparathyroidism 35 per cent presented with stone disease. Of patients presenting with urinary calculi some 10 per cent would be found to have hyperparathyroidism if thoroughly investigated. With a large array of biochemical tests now being carried out on all patients, and with the increasing popularity of regular screening procedures on the healthy population, larger numbers of patients with asymptomatic hyperparathyroidism are being found – 40 per cent of our own series of patients with surgically proven hyperparathyroidism. In fact most of these patients, particularly in the older age groups, will have one or other of a number of rather vague symptoms – lethargy, malaise, polyuria, polydipsia or hypertension – which although not diagnostic of parathyroid disease may be relieved by removing the overactive parathyroid tissue[1].

The incidence of hyperparathyroidism is far higher than was first described and has recently been reported to be approximately 28 new cases per 100 000 population per year, both in the USA[2] and in England[3]; the incidence increasing with age, especially in women, to approximately 188 per 100 000 among women over the age of 60 years[2]. Seventy per cent of our cases were female.

Diagnosis

The diagnosis of hyperparathyroidism is made by the finding of persistent hypercalcaemia, having ensured that the raised calcium is not the result of a high serum albumen, and having excluded all other causes of hypercalcaemia[4]. It is essential that the surgeon undertaking parathyroid surgery works closely with an experienced endocrinologist as there are many pitfalls to trap the unwary into an incorrect diagnosis. Peripheral venous levels of parathyroid hormone are sometimes but not invariably raised in primary hyperparathyroidism. With the older assay techniques any detectable circulating parathyroid hormone was felt to be an indication of parathyroid overactivity. The more recently developed amino terminal assay is more reliable and gives an excellent correlation of peripheral levels of hormone with parathyroid pathology[5]. The steroid suppression test[6] will help to exclude non-parathyroid causes of hypercalcaemia but

again a number of false positive and negative results will be found.

Once a definite diagnosis of hyperparathyroidism has been established, attempts may be made to localize the overactivity to one or other of the parathyroid glands. Unfortunately this is far from easy although many centres are working to improve their ability to localize parathyroid tissue preoperatively. At present we can achieve an 87 per cent chance of predicting the site of a single adenoma using the technique of selective sampling of neck veins for parathyroid hormone[7]. This technique is of particular value in patients in whom previous surgery has failed to find an abnormal gland.

Ultrasound is, in our experience, of some value especially in reoperations on the neck. Computerized axial tomography is of little value in the neck but may find the occasional anterior mediastinal parathyroid adenoma where ultrasound cannot be used. Selective arteriography is effective in expert hands, again particularly in the patient who has been explored previously, but may carry unjustifiable risks in the older patient. Isotope scans of the parathyroids have unfortunately not lived up to their earlier high expectations.

Preoperative localization is therefore at present far from perfect and makes it all the more important that the surgeon has a full knowledge of the various possible pathological abnormalities and anatomical variations of the parathyroid glands and has in his mind a clear plan of the operation he is to undertake to cover all eventualities.

Indications for parathyroid exploration

It is our opinion that all patients with proven hyperparathyroidism should be offered surgery providing they are fit to withstand the anaesthetic and operation. There is of course no argument about the symptomatic patient, but the justification for operating on the many asymptomatic patients is often questioned. It must be remembered that many of these so-called asymptomatic patients have symptoms which may be related to the hypercalcaemia and, although no adequate long-term study of the natural history of mild asymptomatic hyperparathyroidism has been carried out, what evidence there is suggests that some 20 per cent (of 147 patients observed over a 5 year period) will develop complications of the disease which precipitate parathyroid surgery[8]. To have operated on these patients as soon as the diagnosis is made would cure the hyperparathyroidism before more serious and irreversible complications, particularly renal, occur. It is remarkable how frequently these rather vague symptoms improve after surgical correction of the hypercalcaemia, and how the patients feel an improvement in their general health and well-being. It should also not be forgotten that hypercalcaemia is in its own right a lethal condition, particularly in the older patient.

The operation

1

Position of patient and anaesthesia

All patients must have a preoperative inspection of their vocal cords to confirm that both recurrent laryngeal nerves are intact.

The patient is positioned with the neck extended and the head resting on a rubber ring. A small sandbag under the shoulders may help but care must be taken not to overextend the neck. This is not only dangerous in the older patient but may also make the operative exposure less satisfactory. A 20–30° head-up tilt helps to reduce venous bleeding. A general anaesthetic using moderate hypotension down to 70–80 mmHg systolic blood pressure, with the help of an experienced anaesthetist (using a sympathetic blockade, or a sodium nitroprusside technique), is a most useful aid in preventing peroperative bleeding.

The two most important factors in the search for the parathyroid glands are adequate exposure and absence of bleeding in the operative field. Vital staining of parathyroid tissue using a preoperative infusion of methylene blue is sometimes suggested. Most surgeons who carry out large numbers of parathyroid explorations find this technique of altering the colour difference between parathyroid and normal tissue unnecessary, unreliable and sometimes even misleading. It is far more important that the surgeon should become confident in recognizing the subtle differences between the reddish brown colour of the normal parathyroid, the somewhat darker abnormal parathyroid, and the various other colours of the adjacent thyroid, lymph nodes and adipose tissues.

Draping and incision

2

The neck is draped as for a thyroidectomy; four single towels will be found to be simpler than a double head towel. An 8–10 cm long transverse skin crease incision is made approximately midway between the notch of the thyroid cartilage and the suprasternal notch. Care should be taken not to curve the incision too much when the neck is well extended; the incision will appear more curved when the head is positioned normally.

3

It may be found helpful in making a symmetrical incision to press a tightly held suture into the skin in order to impress a line to follow with the scalpel. On no account should vertical skin scratches be made across the line of the incision in order to help subsequent wound alignment; these may leave unsightly scars.

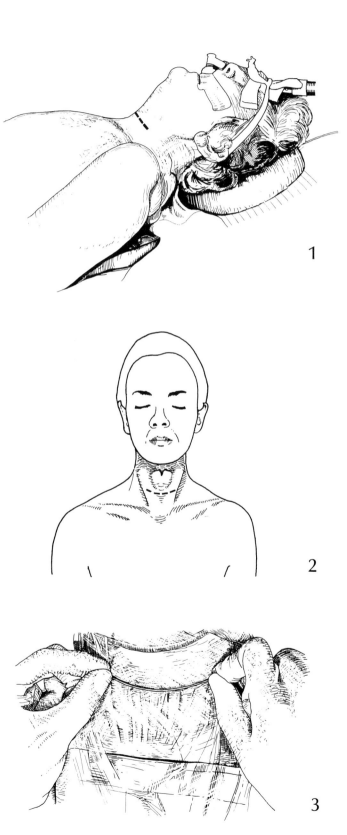

1

2

3

4

The incision is taken through subcutaneous fat and, at either end of the incision, the platysma muscle. The skin, fat and muscle are then separated as one layer from the underlying strap muscles. It is most important for adequate exposure to develop this plane as far up as the thyroid and down to the suprasternal notch. Once the correct plane is found this separation is made easier by using blunt dissection with firm but gentle pressure of the fingers of both hands covered by a gauze swab.

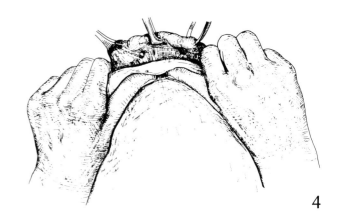

4

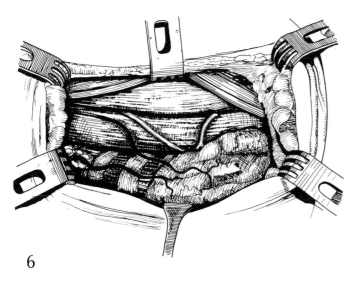

5

Exposure of the thyroid and parathyroids

5

A self-retaining ring retractor, bent to lie over the neck, with 4–6 rake blades will be found to be much more satisfactory than other forms of wound retraction. In this and subsequent illustrations the patient's head is on the right.

6

The strap muscles are separated in the midline. It is never necessary to divide the muscles transversely. These muscles are always thin enough to retract laterally and muscle division causes unnecessary bleeding, which can make adequate parathyroid exploration impossible.

If no gland abnormality has been localized preoperatively each side of the neck must be explored thoroughly in turn. It is the author's practice to start exploring the right side of the neck, standing on the patient's left. The thyroid gland may then be held by one hand while dissection continues with the other, using short fine curved scissors or dissecting forceps. When exploration on one side is complete, the surgeon and assistant change sides to explore the other side of the neck. It must be admitted that some surgeons find this technique awkward and prefer to stand on the same side of the patient's neck they are exploring. The strap muscles are separated from the thyroid gland and the middle thyroid vein ligated and cut.

6

7 & 8

Finding the parathyroid glands

The thyroid gland may now be gently lifted up and the other important landmarks found. These are the inferior thyroid artery and the recurrent laryngeal nerve. The surgeon must be careful not to start looking for parathyroid tissue until this complete exposure of the area has been achieved. *The superior parathyroid* is easier to find than the inferior. It usually lies on the posterior surface of the thyroid gland just cranial to the inferior thyroid artery, always deep to a thin but definite transparent fascial layer under which it can be seen to move, with its associated fatty tissue, when pushed with the scissors or dissecting forceps. It may lie further up the course of the superior thyroid vessels or, if the gland enlarges, may descend deep to the inferior thyroid vessels to lie lateral to, or even behind, the oesophagus. The *mobility* of the gland within its fascial sheath together with its *site*, the typical yellow-brown *colour* and the soft *consistency* of parathyroid tissue compared to the firmer lymph nodes and thyroid gland, are the four all-important factors in the localization of parathyroid glands.

The inferior parathyroid is more variable in position and may sometimes be difficult to distinguish from 'brown fat' present in large amounts in the neck of some patients. The normal parathyroid, although varying in size from 1 to 10 mm in length, always has a definite structure and vascular supply compared to the more amorphous fatty tissue; it is also not infrequently wrapped, at least in part, in a layer of normal yellow fat. The inferior gland is usually found on the posterolateral surface of the thyroid gland caudad to the inferior thyroid artery. It may however be found anywhere down the course of one of the inferior thyroid veins, along the thymus or in the anterior mediastinum – what is sometimes called the 'thyrothymic axis'. It is important to explore this area and to incise the surface of the thymic lobe as far down as the innominate vein if no inferior gland can be found in the neck. A parathyroid gland may lie within the thymus unseen until the thymic capsule is opened.

Either superior or inferior parathyroid gland may occasionally lie further lateral in the neck but no further out than the carotid sheath. Rarely a gland is completely intrathyroid; most supposed intrathyroid glands are in fact sunk into the surface of the thyroid and may be found by careful dissection of the thyroid surface beneath the fascial covering of the gland. The descent of the glands is also variable; occasionally both parathyroid glands on one side are above or both below the inferior thyroid artery, and occasionally three glands may be on one side of the neck and only one on the other. In approximately 10 per cent of our cases more than four glands were found. Unfortunately the positions of the parathyroid glands are not symmetrical on the left and right sides of the neck.

It should be noted that the parathyroid glands of children and adolescents are smaller and lighter in colour than adult glands and may be even more difficult to find because of the relatively larger thyroid and thymus glands.

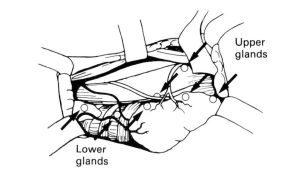

Upper glands

Lower glands

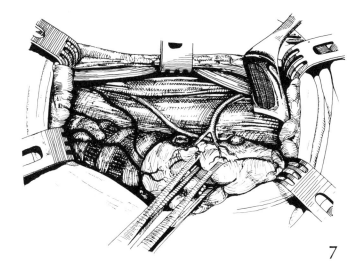

7

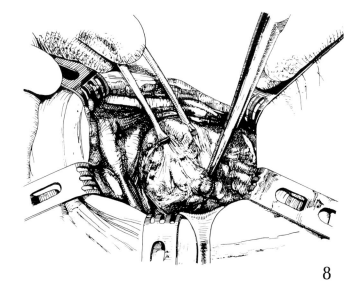

8

Pathology and surgical plan

Adenoma

Eighty-eight per cent of our patients with hyperparathyroidism were found to have a single parathyroid adenoma; 60 per cent of these were situated in the position of one of the inferior glands. In these patients only the adenoma need be removed although it must be emphasized that care must be taken to remove the adenoma completely. Great difficulty is sometimes encountered in separating a large adenoma in the superior gland position from the recurrent laryngeal nerve which may be completely enclosed by the adenoma as the nerve enters the larynx. One cause for the recurrence of hyperparathyroidism after removal of an adenoma is the further enlargement of a deep fragment of the original adenoma which was not removed at the first operation.

Ten per cent of patients are found to have hyperplasia of all parathyroid tissue. For this reason at least one normal parathyroid gland must be identified in those patients in whom a single adenoma has been found, and a small biopsy taken from the end of the gland furthest from its vascular pedicle and sent for immediate frozen section histological examination in order to confirm the diagnosis.

Hyperplasia

Generalized hyperplasia is usually easy to diagnose because all four glands are large and relatively easy to find. When all the glands have been found and confirmed histologically, three glands are removed completely and the distal two-thirds of the remaining gland are also removed leaving behind the third (approximately 50 mg) adjacent to the vascular pedicle. If possible the remaining fragment should be one of the inferior glands and should be carefully marked with a clip or non-absorbable suture in case further surgical removal becomes necessary. It is our practice to mark all remaining parathyroid tissue, normal or hyperplastic, with one or two vasiular clips placed close to, but not upon, the parathyroid tissue.

Nodular hyperplasia

Patients with nodular hyperplasia of the parathyroid present a difficult problem because the glands, although all histologically abnormal, may vary considerably in size, one or more being enlarged and the others being normal in size but containing nodules of hyperplastic tissue. This diagnosis requires a careful and experienced pathologist and fine surgical judgement as to how much parathyroid tissue needs to be removed[9] – further reasons why this type of surgery should not be undertaken by the inexperienced surgeon. Failure to make this diagnosis is a frequent cause of recurrent hyperparathyroidism. All parathyroid glands must be found in these patients and approximately one-half of the most normal gland should be left and carefully marked. All other parathyroid tissue should be removed.

Nodular hyperplasia is the commonest abnormality found in the parathyroids of patients with hypercalcaemia associated with the rare familial multiple endocrine adenopathy. The type I adenopathy patient usually also has a prolactinoma and gastrinoma. The even rarer type II adenopathy is associated with medullary carcinoma of the thyroid and phaeochromocytoma. Familial hyperparathyroidism may also be found as a single abnormality unrelated to generalized adenopathies.

Carcinoma

Carcinoma of the parathyroid is very rare, accounting for 1–2 per cent of cases of hyperparathyroidism. It is usually diagnosed when a case of recurrent hyperparathyroidism is re-explored and local invasion is found. Parathyroid carcinoma is very difficult to recognize from the histological sections alone. There is no satisfactory treatment for this condition but a surgical attempt should be made to remove as much parathyroid tissue as possible before irradiating the neck, although there is little evidence that radiotherapy is effective.

Frozen sections

Immediate frozen section histological confirmation of parathyroid tissue must always be obtained. If this facility is not available the operation should not be carried out.

Specimens sent for frozen section should be numbered, not given anatomical identities which tend to confuse at this stage. While awaiting the histological results it may be found useful to suture a numbered metal marker adjacent to the biopsy site to aid later identification. If possible, the pathologist should be able to enter the operating room, keep a 'map' of the biopsy sites and be involved in the surgical decisions concerning the patient.

Missing gland

If no abnormal gland can be found and if one of the four glands from normal sites is missing full exploration must be undertaken, up to the angle of the jaw, laterally to include the carotid sheath, posteriorly behind the oesophagus, and caudally to include the removal of all thymic tissue down to the innominate vein. If a gland is still not found a total removal of loose areolar tissue on that side of the neck, and then, after full mobilization and inspection of the thyroid, a total thyroid lobectomy on the side of the missing gland should be carried out. The operation should then be concluded. The same procedure should be followed if four normal glands have been found, but in this case no thyroid tissue should be excised unless one of the localization tests has suggested a definite abnormality. A few lymph nodes should always be taken for biopsy in case a diagnosis of sarcoidosis, causing hypercalcaemia, has been missed.

Mediastinal exploration

If hypercalcaemia persists when no abnormal tissue has been found, the anterior mediastinum should be explored through a full-length median sternotomy. Needless to say this should only be carried out by a surgeon with considerable experience of parathyroid surgery and after a careful review of the evidence for a diagnosis of hyperparathyroidism has been made. The neck should be re-explored no more than one week after the first operation, just before carrying out the sternotomy, and under the same anaesthetic. If carried out at this time no difficulty will be found with adhesions and fibrosis in the neck. After the median sternotomy a complete clearance of all adipose and thymic tissue is made down to the origin of the aorta and laterally to the hilum of each lung. Parathyroid glands in the anterior mediastinum do occur but are rare and most abnormal glands in this position, usually within the capsule of the thymus, can be reached retrosternally from the neck without very much difficulty.

9

Closure of incision

Before closing the incision the blood pressure must be allowed gradually to return towards normal; careful haemostasis is then achieved and a fine tube suction drain inserted through the lateral part of the lower skin flap. It is a good idea to allow some of the holes of the drain to lie superficial to the strap muscles in case of bleeding in this plane. The strap muscles are closed with interrupted absorbable sutures. The sandbag under the shoulders is then removed and the head and neck flexed a little to allow the platysma to be closed with interrupted absorbable sutures. Skin clips are used to close the skin. Half of these should be removed at 24 h with the drain, if bleeding has ceased. The remaining skin clips are removed 48 h after the operation.

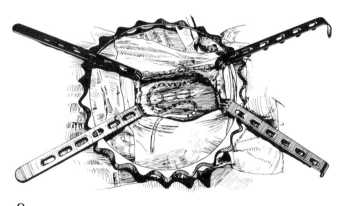

9

Postoperative management

The postoperative course of these patients is usually remarkably uneventful. Daily calcium estimations must be carried out to ensure that hypercalcaemia does not persist and to monitor the fall of calcium to within normal limits usually within 2–3 days of the operation. Daily monitoring of calcium levels must continue for at least one week after surgery to make sure that there is no gradual development of hypocalcaemia, and no delayed recurrence of hypercalcaemia. Temporary hypocalcaemia, with associated paraesthesia and possible tetany, may occur if a large abnormal gland has been removed. This can usually be corrected by means of oral calcium supplements. If there is extensive parathyroid bone disease with associated loss of bone calcium the hypocalcaemia will be more profound and may last several months. In these patients oral calcium supplements and 1,25-dihydroxycholecalciferol (Rocaltrol) should be given orally up to $8\,\mu g$ per day in divided doses until the serum calcium returns to normal levels. The patient is then maintained on approximately $0.5\,\mu g$ per day, with weekly measurements of serum calcium levels until the bones have recalcified and the residual parathyroid tissue has recovered its normal function. If there is no residual parathyroid or no recovery occurs these supplements may need to be continued indefinitely with careful and regular monitoring of calcium levels in order to prevent iatrogenic hypercalcaemia. Associated magnesium deficiency is also sometimes a problem in patients with severe parathyroid bone disease.

Other postoperative complications are identical with those of thyroid operations (see p. 369), haemorrhage with its possible associated tracheal compression being the most serious. Recurrent laryngeal nerve injury should be rare if care is taken always to identify both recurrent laryngeal nerves at operation. Temporary hoarseness is often present after extensive paratracheal and paralaryngeal dissection. Normal function of the vocal cords in these patients can be confirmed postoperatively, as preoperatively, by indirect laryngoscopy.

Recurrent hyperparathyroidism

The surgery for patients with persistent or recurrent hyperparathyroidism after previous exploration is extremely difficult and should only be undertaken at specialist referral centres.

Acknowledgement

I am grateful to Dr Jeffrey O'Riordan for many helpful suggestions during the preparation of this chapter and for providing an invaluable and expert service to our patients.

References

1. Milroy E. J. G., O'Riordan, J. L. H. Investigation and management of urinary calculi of metabolic origin. In: Hadfield, G. J., Hobsley, M., eds. Current surgical practice, Vol. 3, p. 80. London: Arnold, 1981

2. Heath, H., Hodgson, S. F., Kennedy, M. A. Primary hyperparathyroidism. Incidence, morbidity and potential economic impact in a community. New England Journal of Medicine 1980; 302: 189–193

3. Fisken, R. A., Heath, D. A., Somers, S., Bold, A. M. Hypercalcaemia in hospital patients. Clinical and diagnostic aspects. Lancet 1981; 1: 202–207

4. Tomlinson, S., O'Riordan, J. L. H. The parathyroids. British Journal of Hospital Medicine 1978; 19: 40–53

5. Papapoulos, S. E., Hendy, G. N., Manning, R. M., Lewin, I.G., O'Riordan, J. L. H. Amino-terminal labelled antibody assay for human parathyroid hormone. Journal of Endocrinology 1978; 79: 33P–34P

6. Dent, C. E., Watson, L. The hydrocortisone test in primary and tertiary hyperparathyroidism. Lancet 1968; 2: 662–664

7. Dunlop D. A. B., Papapoulos, S. E., Lodge, R. W., Fulton, A. J., Kendall, B. E., O'Riordan, J. L. H. Parathyroid venous sampling: anatomic considerations and results in 95 patients with primary hyperparathyroidism. British Journal of Radiology 1980; 53: 183–191

8. Purnell, D. C., Scholz, D. A., Smith, L. H., Sizemore, G. W., Black, B. M., Goldsmith, R. S., Arnaud, C. D. Treatment of hyperparathyroidism. American Journal of Medicine 1974; 56: 800–809

9. Castleman, B., Roth, S. I. Tumours of the parathyroid glands. Washington D.C.: Armed Forces Institute of Pathology, 1978 (Atlas of tumour pathology, 2nd series, fascicle 14)

Illustrations by Carol J. Pienta

Thymectomy

Francis T. Thomas MD, FACS
Professor of Surgery, Department of Surgery, School of Medicine,
East Carolina University, Greenville, North Carolina

Introduction

The thymus gland has a fascinating lore, but its role as a major architect of the developing immunological system has only recently been discovered. Even today, little is known of its function in pathogenesis of many unusual conditions such as myasthenia gravis, red cell aplasia, collagen disorders and other syndromes which are cured or reversed by thymectomy.

Indications

The two major indications for thymectomy are myasthenia gravis and thymoma, one of the most common mediastinal tumours. Myasthenia gravis is a muscle-weakening disease, presumably involving the motor endplate. About 15 per cent of myasthenic patients will have a thymoma. There is controversy concerning the efficacy of thymectomy in myasthenia gravis, but an operative mortality of less than 2 per cent permits recommendation of this procedure for most patients who cannot be well managed medically. The best results are obtained in young women with a short disease course. All myasthenic patients should have chest X-rays; if there is an indication of thymic enlargement, computerized axial tomography (CAT) can be helpful in locating a tumour.

The thymus gland, which is quite large in childhood, involutes to a small horseshoe-shaped organ during the ages of 10–15 years. In adulthood, thymomas occur in the anterior superior mediastinum. Some are asymptomatic; others cause pain or compression symptoms. All require surgery because of the possibility of malignancy.

1

Anatomy

The gland is an H-shaped organ deriving its blood supply primarily from branches of the internal mammary artery. Venous drainage from the thymus is usually to branches of the innominate veins, which lie directly posterior to the thymus, and to a lesser degree, to some cervical venous branches. Tearing of these branches, or injury to the innominate vein during posterior dissection of the thymus, can bring about troublesome haemorrhage.

Operative approaches

Three approaches may be used to excise the thymus gland, depending upon its size and the degree of exposure required: the transcervical approach, the hemisternotomy and the median sternotomy. The first approach yields the least exposure and the last the greatest.

The *transcervical approach* is indicated primarily in patients with myasthenia gravis when the thymus is normal in size or when a small thymoma is present. This operation carries a fairly low morbidity and mortality risk; it has been criticized, however, because the incomplete exposure it allows sometimes leads to incomplete thymectomy.

The *hemisternotomy approach* can be used to excise small to moderate-sized thymus glands in patients with myasthenia gravis or thymoma. This approach is the author's choice because of the superior exposure compared with that afforded by the transcervical approach and the lesser operative trauma compared with that accompanying full median sternotomy.

Median sternotomy should be used in all cases where a large tumour of the thymus is present, but the surgeon must remember that this extensive procedure carries the highest risk of postoperative morbidity, including sternal

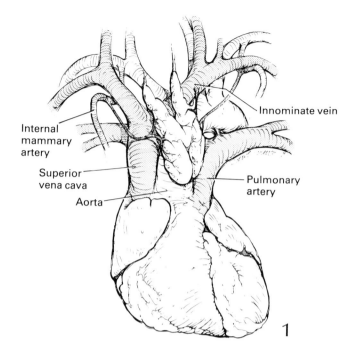

1

dehiscence and respiratory insufficiency. Fear of such potential complications need not deter one from using the incision if it is appropriate, but the surgeon should be well informed about the management of the complications and should not be hesitant to seek help. Those who regularly perform open heart surgery have had considerable experience with this wound and are likely to be of help in management of the complications should they occur.

Close cooperation of a neurologist or internist will be helpful in management of the myasthenic patient. Physiotherapy may be an aid to proper breathing in the postoperative period. Repeated measurement of vital capacity is indicated.

Position of patient

2

The patient to undergo thymectomy is first placed in the supine position with arms at the sides. After intubation and stabilization of the patient, the head is turned and the table is then adjusted to the reverse Trendelenburg position. This position is helpful in minimizing bleeding, especially that of venous origin. Careful monitoring of the blood pressure is required with this position, as in some patients it will produce a fall in blood pressure.

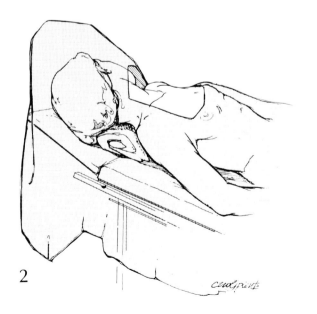

2

The operation

TRANSCERVICAL APPROACH

The patient's head is turned to one side. The anaesthesia machine and anaesthesiologist move to the side to which the head is turned while the surgeon stands opposite.

3

The incision

A standard collar incision is made about 1 cm above the sternal notch.

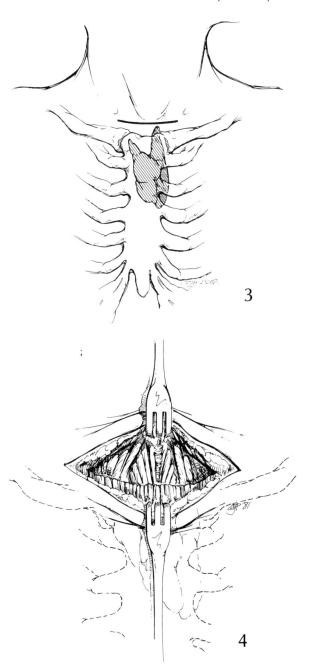

3

4

The incision is then carried through the skin, subcutaneous tissues and platysma.

4

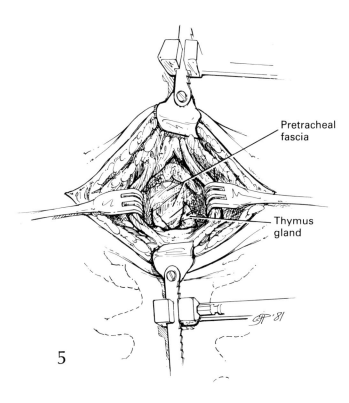

Pretracheal fascia

Thymus gland

5

5

The sternothyroid and sternohyoid muscles are split in the midline along the direction of the fibres and retracted laterally to expose the pretracheal fascia. This fascia is an important landmark for the operation, extending down along the anterior pericardium.

6

Retraction of the muscles permits entry into the pre-tracheal space and mediastinum. With a self-retaining retractor providing exposure in the pretracheal space, the two cervical tails of the thymus are usually readily identifiable.

The thymus tissue is light brown in colour and denser than the cervical mediastinal fat tissue. The surgeon should keep in mind that in the adult the thymus is largely atrophic and identification is therefore often difficult.

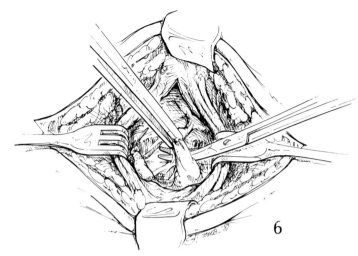

7

Once the tails of the thymus have been identified, the surgeon frees the thymus up outside the capsule, by means of blunt and sharp dissection, maintaining traction on the specimen and bringing it up into the cervical space.

The greatest single problem with thymectomy by the cervical approach is the likelihood of incomplete removal of the gland. For this reason, traction is employed, to improve delineation of the capsule and ensure more complete excision of the thymic tissue. Mediastinal fat should be brought along with the thymus. Dissection can then be continued posteriorly. A careful search should be made at this point for medium-sized veins coming from the innominate veins to the thymus.

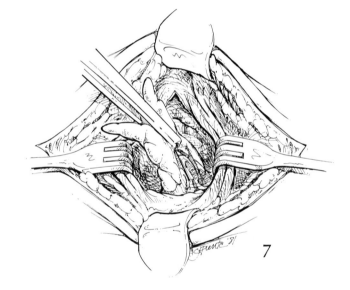

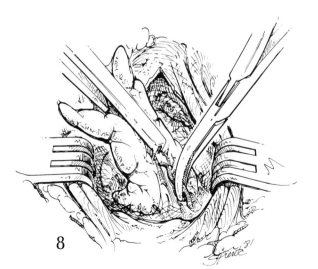

8

The thymic blood supply should be thoroughly secured by clamping of any feeding neck vessels.

Thymomas or large thymic glands may acquire a blood supply from internal mammary branches, and these can usually be identified and clamped as they enter the gland. Gauze pressure is necessary for the venous branches to the innominate. A drain is not needed.

PARTIAL OR HEMISTERNOTOMY

9

The incision

The incision for superior hemisternotomy begins in the midline at the suprasternal notch and extends down to the third or fourth intercostal space.

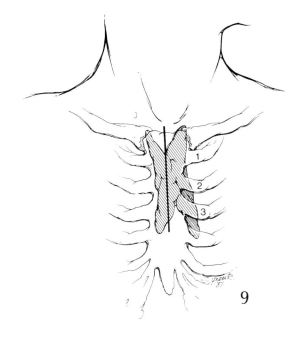

9

10

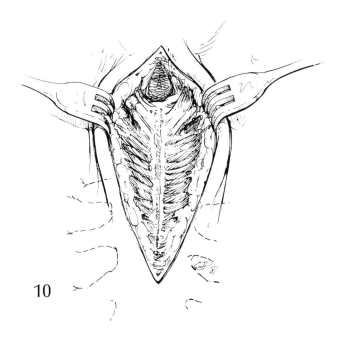

10

The subcutaneous tissue is opened. The pectoral fascia is opened in the midline of the sternum, which may be identified by palpation of the intercostal spaces on either side of the lateral sternum.

Haemostasis is usually achieved with the electrocautery. Once the sternum is exposed, its midline may be marked with the electrocautery, to make sure that the split will be precisely centred.

11

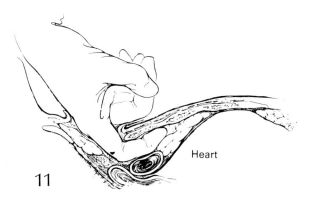

Heart

11

The incision should be begun in such a way that the skin can be retracted upward to allow dissection around the top of the sternum. A small skin retractor is used to retract the skin superiorly and, by blunt dissection, using a clamp and a finger, one can go around to the suprasternal notch and dissect bluntly along the posterior sternum, to push tissue off the bone.

12

The split is then carried out with the sternal saw, the surgeon taking care to hold the foot of the saw firmly against the posterior table of the sternum, simultaneously advancing the saw and maintaining the firm contact in order to protect the heart.

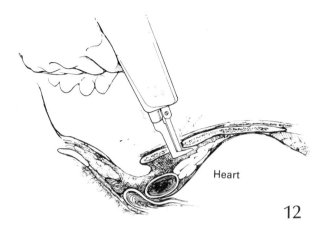

Heart

12

13

Once the sternum is partially transected, a blunt retractor can be used to wedge the sternum open. Wedging the sternum open in this fashion can sometimes produce fractures, however, and therefore it may be desirable to angle the cut laterally to either side, at the lower edge of the sternal wound, so that the area of fracture is minimized. The anterior and posterior sternal tables may be electrocoagulated and the sternal bone treated with bone wax for haemostasis.

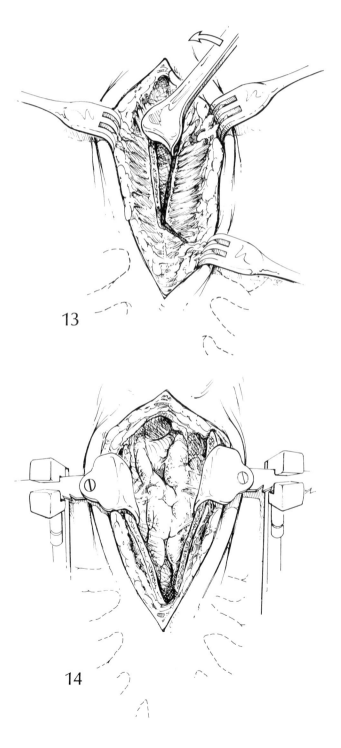

13

14

14

The cut sternal edges can now be separated with a single-blade self-retaining retractor which is opened enough to provide good exposure of the thymus. After careful palpation and blunt dissection, to make sure that the vascular supply to the thymus will not be disrupted, excision of the thymus may then be carried out as described for the transcervical approach.

This is the best moment for judging whether a mediastinal tumour is benign or malignant. This decision must be made by the surgeon at operation since the pathologist is unable to differentiate histologically between benign and malignant thymomas. Operative findings are the most valuable guide to judgement about malignancy of the tumour: fixation and ingrowth into adjacent structures are hallmarks of malignancy. If the surgeon feels the tumour is malignant, he should carry out a wide resection of the tumour, including the anterior pericardium and other tissues through the anterior mediastinum. It is good practice to identify the phrenic nerves and resect the tumour together with the anterior pericardium between the right and left phrenic nerves. The innominate vein can be sacrificed if it is adherent to pericardium or tumour.

15

Following excision of the thymus, haemostasis is secured, and a drainage tube (usually a Hemovac) is placed through a stab wound in the medial or lateral neck and attached to suction drainage.

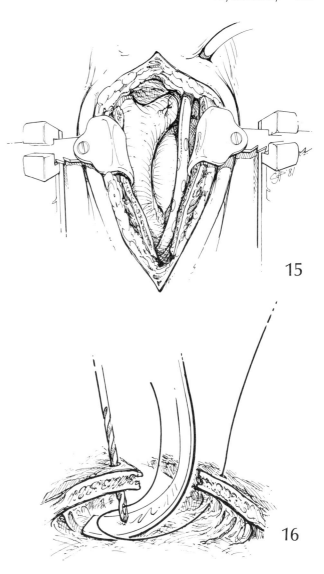

15

16

Closure of the sternum is accomplished with No. 18 gauge wire or No. 5 monofilament suture, inserted through holes created in the sternum by an orthopaedic hand drill. It is important for the tip of the drill to be shielded from the vulnerable cardiac surface by a malleable retractor. Special drill tips with an eye greatly simplify threading of the wire through the sternum.

16

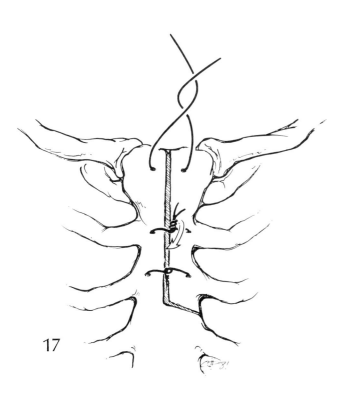

17

17

Alternatively, the wire or suture may be placed to encircle the sternum, with swaged-on large needles. In passing the sutures around the edges of the sternum, the surgeon must keep in mind that the internal mammary artery lies within 1–2 cm of the suture; if it is punctured, massive bleeding may result.

Once the wires are placed, they are drawn up and tightened with pliers or a stout needle holder. When the proper tension has been effected, the ends are twisted, cut and turned under.

The pectoral fascia is closed with 2/0 or 3/0 chromic and the skin is closed with staples or interrupted vertical mattress sutures.

MEDIAN STERNOTOMY

18

The procedure of choice for all large thymomas is the median sternotomy. This longitudinal incision is made from the suprasternal notch the full length of the sternum to below the xiphoid process.

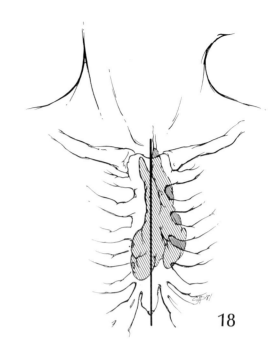

18

19

Used for maximum exposure, this incision should be begun in such a way that the skin can be retracted upward to allow dissection around the top of the sternum. Should tracheostomy be necessary in the postoperative period, it can thus be performed without entering the area of sternal and mediastinal dissection. This measure is taken to minimize the possibility of infection in that area.

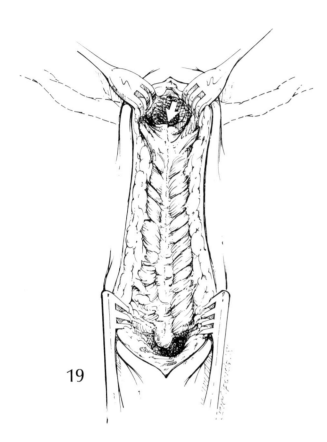

19

20

A small skin retractor is used to retract the skin superiorly and, by blunt dissection, using a clamp and a finger, one can go around to the suprasternal notch and dissect bluntly along the posterior sternum, to push tissue off the bone. Inferiorly, in similar manner, a blunt plane is developed directly on the posterior sternum and the finger used to dissect bluntly tissues of the mediastinum off the posterior table of the sternum. Often the tissue can be pushed off completely by working from above and below.

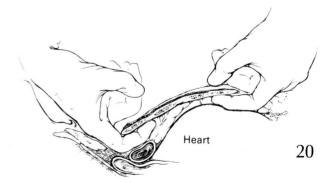

Heart

20

21

Before beginning transection of the sternum, it is good practice to mark the midline with the electrocautery, to ensure that the sternal split will be exactly in the centre. A large scissors may be used to begin the sternal incision from below, cutting the cartilage portion of the xiphisternum in the midline and providing an accurate entrance point for the sternal saw.

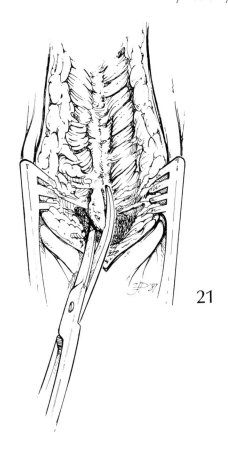

21

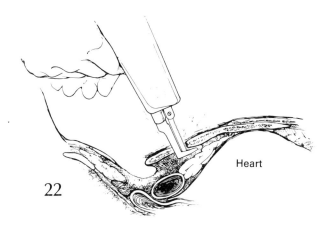

22

Heart

22

The surgeon must simultaneously advance the saw and pull it upward, so that the foot is engaged against the posterior table of the sternum, to avoid damage to the heart.

23

Once the sternum has been completely transected, the cut edges are packed with bone wax for haemostasis; electrocautery may be used where necessary. Retractors are placed to accomplish full exposure of the thymus.

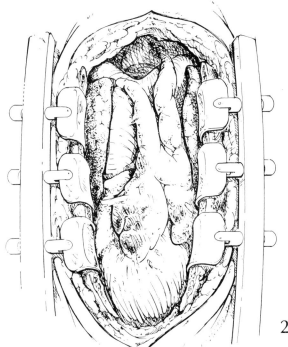

23

24

The thymoma may then be removed as described earlier, with careful blunt dissection to avoid vascular disruption.

The sternum is then closed with transfixion wires around the lateral edges, as shown in *Illustrations 16* and *17*.

One or two mediastinal drainage tubes (No. 32 or 36) may be placed through a separate subxiphoid skin incision and laid along the entire length of the wound. The pectoral fascia may then be closed over the anterior sternum with a strong suture such as 2/0 or 0. Subcutaneous tissue is closed with running suture of 2/0 or 3/0 chromic catgut and the skin is closed with staples or interrupted vertical mattress sutures.

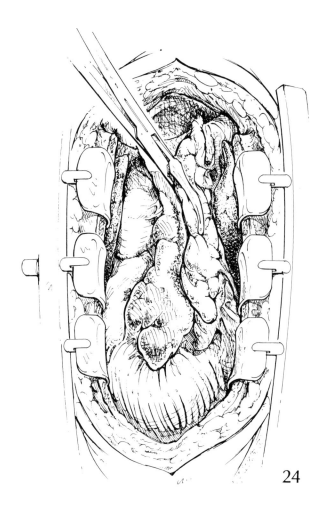

24

Postoperative care

Of the three approaches the median sternotomy incision produces significant respiratory embarrassment and thus requires the closest postoperative monitoring of respiratory function. Attempts should be made to maintain a nasotracheal tube in position if necessary; tracheostomy should be avoided if at all possible because of the potential for wound contamination. Culliford *et al.*[1] have had a large experience with median sternotomies and have developed some ingenious techniques for management of complications. Infection or dehiscence can be lethal and the surgeon should be prepared to deal with such complications.

Respiratory insufficiency in myasthenics can be treated by a combination of medical treatment and mechanical ventilation, preferably using a non-reactive nasoendotracheal tube to improve respiratory muscle function.

Reference

1. Culliford, A. T., Cunningham, J. N., Zeff, R. H., Isom, O. W., Teiko, P., Spencer, F. C. Sternal and costochondral infections following open-heart surgery. A review of 2594 cases. Journal of Thoracic and Cardiovascular Surgery 1976; 72: 714

Further reading

Bernatz, P. E., Khonsari, S., Harrison, E. G., Taylor, W. F. Thymoma: factors influencing prognosis. Surgical Clinics of North America 1973; 53: 885–892

Buckingham, J. M., Howard, F. M., Bernatz, P. E. *et al.* The value of thymectomy in myasthenia gravis. A computer-assisted matched study. Annals of Surgery 1976; 184: 453–458

Crowe, J. K., Brown, L. R., Muhm, J. R. Computed tomography of the mediastinum. Radiology 1973; 128: 75–87

Illustrations by D. D. Simmonds

Operations on the adrenal glands

R. B. Welbourn MA, MD(Cantab.), HonMD(Karolinska),
FRCS, FCS(West Africa), HonMRCS(Denmark)
Professor of Surgical Endocrinology, Royal Postgraduate
Medical School and Hammersmith Hospital, London

Introduction

One or both adrenal glands are removed either because they secrete excessive quantitites of hormones, which cause distress, or because they are the sites of tumours, or for both these reasons. Before the advent of cortisone in about 1950 and its use for providing replacement therapy during and after operation[1], radical adrenalectomy and removal of adrenal tumours from patients with Cushing's syndrome were fraught with danger and often proved fatal.

Removal of phaeochromocytomas was similarly hazardous until it was appreciated that many patients were hypovolaemic and before long-acting α-blocking agents and β-blocking drugs were available[2].

Recent developments in the biochemical diagnosis of syndromes and the anatomical localization of tumours have rendered exploratory operations almost obsolete. The surgeon usually knows before operation the nature and site of the lesion that he will find and can plan his approach accordingly.

Operations and indications

Bilateral total adrenalectomy

This is now used mainly for Cushing's syndrome, caused by bilateral adrenal hyperplasia or adenomatous hyperplasia. Several alternative forms of treatment are now available for this condition, including operations on, or irradiation of, the pituitary and the use of drugs. However, they have not yet been shown to be superior to adrenalectomy in the long term. The operation is also required for removal of bilateral phaeochromocytomas. These are particularly common in association with medullary carcinoma of the thyroid (multiple endocrine adenopathy type II). Even if cortical tissue can be preserved to obviate the need for permanent steroid replacement therapy, it is probably wise to remove both glands completely, because any remaining medullary tissue may become tumorous later. In this syndrome the adrenals, if involved, should always be treated before the thyroid so as to prevent vascular accidents, which may be fatal.

Bilateral adrenalectomy was formerly undertaken for primary aldosteronism caused by bilateral hyperplasia, but the results were poor and the operation has been largely superseded by medical treatment with spironolactone. The procedure was also used for treating selected patients with advanced cancer of the breast or prostate, but other forms of endocrine therapy and chemotherapy are now usually preferred.

Subtotal adrenalectomy

This was undertaken formerly for patients with Cushing's syndrome[1] and for those with primary aldosteronism caused by bilateral hyperplasia, in the hope of restoring normal adrenal function. The results, however, were unpredictable and the operation is now rarely used.

Removal of neoplastic glands

Except for about 10 per cent of phaeochromocytomas and a few neuroblastomas, neoplastic glands are nearly always unilateral. Removal is undertaken for the following.

1. *Cortical tumours* (benign or malignant), associated with
   (a) Cushing's syndrome;
   (b) Conn's syndrome (primary aldosteronism);
   (c) virilization;
   (d) feminization;
   (e) mixed syndromes; or
   (f) no endocrine features.

2. *Medullary tumours*
   (a) phaeochromocytoma (usually benign);
   (b) neuroblastoma (malignant);
   (c) ganglioneuroma (benign).

When the tumour is benign and small, non-tumorous cortical tissue is preserved, if possible, except in Conn's syndrome, when it is preferable to remove the whole gland because it may be the site of hyperplasia in addition to neoplasia. When the tumour is malignant, the whole gland is removed as widely as possible, together with adjacent invaded structures, particularly the kidney.

Approaches

Three approaches – posterior, anterior and lateral – are available, and each is ideal in certain circumstances[3]. The posterior route is recommended in most cases for removal of hyperplastic or normal glands or of small tumours. The anterior approach is advised for most patients with phaeochromocytomas and the lateral for all those with large tumours, whether these are cortical or medullary. The lateral approach is also recommended if any special difficulty is anticipated as in reoperations on the adrenal gland.

Special care before, during and after operation

Preoperative

1. Congestive cardiac failure, hypokalaemia, diabetes, infection or psychosis may require emergency treatment in patients with Cushing's syndrome. Metyrapone inhibits the synthesis of cortisol, induces remission and (like antithyroid drugs in toxic goitre) is valuable preoperatively. It is given in a dose of 250 mg 6 hourly, increasing if necessary to 750 mg 6 hourly, until the optimal effect has been achieved. This usually requires 3–6 weeks. Breakdown and infection of wounds were common in Cushing's syndrome, but can be largely prevented by this regimen and also by vitamin A and antibiotics. The former counteracts the adverse effects of cortisol excess on wound healing. Fifty thousand iu per day should be given by mouth for a week before operation, by intramuscular injection until the patient can swallow after operation, and then by mouth again until healing is complete. Appropriate preoperative prophylactic antibiotics should be given. Venous thromboembolism is not uncommon postoperatively, and intermittent pneumatic compression of the legs or other methods should be used to prevent it.
2. In patients with Conn's syndrome, congestive cardiac failure and hypokalaemia may require emergency treatment. Potassium deficiency must always be corrected with spironolactone and potassium supplement before operation.
3. A reliable intravenous infusion must be set up before operation.
4. Bleeding may be profuse in patients with large tumours, and blood must be readily available for transfusion.
5. X-rays showing the lower ribs should be present in the theatre if the posterior or lateral approach is to be used.

Replacement of steroids

The adrenal cortex is essential to life, and death follows within a few hours of bilateral adrenalectomy unless adequate replacement of steroids is provided. Steroids are not usually required in the removal of unilateral tumours, except in patients with Cushing's syndrome. However, if signs of adrenal insufficiency develop, they must be started without delay.

The following schedule is recommended for adults having bilateral total adrenalectomy, except for those with Cushing's syndrome.

Night before operation Cortisone acetate 100 mg by intramuscular injection (50 mg into each buttock).

Day of operation A reliable intravenous infusion is set up shortly before induction of anaesthesia and maintained until the blood pressure has been stable for 48 h after operation. Hydrocortisone succinate is added to the infusion and run in at a rate of 4–5 mg/h, so that 100 mg are given in the first 24 h. If bilateral adrenalectomy was not anticipated (e.g. in patients with bilateral phaeochromocytomas), the hydrocortisone drip may be started and the intramuscular cortisone given during the operation.

First postoperative day Hydrocortisone succinate in the infusion, 100 mg in 24 h.

Second day Hydrocortisone by mouth (or intravenously), 20 mg 6 hourly.

Third to fifth days Hydrocortisone by mouth, 20 mg 8 hourly.

Sixth to ninth days Hydrocortisone by mouth, 20 mg twice daily.

Tenth day and thereafter Hydrocortisone 10 mg thrice daily, and fludrocortisone, 0.1 mg once daily, both by mouth. Some patients need more hydrocortisone and some manage well on less.

If the systolic blood pressure falls below 100 mmHg during the first 48 h (and if bleeding or other causes can be excluded), the rate of infusion of hydrocortisone should be increased. If the pressure falls suddenly, 100 mg of hydrocortisone should be injected intravenously. Within the next few days, if the patient develops anorexia, nausea, abdominal discomfort, tachycardia or slight pyrexia, subacute adrenal insufficiency should be suspected and the dose of hydrocortisone increased.

Replacement of steroids in patients with Cushing's syndrome

The management is similar to that just described, except that larger doses are needed, even if only one hyperplastic gland is removed. The following doses are recommended.

Night before operation   Cortisone acetate, 100 mg by intramuscular injection.

Day of operation   Hydrocortisone succinate by intravenous infusion, 300 mg in 24 h.

First and second postoperative days   Continue infusion at this rate and change to hydrocortisone by mouth, 80 mg 8 hourly, as soon as possible.

Third to fifth days   Hydrocortisone acetate by mouth, 60 mg 8 hourly.

Sixth day   Hydrocortisone by mouth, 40 mg 8 hourly.

Seventh and eighth days   Hydrocortisone by mouth, 40 mg 12 hourly.

Ninth and tenth days   Hydrocortisone by mouth, 20 mg 8 hourly.

Twelfth day onwards   Hydrocortisone by mouth, 20 mg 12 hourly.
Sometimes a higher dose is needed for a long time, but eventually it can usually be reduced to about 10 mg 8 hourly.

Patients who have undergone unilateral adrenalectomy for tumours eventually recover normal adrenal function in the remaining gland and manage without replacement therapy. Those with carcinomas usually do so in a few weeks, while those with adenomas sometimes require much longer.

Dosage in children

Up to the age of about 5 years the doses should be one-third of those used in adults and up to about 15 years, two-thirds. Older children require adult doses. The maintenance dose of hydrocortisone in those requiring permanent replacement must be adjusted regularly with great care, because any excess stops growth.

Medullary tumours

Patients with phaeochromocytomas and other medullary tumours with hypertension and/or excessive secretion of catecholamines must be prepared for a week or more with the α-blocking agent phenoxybenzamine by mouth to prevent excessive hypertension when the tumour is handled and severe hypotension when it is removed. The β-blocking agent propranolol is used in the presence of tachycardia or cardiac arrhythmias. Labelatol has been used as a combined α- and β-blocking drug, but it is not effective.

During operation the blood pressure is measured continually. Both adrenal glands and any suspicious masses within the abdomen are squeezed gently and the effect on the blood pressure is noted, for squeezing a phaeochromocytoma causes the pressure to rise sharply. Tumours should be handled as gently as possible during removal and their vessels should be controlled as early as convenient. Any excessive rise in blood pressure is controlled with the fast-acting α-blocker phentolamine, or sodium nitroprusside injected into the infusion. Cardiac arrhythmias are treated similarly with propranolol. Any blood which is lost during operation is restored quantitatively. In addition plasma, up to about 2 litres, is usually necessary, as soon as the tumour has been removed, to maintain the systolic blood pressure at about 120 mmHg. The arterial pressure is a better guide to transfusion of the plasma than the central venous pressure. These measures, together with preoperative α-blockade, usually prevent any excessive fall of pressure after operation. When a tumour has been removed, a careful search must be made for another before the abdomen is closed.

Postoperative blood pressure

All patients undergoing adrenalectomy, and especially those with Cushing's syndrome and phaeochromocytoma, should have their blood pressure and pulse rate measured continually, or at least every 15 min, until both have been stable for 48 h. The plasma electrolytes should be estimated daily during this time.

Surgical technique

Although exploratory operations are rarely needed, it may be necessary to inspect both glands or to examine the whole abdomen before either adrenal is removed. The posterior and anterior approaches allow both glands to be assessed before removal of either, but only the anterior approach permits examination of the whole abdomen. The lateral approach gives the best exposure, but allows one gland only to be examined fully.

General anaesthesia is essential.

1

Identification of adrenals

The adrenal glands lie in the perinephric fat above the kidneys. They have close and important relationships to the lower ribs, the pleura and the great vessels. The amount of perinephric fact varies greatly. In patients with Cushing's syndrome, it is usually excessive, sometimes gross, and has a firm consistency, like suet. Some of it may be removed by hand to provide access.

The right adrenal sits like a cap on the upper pole of the kidney and is closely applied medially and anteriorly to the inferior vena cava. Its vein is very short and runs directly into the vena cava. Occasionally there are two, or even three, veins.

The left adrenal lies over the upper pole of the kidney and extends down its medial side, almost to the hilum. Medially, it is separated from the aorta by the crus of the diaphragm. Its vein is longer than that on the right and runs from the lower pole of the gland to join the left renal vein.

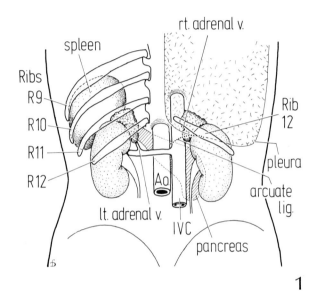

1

Recognition of pathological states

Normal adrenals weigh 5–6 g each, and have smooth surfaces. Single *cortical adenomas* or *carcinomas* whose colour is the same as that of the normal cortex and *adrenal medullary* tumours are usually recognized without difficulty. Small tumours (up to about 3 cm in diameter) arise from normal-looking glands, while larger ones usually replace all the normal tissue. Carcinomas are often 10 cm or more in diameter, are very vascular, often invade adjacent structures, including the kidney or inferior vena cava, and may involve the liver by direct invasion or by metastasis.

In *Cushing's syndrome*, hyperplastic glands are often twice, and occasionally up to five times, as large as normal. The two glands are usually, but not always, about the same size. They often contain micronodules, up to 2 or 3 mm in diameter, and occasionally larger nodules, which may be single or multiple (adenomatous hyperplasia). Benign adenomas are single, usually 2–3 cm in diameter, and occasionally larger. The non-tumorous parts of the adrenals are atrophic.

In *primary aldosteronism* one, or sometimes more, adenomas, 1–3 cm in diameter, and occasionally smaller, are usually found (Conn's syndrome). A small one, which has been demonstrated preoperatively, may not be apparent until the gland has been removed.

POSTERIOR APPROACH

Bilateral posterior incisions, with the patient face-downwards, allow both adrenals to be examined before either is removed. Normal and hyperplastic glands and tumours up to about 5 cm in diameter can be excised readily. The postoperative course is much smoother than that following the other two approaches and, if wounds become infected, any abscess drains readily. This route is advised for bilateral total adrenalectomy unless there are special reasons for entering the abdomen, and for removal of small cortical tumours.

2

Position of patient

The patient is laid face down on the table with the break under the twelfth rib. Firm pillows are placed under the chest and pelvis, so that there is no pressure on the abdomen, and a soft pillow is put under the shins to bend the knees slightly and raise the feet. A strap is fastened round the pelvis. The table is broken to abolish the lumbar lordosis.

One or both glands may be explored and either or both removed. The approach to each side is identical, but the techniques of removal are different. The surgeon stands on the side on which he is operating.

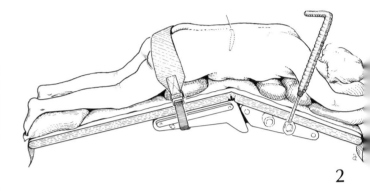

2

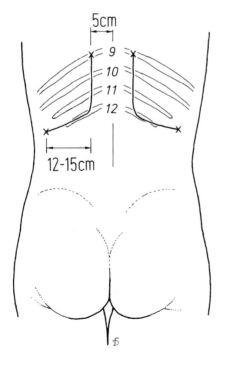

3

3

The incision

The skin incision starts at the level of the ninth rib, about 5 cm from the midline, runs vertically (for 12–15 cm) to the twelfth rib, then takes a sharp turn, running obliquely (for 12–15 cm) along the rib to its tip and finally laterally onto the abdominal muscles. In fat patients the incision must be extended at both ends. The subcutaneous fat is divided and the latissimus dorsi muscle and the sacrospinalis fascia are exposed.

Resection of rib

The twelfth rib is palpated and the incision is deepened through the muscles and fascia, down to the periosteum, and to the lumbar fascia and external oblique muscle. (If the twelfth rib is rudimentary, better access is obtained by resection of the eleventh rib.)

4

The sacrospinalis muscle is retracted medially, and the periosteum is incised and then cleared totally from the rib with raspatories. In Cushing's syndrome fractures and callus are often found and the ribs may be extremely friable. The rib is cut with shears, close to the vertebral body, and removed, its lateral attachments being divided with scissors.

The deep layer of periosteum and the renal fascia are then incised together, exposing the perinephric fat. Care is taken to preserve the subcostal neurovascular bundle.

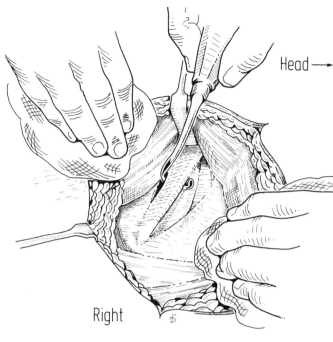

4

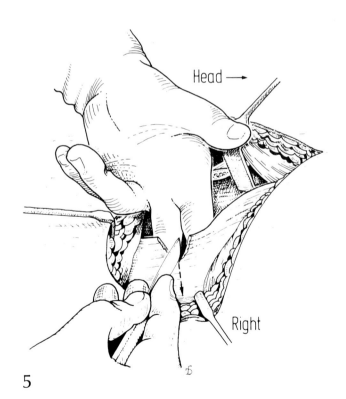

5

5

Incision of flank muscles

Two fingers are then inserted, beyond the tip of the rib, between the lumbar fascia and abdominal muscles superficially and the peritoneum deeply, and the muscles and fascia are divided transversely.

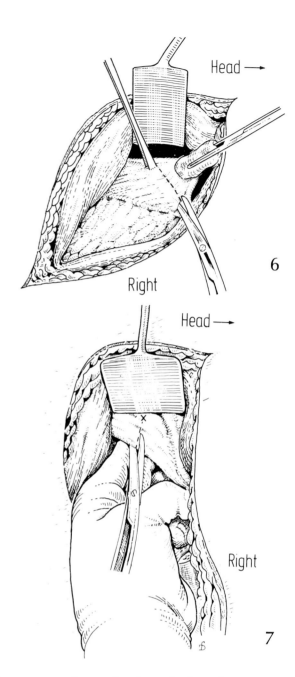

6

7

6 & 7

Incision of diaphragm

Retraction upwards of the eleventh rib now exposes the reflection of the pleura and the lateral arcuate ligament of the diaphragm, which are joined by loose connective tissue. The pleura is freed and reflected upwards, partly with scissors and partly by gauze dissection, and the diaphragm is incised vertically up to the eleventh rib. If the pleura is opened, no harm is done, but the lung must be expanded and the pleura sutured before closure of the wound.

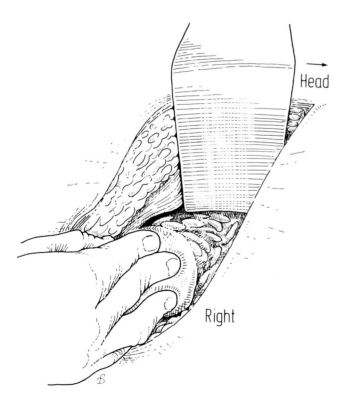

8

Exposure and examination of adrenal

8

The upper pole of the kidney can be felt with the fingers through the perinephric fat. Dissection soon exposes it, and it is cleared and retracted downwards by the assistant's hand. The eleventh rib, pleura, diaphragm and underlying abdominal viscera are now retracted upwards in the costovertebral angle, exposing the perinephric fat above the kidney.

Usually the exposure is adequate, but occasionally the eleventh rib obscures the gland and renders adrenalectomy difficult. If so, the periosteum is cleared from its posterior end, 1 or 2 cm of bone are resected with shears, the rib is retracted further upwards, and the diaphragm is divided a little higher.

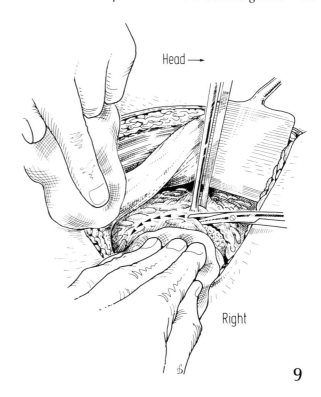

9

9, 10 & 11

The adrenal is found by dissection with scissors and forceps in the perirenal fat. It is readily distinguished by its orange-yellow colour and firm, compact structure. It is mobilized partly by sharp and blunt dissection with scissors and partly by blunt dissection with the fingers. The small vessels which enter the periphery of a normal or hyperplastic gland rarely bleed much and can be controlled with diathermy. The main vein, however, is relatively large and must be preserved until it has been mobilized. The gland is inspected and palpated carefully between fingers and thumb.

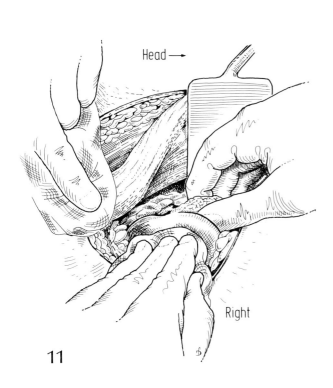

11

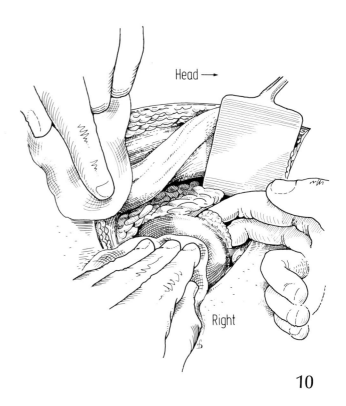

10

Removal of the adrenal

12, 13 & 14

The adrenal is grasped with modified Duval's lung forceps (whose jaws are 6mm apart when the first teeth of the ratchets engage) and dissection is continued all round the periphery. The main vein is divided with care between ligatures or clips. If, as may happen occasionally on the right, a hole is torn in the vena cava, bleeding is profuse and the hole must be grasped quickly with sponge-holding forceps. If this does not control the bleeding at once, a large pack is inserted firmly and left for 5min before the forceps is applied again. A Cooley or De Bakey clamp is then applied to the vena cava and the hole is sutured.

When all the surrounding fat and vessels have been divided, the gland is free and can be removed. There are sometimes ectopic nodules of adrenocortical tissue near the glands. If adrenalectomy is to be total, they must be looked for and removed. In hypertensive states (Cushing's and Conn's syndromes and phaeochromocytoma) renal biopsies may be taken. The adrenal beds are usually dry and fill with fat when the retractors are removed.

Closure of incision

The table is straightened and the wound closed. If the pleural cavity has been opened, the lung must be ex-panded before it is sutured, and an underwater chest drain may be desirable for a day or two.
    Drainage of the adrenal bed is rarely necessary.
    The wound is sutured in three layers:

1. medially, the intercostal muscles above and the lumbar fascia and quadratus lumborum below; and, laterally, the external oblique muscle and lumbar fascia above and below;
2. latissimus dorsi muscle and the sacrospinalis fascia;
3. skin and subcutaneous tissue.

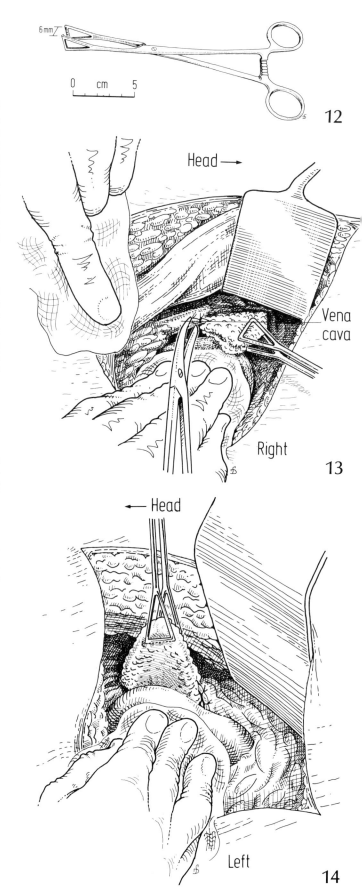

ANTERIOR APPROACH

An anterior abdominal incision allows both glands to be palpated, inspected and removed and the whole of the para-aortic region to be explored. Great difficulty may be experienced on the right side if the patient is very fat or deep-chested or if the liver is enlarged. A tumour more than about 5 cm in diameter on the *right* also presents difficulties because of its relationship (and that of its vein) to the inferior vena cava. This route is advised mainly in patients with phaeochromocytoma. It may be used in those with Conn's syndrome, but the posterior approach is preferable. It is not advised in patients with Cushing's syndrome, unless a primary or secondary ectopic ACTH-secreting tumour is suspected within the abdomen, because postoperative infection may result in the formation of a subphrenic abscess. Nor is it advised in those who have had previous upper abdominal operations or inflammatory disease, because of the likelihood of adhesions.

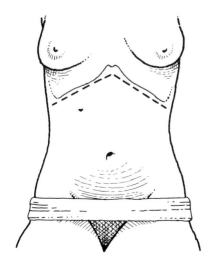

15

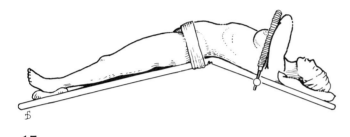

16

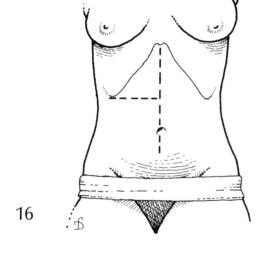

17

15

Position of patient

The patient lies supine with the twelfth thoracic vertebra overlying the bridge or the break in the table. A strap should secure the pelvis so that the table can be tilted to either side. The operation starts with the bridge up or the table broken and with the patient flat.

The incisions

16

Midline

Usually, and particularly if the subcostal angle is narrow or the patient thin, a midline incision is made from the xiphisternum to 2 cm or so below the umbilicus. If access to either or both glands is inadequate, the incisions may be extended laterally (in either or both direction), at the level of the costal margins.

17

Roof top

If the subcostal angle is wide and the patient is fat, two long subcostal incisions are made and joined in the centre by a curve to make a 'roof top'. They are made one finger's breadth below the costal margins and extend to the tips of the tenth ribs laterally.

The incision is deepened through the subcutaneous fat and then through the muscles of the abdominal wall. The superior epigastric vessels are secured deep to the rectus muscles. The peritoneum is incised and the falciform ligament divided between ligatures. This incision gives the best possible access from the front, but takes a long time to close.

Abdominal exploration

The abdominal contents are explored. In patients with phaeochromocytomas the whole para-aortic region and pelvis are examined carefully for tumours.

Exposure of left adrenal

18

The surgeon stands on the patient's right. It is sometimes helpful for the table to be tilted about 30° towards him. The viscera are controlled with packs.

The spleen is grasped with the left hand, and the peritoneum behind it is divided with scissors so that it can be mobilized and drawn forwards and to the right, together with the tail of the pancreas, the splenic vessels and the greater curvature of the stomach. (Alternative routes to the left adrenal, through the lesser omentum or the gastrocolic omentum, are much less satisfactory.)

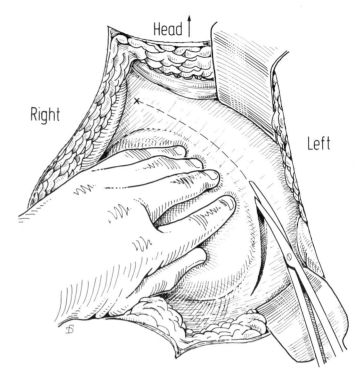

18

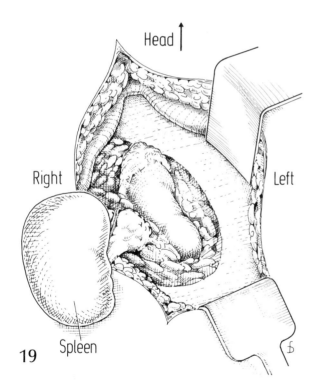

19 Spleen

19

The spleen is retracted by an assistant's hand over a gauze pack. In a thin patient the adrenal is seen clearly just above the kidney and deep to the renal fascia, lying in front of the left crus of the diaphragm. If there is much fat, the kidney must be felt through it and the adrenal found by dissection in the perinephric fat at its superomedial border.

Removal of left adrenal

Dissection, palpation and removal of the gland have been described already. Ligation and division of the vein may be left to the end, so that it forms a pedicle for the gland.

20

Exposure of right adrenal

The surgeon remains on the patient's right side and, if necessary, the table is tilted about 30° towards the left. The liver is retracted gently upwards and the hepatic flexure of the colon downwards. The duodenum is retracted downwards and to the left, while the peritoneum above it is incised. There is no need to mobilize the duodenum by incision of the peritoneum around it.

21

The inferior vena cava is now exposed and the adrenal is seen, or found, lying close to its right side, behind the renal fascia, above the kidney and below the liver.

Removal of right adrenal

The kidney is retracted downwards by an assistant's hand over a gauze pack, and the adrenal comes down with it.

The adrenal vein should be sought immediately, between the gland and the vena cava. This vein, which is short and runs directly into the cava, may be torn and cause serious bleeding unless it is controlled at this stage. Rotation of the vena cava to the left with a small gauze dab, held in long forceps, aids this manoeuvre.

22

The upper pole of the gland is sited very deeply and may be difficult to expose behind the liver. It is attached closely to the vena cava by a tough bundle of connective tissues which must be cut very carefully with scissors.

Change of approach

If removal of a gland or tumour is impracticable from the front, the incision should be closed and the operation completed by the posterior or lateral route, either at once or later.

Closure of incision

The table is straightened and flattened and the abdomen closed in three layers:

1. peritoneum, posterior rectus sheath (and deep lateral muscles);
2. anterior rectus sheath (and external oblique);
3. skin and subcutaneous fat.

(The structures mentioned in brackets are sutured when the roof top incision is used or when a vertical incision is extended laterally.)

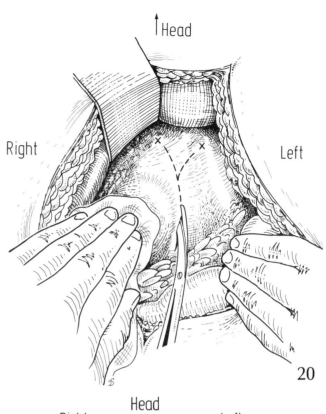

20

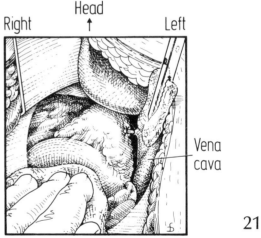

21

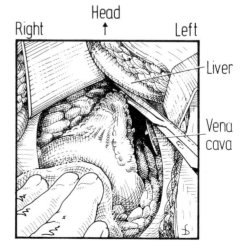

22

LATERAL APPROACH

An oblique thoracoabdominal incision with resection of a rib gives the best possible exposure of one adrenal. With both the other routes the adrenal is exposed by downward retraction of the kidney, while with this one the gland lies in the middle of the operative field. The opposite gland and ectopic phaeochromocytomas can be palpated *via* the peritoneal cavity, but they cannot be seen or removed.

This route is recommended for nearly all tumours larger than about 5 cm in diameter. The only exception is a left-sided phaeochromocytoma up to about 10 cm, which may be removed from the front. It is also recommended for reoperation for local recurrence of a tumour or for removal of an enlarged adrenal remnant after subtotal adrenalectomy for Cushing's or Conn's syndromes.

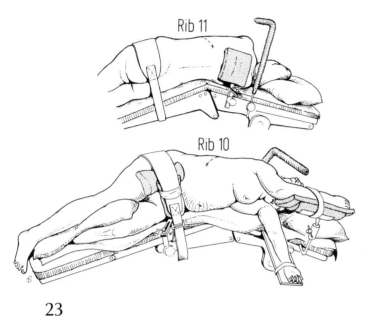

23

23

Position of patient

The patient is placed in the lateral position (without any tilt forwards or backwards) with the side to be explored uppermost and the tenth and eleventh ribs lying over the break in the table. The table is broken to expand the lower chest. Great care should be taken with this manoeuvre, since vertebrae and ribs are often fragile in Cushing's syndrome. The surgeon stands behind the patient.

Left adrenalectomy

The incision

The eleventh rib is found by palpation and a straight incision is started where it emerges from the lateral border of the sacrospinalis. The incision is extended along the line of the rib well into the abdominal wall. The rib and abdominal muscles are exposed and the rib is resected subperiosteally as far back as its angle.

24

Incision of abdominal muscles and lumbar fascia

A finger is burrowed between the abdominal wall and the peritoneum, and the abdominal muscles and lumbar fascia are incised in the line of the incision. The intercostal nerve and vessels are preserved carefully. The colon, which lies anteriorly, must not be damaged. The bed of the rib is incised, the pleura is retracted upwards with care and the diaphragm is divided in line with the incision. No harm is done if the pleural cavity is opened inadvertently.

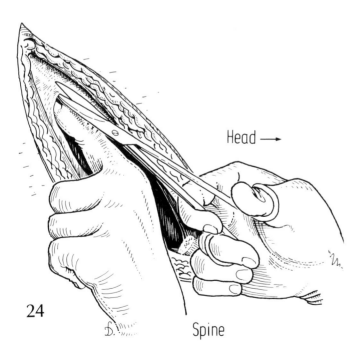

24

25

Exposure and removal of adrenal

Retractors are inserted, the kidney is found by palpation and the renal fascia is incised widely to expose it. The kidney is retracted downwards and the adrenal is identified. The tail of the pancreas, which lies anterior and inferior to the adrenal, must not be mistaken for it. If the abdominal cavity is to be explored, the peritoneum is incised in front of the colon and a hand is inserted. Dissection and removal of the gland have been described already. Ligation and division of the vein may be left to the end, as in the anterior approach.

Closure of incision

The table is straightened and the incision closed. If the pleura has been opened, care is taken to expand the lung fully before closure. The peritoneum is sutured with continuous catgut, if it has been opened. The wound is closed in three layers:

1. rib bed behind and the lumbar fascia in front;
2. superficial muscles;
3. skin and subcutaneous fat.

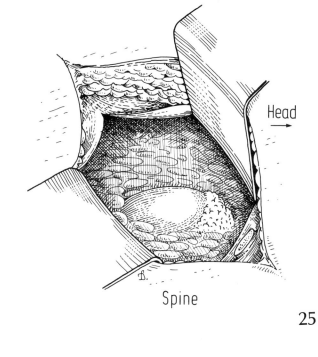

25

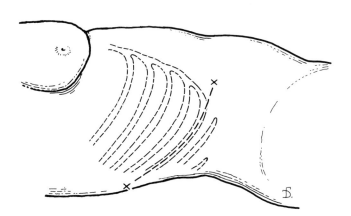

26

Right adrenalectomy

26

The incision

The tenth rib is palpated and an incision made along it from the point where it emerges from the lateral border of the sacrospinalis muscle to 2 or 3 cm beyond the costal margin.

27

Incision of diaphragm

The ribs are held apart by a self-retaining retractor and the kidney is palpated through the diaphragm. An incision about 10 cm long is made *posteriorly* in the diaphragm, approximately at right angles to the skin incision and over the upper pole of the kidney. It should be about 1 cm from the insertion of the diaphragm so that there is sufficient tissue posteriorly to hold stitches when the diaphragm is repaired. Bleeding points in the cut edge of the muscle are sealed with diathermy or ligated.

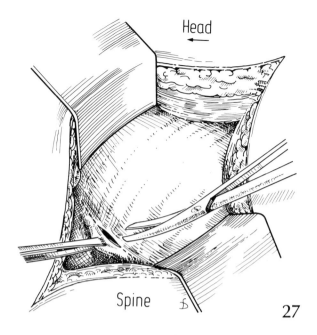

27

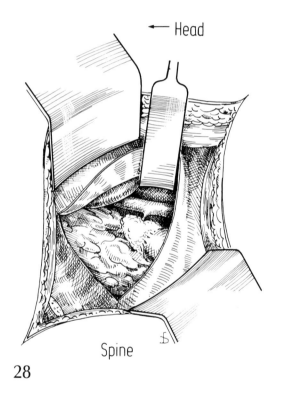

28

28

Exposure and removal of adrenal

The lung is retracted upwards and the liver forwards. The renal fascia is incised widely and the adrenal, which lies in the centre of the field, is located in the perirenal fat at the upper pole of the kidney, close to the inferior vena cava. The peritoneal cavity may be explored, if necessary, through an incision in front of the colon, as on the left side. The gland is removed, as described already.

Closure of incision

The table is straightened and the peritoneum (if it has been opened) and the diaphragm are closed with continuous catgut sutures. An underwater, intercostal drain (through the seventh or eighth space in the mid-axillary line) is advisable for 1 or 2 days. The incision is closed in three layers:

1. rib bed;
2. superficial muscles; and
3. skin and subcutaneous fat.

29

REMOVAL OF SMALL BENIGN TUMOURS

Small tumours can be removed by any route. However, the posterior approach is advised for cortical adenomas and the anterior for phaeochromocytomas. They are removed in the same way as non-tumorous glands, except that more vessels may require ligation. In Cushing's syndrome as much normal adrenal tissue as possible should be left behind, but in other conditions the gland should be removed completely.

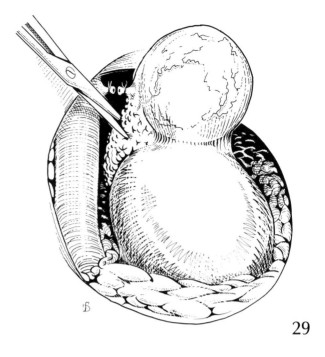

29

REMOVAL OF LARGE TUMOURS

30

The lateral approach gives the best exposure, but the incision must be enlarged forwards and downwards as far as necessary.

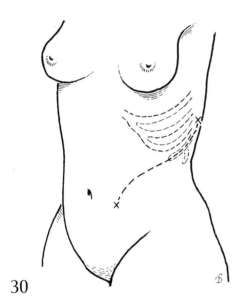

30

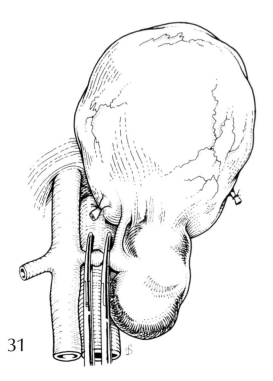

31

31

Direct invasion of surrounding tissues may preclude complete or even subtotal removal, but very large malignant tumours are often resectable. If the kidney alone is invaded, it is removed together with the tumour. A plane of cleavage is found outside the capsule of the tumour, and dissection is made on each side in turn until the main vessels are reached. Bleeding, which may be severe, is best controlled by pressure with abdominal packs. There are often several arteries supplying the tumour, but only one vein (the enlarged adrenal vein) draining it. These vessels are divided and ligated as soon as they are found. Tumour may pack the vein and extend into the vena cava. In this case the cava may be clamped below and above, opened and the tumour withdrawn. It is then closed with a fine arterial suture.

ADRENALECTOMY IN CHILDREN

The indications are the same as those in adults, but malignant tumours are relatively more common. Operations for neuroblastoma are described in the *Paediatric Surgery* volume.

Tumours are best approached by a lateral incision and that through the bed of the eleventh rib gives good access on each side. For bilateral adrenalectomy the posterior and anterior approaches may provide inadequate access, even in teenagers, and the bilateral eleventh rib approach is advised. The two operations can usually be undertaken on one occasion, the child being turned from one side to the other.

The smaller doses of steroids required for replacement during and after operation have been described already.

Results

With suitable preparation and care, the operative mortality for removal of benign lesions of the adrenals is now about 1 or 2 per cent. That for patients with large malignant lesions of the cortex or the medulla is appreciably higher.

Survival figures

These are approximately as follows.

Cortical lesions

1. Benign
   (a) Cushing's syndrome[4]
       10 years 66 per cent
       20 years 50 per cent
   (b) Conn's syndrome[5]
       Good, but no long-term details of large series have been published
2. Malignant[4]
   Almost all patients die within 5 years

Medullary lesions

1. Phaeochromocytoma[6,7]
   10–20 years 66 per cent
2. Neuroblastoma[8]
   (a) Infants (<1 year old)
       (i) Stages I, II and IVS
           2 years 90 per cent
           5 years 80 per cent
       (ii) Stages III and IV
           2 years 30 per cent
   (b) Children (>1 year old)
       2 years 15 per cent

References

1. Priestley, J. T., Sprague, R. G., Walters, W., Salassa, R. M. Subtotal adrenalectomy for Cushing's syndrome. A preliminary report of 29 cases. Annals of Surgery 1951; 134: 464–475

2. Ross, E. J., Prichard, B. N. C., Kaufman, L., Robertson, A. I. G., Harries, B. J. Preoperative and operative management of patients with phaeochromocytoma. British Medical Journal 1967; 1: 191–198

3. Edis, A. J., Ayala, L. A., Egdahl, R. H. Manual of endocrine surgery. Berlin: Springer-Verlag, 1975

4. Welbourn, R. B. Some aspects of adrenal surgery. British Journal of Surgery 1980; 67: 723–727

5. Ferriss, J. B., Beevers, D. G., Boddy, K. et al. The treatment of low-renin ('primary') hyperaldosteronism. American Heart Journal 1978; 96: 97–109

6. Modlin, I. M., Farndon, J. R., Shepherd, A. et al. Phaeochromocytomas in 72 patients: clinical and diagnostic features, treatment and long term results. British Journal of Surgery 1979; 66: 456–465

7. Remine, W. H., Chong, G. C., Van Heerden, J. A., Sheps, S. G., Harrison, E. G. Current management of pheochromocytoma. Annals of Surgery 1974; 179: 740–748

8. Grosfeld, J. L., Schatzlein, M., Ballantine, T. V. N., Weetman, R. M., Baehner, R. L. Metastatic neuroblastoma: factors influencing survival. Journal of Pediatric Surgery 1978; 13: 59–65

Illustrations by Oxford Illustrators

Operations on the pancreas for insulinoma

L. P. Le Quesne DM, MCh, FRCS, HonFRACS
Professor of Surgery and Director of Surgical Studies,
The Middlesex Hospital, London

Introduction

An insulinoma (or insulin tumour) arises from the β-cells of the islets of Langerhans. The great majority of these tumours are solitary and benign, but approximately 10 per cent are multiple, some 10 per cent are malignant, and rarely the tumour forms part of the multiple endocrine adenoma syndrome. The tumour causes symptoms as the result of excessive, inappropriate secretion of insulin (organic hyperinsulinism) resulting in attacks of hypoglycaemia. In the adult this condition is almost invariably due to a tumour of the islets and only very rarely to islet-cell hyperplasia, but in children such tumours are rare and the condition is commonly caused by a particular type of hyperplasia (nesidioblastosis). Solitary adenomas are usually small (less than 2 cm) and are evenly distributed throughout the pancreas; on conventional microscopy they are indistinguishable from other functioning tumours arising from the islets, but electron microscopy reveals the presence of proinsulin crystals within the cells.

Good results in the surgical management of patients with an insulin-secreting tumour of the pancreas are absolutely dependent upon an accurate preoperative diagnosis. This is usually indicated in the first instance by the clinical history and the demonstration of hypoglycaemia during the attacks. This in itself is inadequate evidence to justify the diagnosis, and it is essential to demonstrate that the hypoglycaemia is due to organic hyperinsulinism. The absolute level of the plasma insulin concentration may well be within normal limits, and the essential diagnostic step is to demonstrate an inappropriately high level of insulin concentration in the face of an abnormally low (hypoglycaemic) blood glucose concentration. This is usually done by the simultaneous measurement of plasma insulin and glucose concentrations after the provocation of hypoglycaemia by a period of starvation, a 12 h, overnight fast usually sufficing. In some circumstances a more prolonged fast and/or the measurement of C-peptide levels may be required to establish the diagnosis. *It must be emphasized that the abdomen should not be opened in search of an insulin tumour in the absence of convincing evidence of inappropriate insulin secretion in the presence of hypoglycaemia.*

The majority of insulin tumours can be detected at laparotomy, but in some 10 per cent the surgeon is unable to locate the tumour even on careful palpation of the fully mobilized pancreas. This has focused attention on the possibility of preoperative localization of the tumour. Usually the tumours are too small to be identified by ultrasound or CT scanning. Arteriography has been widely used in an attempt to demonstrate the position of islet-cell tumours. Depending on the exact technique used, a success rate varying from 40 to 80 per cent is claimed for this examination, but there is no convincing evidence that arteriography can locate those tumours, usually small, which the surgeon is unable to identify at operation. The site of an insulin tumour may also be indicated by percutaneous, transhepatic catheterization of the portal and splenic veins, with measurement of the insulin concentration in samples of blood taken at known sites in relation to the pancreas, especially at frequent intervals along the splenic vein, the site of a tumour being indicated by an abrupt peak in the insulin concentration. By this technique a tumour can certainly be localized in some patients, but further experience is needed to assess its overall value.

Principles of treatment

The essential step in treatment is to locate the tumour in the pancreas and then to remove it; removal is usually best achieved by enucleation of the tumour, but if the tumour is in the distal half of the pancreas it may be safer to perform a limited excision of the distal pancreas. Patients with an insulin tumour are often obese, as the result of a high carbohydrate intake to prevent hypoglycaemic attacks, and this increases the technical difficulties of operation.

Prior to operation it is wise to evaluate the patient's response to diazoxide, a substituted benzothiadiazine which inhibits insulin release, and in particular to determine whether or not it causes a dangerous degree of water retention. By the use of this drug the patient's condition can be stabilized, and a knowledge of the patient's response to it may be of value when faced by certain circumstances during the operation (see below).

Three particular problems in treatment require mention.

Multiple tumours

In about 10 per cent of patients there is more than one tumour, so that even if a tumour is identified early in the operation, the remainder of the gland should be palpated carefully. It has been suggested that repeated estimation of the blood glucose concentration over a period of 20–40 min after the removal of an adenoma will indicate whether a further tumour is present, in that removal of a solitary adenoma, or of all tumours in the gland, is followed by a rise in the blood glucose concentration. This is certainly true, but such a rise may not be apparent for a number of hours, and it is not certain that repeated measurements over a short period give conclusive evidence as to whether or nor there are further tumours in the gland[1].

Failure to identify a tumour at operation

In some 5–10 per cent of patients with an undoubted insulinoma the surgeon is unable to identify the tumour at operation. This presents a difficult problem, and underlines the importance of a firm preoperative diagnosis. The standard solution to the problem is to perform an extensive distal pancreatectomy, that is to say an excision of the pancreas from the tail to the right-hand edge of the superior mesenteric vessels, leaving the head and uncinate process of the gland in situ. However, the success rate of this procedure, as judged by removal of the tumour, is only about 50 per cent[2,3]. An alternative approach is to leave the gland intact and treat the patient with diazoxide; hence the importance of establishing the patient's response to this drug prior to operation. If, at a later date, the patient's symptoms are no longer controlled by this drug then a further laparotomy can be performed, preceded by studies to locate the tumour. Faced with this problem, there is at present no clear evidence as to the correct procedure. The decision will be influenced by whether or not the patient's response to diazoxide is known, and whether or not a percutaneous, transhepatic portal vein catheterization study has been performed.

Management of a metastasizing tumour

On histological grounds it is difficult, often impossible, to determine whether an insulinoma is benign or malignant, and in general the only clear evidence of malignancy is provided by the development of metastases. If, at laparotomy, metastases are detected, as much as possible of the tumour should be removed, including the removal of hepatic deposits where feasible. Thereafter the patient should be treated with diazoxide to control the symptoms, and with the antimitotic drug streptozotocin in an attempt to control the tumour.

(For a full discussion of the problems involved in the management of patients with an insulinoma see Le Quesne et al.[4] and Daggett et al.[5]).

Preoperative preparation

Apart from the usual preoperative measures required in any patient who is to undergo a major abdominal operation, the blood glucose concentration requires special attention to avoid the development of hypoglycaemia both before and during operation. An intravenous infusion is set up to deliver 10 per cent dextrose at a rate aimed to maintain the blood glucose concentration at 6.6–10 mmol/l (120–180 mg/100 ml). If the patient's blood glucose level is well controlled by diazoxide this infusion need not be started until just before the operation, but if such is not the case it should be started the evening before operation. Repeated blood glucose estimations should be performed over the operative period to ensure that satisfactory levels are maintained.

The operation

The operation is performed with the patient supine, under general anaesthesia. The principle of the operation is to expose and mobilize the pancreas in such a way that it can be carefully palpated throughout its extent, the most difficult portion of the pancreas to examine carefully being the uncinate process.

1

The incision

A number of incisions (midline; paramedian) can be used, but the most suitable for exploration of the entire pancreas is a curved transverse incision, convex towards the head, in the upper abdomen. It should extend well lateral to the linea semilunaris on each side. The recti abdominis are divided. A general laparotomy should be performed and special attention paid to the liver which may be the site of metastases from a malignant insulinoma.

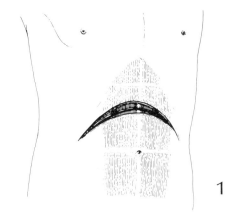

1

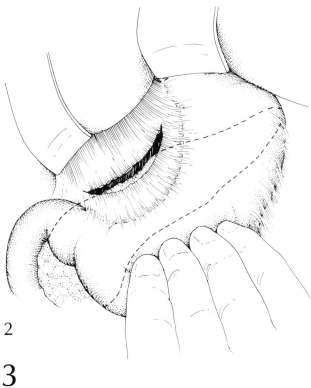

2

2

Division of lesser omentum

The lesser omentum is divided, so that the anterior surface of the body and tail of the pancreas can be inspected and palpated after the stomach has been retracted downwards and to the left.

3

Exposure of anterior surface of pancreas

To expose the whole of the anterior surface of the pancreas the greater omentum is separated from the transverse colon and lifted up with the stomach. On the left this dissection should extend to the spleen, care being taken to divide the peritoneal folds running to its tip, so as to avoid tears in the capsule of the spleen. On the right the dissection should extend to the hepatic flexure, which is reflected downwards off the anterior surface of the pancreas and second part of the duodenum.

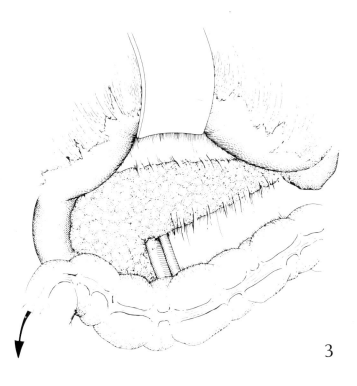

3

4

Mobilization of head and proximal body of pancreas

The peritoneum lateral to the second part of the duodenum is divided from the common bile duct above to the junction of the second and third portions of the duodenum below, followed by mobilization of the duodenum and head of the pancreas (Kocher's manoeuvre). This mobilization, which is carried out in an essentially avascular plane, must be thorough, and should extend across the inferior vena cava to expose the anterior surface of the aorta and the left renal vein.

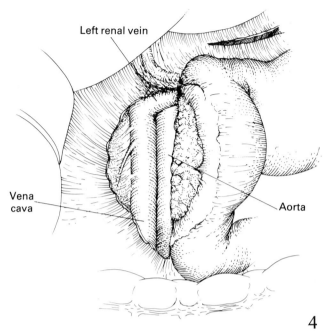

4

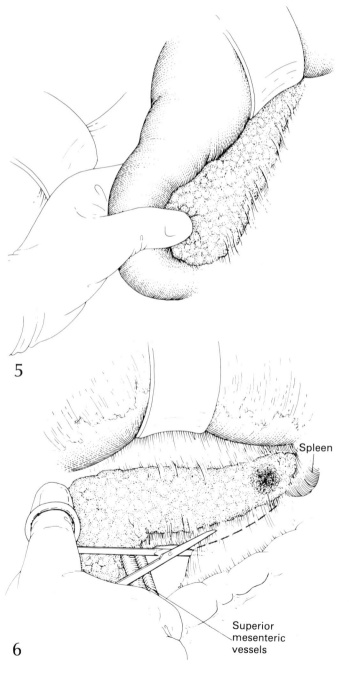

5

6

5

Palpation of head of pancreas

When this mobilization has been completed it is possible to palpate the head and most of the body of the pancreas between the thumb and fingers of the left hand. The tumour may be seen projecting from the surface of the gland. If embedded in the gland it is felt as a smooth, firm lump, usually 1–2 cm in diameter.

6

Mobilization of distal body and tail of pancreas

The peritoneum along the inferior border of the pancreas is divided from the superior mesenteric vessels medially to the spleen laterally, allowing the distal body and tail of the pancreas to be lifted from its bed and palpated between fingers and thumb. Care should be taken to extend the mobilization to the tip of the pancreas, as it is easy to overlook a tumour lying close to the hilum of the spleen. It is essential that the whole pancreas is palpated carefully, as there may be more than one tumour.

7

Enucleation of a tumour in head of pancreas

The peritoneum over the tumour is incised, together with the usually thin layer of pancreas covering the tumour. Insulinomas have only a tenuous capsule, with a poor plane of cleavage surrounding them. Their enucleation is achieved by a mixture of gentle blunt and sharp dissection, care being taken to keep close to the tumour so as to avoid damage to small pancreatic ducts. Unless the tumour is deeply placed in the gland there is little danger of damage to a major duct, but on occasions insertion of a bougie into the common bile duct may be helpful. Bleeding is best controlled by accurate use of the cautery. Following enucleation the small, cup-shaped depression in the gland is left open; a suction drain, brought out through a stab in the flank (not through the main incision), is accurately placed down to the site of the tumour.

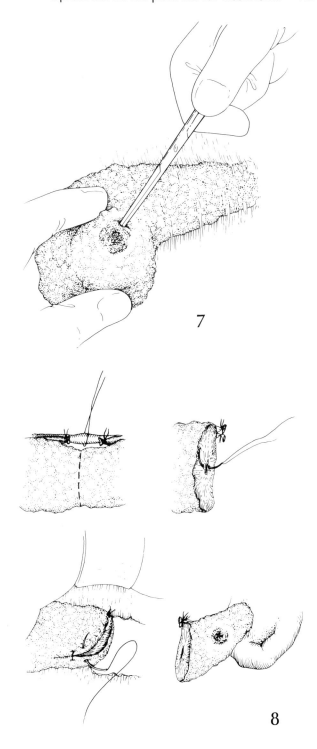

7

8

Distal pancreatectomy

Tumours on the surface of the body and tail of the pancreas can safely be treated by enucleation. However, if they are deeply embedded in the gland distal pancreatectomy is a preferable procedure, to avoid injury to the pancreatic duct. In addition to the distal pancreas the operation involves removal of the spleen. The splenic vessels, running along the upper border of the pancreas, are divided between ligatures at the line of section of the pancreas. The pancreas is divided just to the right of the tumour, and the distal pancreas and spleen removed, after division and ligation of the short gastric vessels. The divided pancreatic duct is transfixed and ligated with a fine synthetic absorbable (Dexon) suture, and the cut edges of the gland are apposed with a series of similar sutures. The cut end of the pancreas and splenic bed are drained with a tube drain brought out through a stab in the left flank.

If, after careful palpation of the whole gland, the tumour cannot be identified and it is decided to perform a blind distal pancreatectomy (see above) the gland is divided through its neck, immediately in front of the superior mesenteric vessels. In this procedure the splenic vein is divided at its junction with the superior mesenteric vein to form the portal vein, and care must be taken to secure both ends of the vein prior to its division.

8

Closure

To keep the stomach empty in the initial postoperative period a gastrostomy tube, brought out through the left side of the epigastrium, may be inserted in preference to a nasogastric tube. The incision is closed in the usual fashion. As previously indicated, drains should be brought out through small, separate incisions, not through the main wound, because of the possibility of the development of a pancreatic fistula. This is an unusual postoperative complication, but if it occurs it is more easily controlled if the pancreatic juice is escaping through a track separate from the main wound.

Postoperative care

In addition to the problems which may occur after any major abdominal operation, and which should be managed in the usual fashion, removal of an insulin tumour, as with any operation on the pancreas, may be followed by pancreatitis. This complication, at least in a clinically significant form, is uncommon, but it is wise to check the serum amylase level for some 48–72 h after operation. To prevent the complication the pancreas should be kept at rest for some 72 h following operation; this is achieved by withholding oral fluids, and keeping the stomach empty by the use of a nasogastric or gastrostomy tube. If at the end of this period the patient's abdomen is soft and the serum amylase within normal limits, oral fluids can be started and the return to a normal oral intake guided by the usual observations. To prevent the development of pancreatitis the administration of either glucagon or aprotonin (Trasylol) has been recommended, but there is no clear evidence that either is of benefit.

If a pancreatic fistula develops from a drain site, the discharge should be controlled by a suction drain, with protection of the surrounding skin, and oral fluids withheld. The fistula usually closes within a few days, but if it does not intravenous feeding may be required until closure occurs. A further operation to close the fistula is rarely required.

The excessive, inappropriate secretion of insulin from the islet-cell tumour results in suppression of β-cell function in the normal islets. After removal of the tumour this function is rapidly regained, but for some 24–48 h after operation there is a transient diabetic state. This is indicated by raised blood glucose levels and glycosuria, but the condition is usually mild and ketosis rarely occurs. In most patients no active treatment is required and normal glucose homeostasis is restored within 2–3 days, but occasionally insulin may be required for a few days.

References

1. Harrison, T. S., Child, C. G., Fry, W. J., Floyd, J. C., Fajans, S. S. Current surgical management of functioning islet cell tumours of the pancreas. Annals of Surgery 1973; 178: 485–495

2. Mengoli, L., Le Quesne, L. P. Blind pancreatic resection for suspected insulinoma; a review of the problem. British Journal of Surgery 1967; 54: 749–756

3. Stefanini, P., Carboni, M., Patrassi, N., Basoli, A. The surgical treatment of occult insulinomas; a review of the problem. British Journal of Surgery 1974; 61: 1–4

4. Le Quesne, L. P., Nabarro, J. D. N., Kurtz, A., Zweig, S. The management of insulin tumours of the pancreas. British Journal of Surgery 1979; 66: 373–378

5. Daggett, P. R., Goodburn, E. A., Kurtz, A. B., Le Quesne, L. P., Morris, D. V., Nabarro, J. D. N., Raphael, M. J. Is preoperative localisation of insulinomas necessary? Lancet 1981; 1: 483–486

Gastrointestinal endocrine tumours

R. B. Welbourn MA, MD(Cantab.), HonMD(Karolinska),
FRCS, FCS(West Africa), HonMRCS(Denmark)
Professor of Surgical Endocrinology, Royal Postgraduate
Medical School and Hammersmith Hospital, London

R. C. G. Russell MS, FRCS
Consultant Surgeon, St John's Hospital for Diseases of the Skin
and The Middlesex Hospital, London

Editor's note

There are no standard surgical approaches to gut endocrine tumours, many varieties of resection being required. Thus the techniques necessary to deal with individual lesions will be found scattered through this series, but particularly in the volumes on *Abdomen* (3rd edition) and *Upper Gastrointestinal Tract* (4th edition). Here we include a brief overall account for reference purposes.

Introduction

The alimentary tract is a major endocrine organ; it contains at least 18 different types of endocrine cell, more than any other organ in the body. Those in the stomach and intestines are distributed among the mucosal cells on the luminal surface and crypts, while most of those in the pancreas are grouped in clumps in the islets of Langerhans. The cells belong to the apud series (with a high *A*mine content and the capacity for amine *P*recursor *U*ptake and *D*ecarboxylation), specialized for the secretion of peptides and amines, and may produce more than one substance. They do not take up conventional histological stains, but some (the enterochromaffin cells) are argentophil and most of the remainder are argyrophil.

The products of these cells may be true hormones (e.g. insulin, gastrin and glucagon), which enter the circulation and exert remote control on bodily functions; or local, paracrine substances (e.g. somatostatin), which exert their control on adjacent cells. A third group of products, neurocrine substances (e.g. vasoactive intestinal polypeptide (VIP) and substance P), are found in nervous tissue as well as the gut, and act as neurotransmitters at synapses.

Of surgical importance are those cells which in diseased states secrete peptides and amines in excess, causing characteristic metabolic and clinical disturbances. These lesions, arising from apud cells, are known as apudomas, and are classified as follows.

Hyperplasia	Neoplasia
	Adenoma
	Adenomatous hyperplasia
	Carcinoid
	Carcinoma

In the gut, hyperplasia is much less common than neoplasia. The secretory capacity of these lesions is great, and single tumours may produce more than one humoral agent. When they do so, one usually determines the metabolic and clinical features at any one time. These features depend more on the products of the lesions than on their nature; however, malignant tumours metastasize to local lymph nodes and the liver, and eventually disseminate widely, but they often take a long time to do so. These tumours may be associated with other endocrine syndromes as part of a familial multiple endocrine adenopathy (MEA), first described in 1953 and 1954.

Gut endocrine tumours are rare. Carcinoids are the commonest, insulinomas and gastrinomas are intermediate (with a combined incidence of about one per million of population per year), and the other tumours are very rare indeed. Diagnosis thus depends on clinical awareness of the syndromes and appropriate clinical investigation, which usually includes direct measurement of the specific hormone by radioimmunoassay. Varying proportions of all endocrine tumours of the gut (including carcinoids) secrete pancreatic polypeptide (PP), which does not exert recognizable features, but which can be measured in the blood, where its excess provides a useful tumour marker.

421

Carcinoid tumours

Carcinoid tumours, which were so named in 1907, are also called argentaffinomas and arise from the enterochromaffin (EC or Kulschitsky) cells in the gut and its derivatives. About one-third of these tumours are found in the appendix, where they are benign, one-third in the jejunum and ileum, where they usually display a low grade of malignancy, and the remainder in other parts of the gut (including the pancreas) and in the bronchus, where they may be benign or malignant. The clinical features vary with the site of the tumour, whether or not it has metastasized and what products it secretes. Appendiceal carcinoids are usually diagnosed at operations for suspected appendicitis. Jejunal and ileal tumours often cause intestinal obstruction and are likewise diagnosed at operation. Those elsewhere are found either incidentally or as a result of their secretions.

Carcinoid tumours, especially if malignant and arising in the midgut, secrete 5-hydroxytryptamine and kallikrein, an enzyme which causes the synthesis of bradykinin from a plasma globulin. These are mainly responsible for the malignant carcinoid syndrome, which was first described in 1930. Both these substances are metabolized and removed from the circulation by the liver, so that the carcinoid syndrome does not develop unless there are functioning liver metastases, or the rate of secretion is greater than the ability of the liver to metabolize the substances, or they gain direct entry to the general circulation by some other route.

The syndrome includes acute features, which occur in episodes and worsen with the passage of time, and chronic features, which are steadily progressive. The episodic attacks may be provoked by food (especially cheese) or alcohol, and include facial and bodily flushing, watery diarrhoea in nearly all patients, and bronchospasm in a few. The chronic features are right-sided cardiac failure, valvular stenoses, telangiectases and oedema, all of which are common, and pellagra, arthralgia and scleroderma, which are rare.

The diagnosis is made by finding an excess (which may be gross) of 5-hydroxyindolacetic acid in the urine (5-HIAA; normal level 2–15 mg/24 h).

Treatment

Primary tumours should be removed surgically. Simple appendicectomy cures nearly all appendiceal carcinoids, but if there is any suggestion of malignancy (e.g. local spread or involvement of the caecum), a right hemicolectomy should be undertaken. Tumours of the small intestine should be excised widely, together with adjacent lymph nodes. The 5 year survival rate is about 70 per cent for patients with resectable lesions, 40 per cent for those with unresectable tumours and 20 per cent for those with liver metastases.

Treatment of patients with the malignant carcinoid syndrome involves avoidance of aggravating factors, symptomatic relief with drugs, destruction or removal of metastases, and cytotoxic drugs. No method is curative, but palliation is good. Drugs that are of value include methysergide for the control of diarrhoea and bronchospasm, p-chlorophenylalanine for diarrhoea, α-methyldopa and prednisone for flushing, and isoprenaline for bronchospasm. Liver metastases can be managed by embolization of the hepatic artery and its branches under radiographic control. Surgical removal of large masses of tumour in lymph nodes, the liver or elsewhere may provide symptomatic relief. Good palliation has been described with cyclophosphamide and methotrexate, 5-fluorouracil and streptozotocin, and with 5-fluorotryptophan.

The pancreatic endocrine tumours

These apudomas are usually named after their principle secretions which cause the metabolic and clinical features.

Insulinoma

This tumour, arising from the B or β cells of the islets, was the first pancreatic endocrine tumour to be described, in 1927. It is the commonest and best known, and is described fully elsewhere (see chapter on 'Operations on the pancreas for insulinoma', pp. 415–420).

Gastrinoma

A clinical syndrome consisting of: fulminant peptic ulceration, which recurred despite normally adequate gastric operations; basal gastric hypersecretion; and a non-β islet-cell tumour of the pancreas was described in 1955 by Zollinger and Ellison and was known by their names. The role of gastrin was not appreciated until later. Today the majority of patients present with a history, physical findings and X-ray studies typical of an ordinary duodenal ulcer. The mean age of onset is about 40 and the range under 10 to over 80 years. Nearly 80 per cent have had symptoms for more than one year and 20 per cent have suffered for more than 5 years.

The possibility of a gastrinoma should be *considered* in every patient with duodenal ulcer, but suspicion should be raised by a fulminant course, the presence of diarrhoea, the association with another endocrine abnormality, especially hyperparathyroidism, which is present in about 25 per cent, and a barium meal which shows large gastric folds in the body and fundus of the stomach, dilatation and mucosal oedema in the duodenum and jejunum with flocculation of barium and rapid transit. Jejunal ulceration or perforation is almost pathognomic of a gastrinoma.

Investigations should start with measurement of gastric acid secretion, which is raised, and measurement of the fasting serum gastrin, which is usually at least twice the upper limit of normal. If there is hyperacidity and hypergastrinaemia, the following possibilities, apart from a gastrinoma, should be considered: G-cell hyperplasia, hyperparathyroidism, a retained excluded antrum after gastrectomy, and chronic renal failure. These conditions can usually be excluded by the intravenous injection of secretin, which inhibits gastrin release in these conditions and often increases it in gastrinoma. Biopsy of the antrum for G-cell population counts will exclude hyperplasia of the antral G cells. Calcium and phosphate estimation will exclude the presence of hyperparathyroidism, and X-ray of the pituitary fossa, together with measurement of prolactin in the blood, will alert the clinician to the possibility of a pituitary tumour.

Vipoma

This syndrome was described by Verner and Morrison in 1958 as a combination of *W*atery *D*iarrhoea, *H*ypokalaemia and *A*chlorhydria, associated with a non-β islet-cell tumour of the pancreas. These features led to the abbreviation 'WDHA syndrome', and the appropriate terms 'Verner-Morrison syndrome' and 'pancreatic cholera' were used also. In fact *hypo*chlorhydria is commoner than achlorhydria, but either feature helps to distinguish the condition from the *hyper*chlorhydric Zollinger-Ellison syndrome, which was described 3 years earlier, in which diarrhoea may also be a prominent feature. The pathogenetic role of VIP was not recognized for many years. However, it is secreted by most tumours causing this syndrome and also by some ganglioneuroblastomas with similar features, and is the cause of the metabolic and clinical disturbances. A high level of VIP in the blood is diagnostic of pancreatic or neural vipomas. Pancreatic polypeptide levels are high in about 80 per cent of patients with the former, but are not found in the latter. A few patients with the same general features, either with or without pancreatic tumours, have normal VIP levels in the blood, and the cause of their abnormalities is not known.

Glucagonoma

This tumour and its resulting clinical features were first described fully in 1966, but did not achieve wide recognition until 1973. The tumour arises from the A or α cells of the pancreatic islets. The excessive quantities of glucagon secreted cause severe migratory necrolytic erythema associated with painful glossitis and angular stomatitis. Protein catabolism causes severe loss of weight and deficiency of amino acids in the blood. Diabetes, anaemia and mental depression are usual, and a few patients suffer diarrhoea. Deep venous thrombosis, sometimes with fatal pulmonary embolism, is common and prophylactic low dosage heparin is advisable until effective therapy has been provided. The diagnosis is made on the basis of a raised blood glucagon level.

Other pancreatic tumours

Rare tumours, described intermittently over the years, include corticotrophinoma, which causes the ectopic corticotrophic variety of Cushing's syndrome. Others, recognized only recently, include somatostatinoma, which causes diabetes and malabsorption, and pancreatic polypeptidoma (PP-oma), which has no specific features and is usually found incidentally. Some tumours which secrete more than one peptide may alter their characters, either under the influence of drug therapy or when they recur after a surgical operation.

Treatment of pancreatic endocrine tumours

Surgical excision is the procedure of choice. It is helpful for the surgeon to know the site of the tumour before operation and whether more than one is present. Selective arterial angiography is probably the best method of localization available at present and, in expert hands, is very reliable except in the case of gastrinomas, which are often difficult to demonstrate. Selective venous sampling is also available, giving excellent results in a very few centres. Scintigraphy and ultrasonography are not helpful and the roles of computerized tomography and other new techniques have still to be determined.

Insulinomas are the most satisfactory tumours to treat, since some 90 per cent are single, benign and cured by one operation. Of the other principal tumours, about two-thirds of vipomas, one-quarter of glucagonomas and probably no more than one-fifth of gastrinomas are similarly amenable to surgical excision. The operative procedure is identical to that described for insulinomas (see chapter on 'Operations on the pancreas for insulinoma,' pp. 415–420) with thorough exploration of the whole abdomen to exclude secondary deposits, extensive mobilization, inspection and palpation of the whole pancreas, enucleation of the tumour and careful closure of any damaged duct. Benign tumours of the body and tail are probably best treated by distal pancreatectomy.

Some surgeons advocate and practise more extensive resections for malignant tumours which have spread locally. However, the operative morbidity and mortality are increased, the chances of cure are slight and, unlike carcinomas of the exocrine pancreas, these lesions tend to grow very slowly. Several other methods are available for their palliation.

Patients with incurable malignant tumours, whose symptoms cannot be controlled by other means, may be treated with cytotoxic drugs. The best for pancreatic tumours is streptozotocin; objective regression is obtained in 90 per cent of vipomas, and 25 per cent of glucagonomas and gastrinomas. Other measures include zinc, which controls the dermatitis of glucagonoma, and long-acting analogues of somatostatin, which are being developed. Embolization of the hepatic artery and 'debulking' operations are also indicated occasionally as in the treatment of the malignant carcinoid syndrome.

Gastrinomas

Few gastrinomas are curable by surgical excision and, until the advent of H_2 inhibitors, the treatment of choice for most patients was total gastrectomy. About 60 per cent of gastrinomas are malignant. Of these some 80 per cent are found to be associated with metastases at operation. Only two-thirds of gastrinomas are situated in the pancreas, and only one-quarter of these are single localized tumours. About one-sixth are in the duodenum, half of which are localized, and some 10 per cent are at unknown sites presenting with metastases. In about 5 per cent of cases islet-cell hyperplasia may present alone and in a similar proportion it may accompany a duodenal or pancreatic tumour. Whatever the nature of the gastrinoma, good results are being achieved with cimetidine (up to 3.6 g/ day). Thus the first step in the management is to treat the patient with cimetidine, to heal the ulcer and to rehabilitate the ill patient. This enables investigation to determine the site of the tumour, which may be difficult or impossible, and to exclude the presence of liver metastases by imaging techniques. If a tumour is located, the abdomen should be explored with the objective of removing it or excising the tail of the pancreas for immunohistochemistry to exclude hyperplasia of the islets. After successful removal of the tumour, cimetidine can be withdrawn only if serial gastrin measurements confirm the success of the procedure by a return to normal levels.

If the tumour cannot be located or extirpated, cimetidine should be continued, and the patient's progress frequently assessed. If there is evidence that the cimetidine or other H_2 blockers are not controlling the hypersecretion, then total gastrectomy is the procedure of choice. This must be performed meticulously with transection of the oesophagus 2 cm or more above the oesophagogastric junction, and a long loop (at least 40 cm), end-to-side oesophagojejunostomy performed.

Prognosis, despite the presence of metastases, is good for malignant gastrinomas, with a survival of over 50 per cent at 5 years and over 40 per cent at 10 years.

Patients with MEA type I usually have hypergastrinaemia and a tendency to peptic ulceration, whether or not they have gastrinomas. In those (the majority) with hyperparathyroidism, the gastrin level depends directly on the calcium level, and parathyroidectomy should always be tried. It may control the ulceration, sometimes for years. It should not, however, preclude an attempt to remove a gastrinoma. Associated lesions, particularly pituitary tumours, must be treated appropriately.

Patients with proven G-cell hyperplasia of the pyloric antrum should be treated by distal gastrectomy (total antrectomy).

Conclusion

With gut endocrine tumours, the surgeon must be aware that he may be dealing with only part of a multi-endocrine abnormality. Without adequate endocrinological and laboratory help, the patient's best interests may not be served and the high perioperative morbidity and mortality associated with the surgical treatment of these complex conditions continue unabated. However, with proper care, many patients are cured or live in reasonable health for years.

Further reading

Bloom, S. R., Polak, J. A., Welbourn, R. B. Pancreatic apudomas. World Journal of Surgery 1979; 3: 587–595

Edis, A. J., Ayala, L. A., Egdahl, R. H. Manual of endocrine surgery. Berlin: Springer-Verlag, 1975

Friesen, S. R., ed. Surgical endocrinology: clinical syndromes. Philadelphia: Lippincott, 1978

Modlin, I. M. Endocrine tumors of the pancreas. Surgery, Gynecology and Obstetrics, 1979; 149: 751–769

Welbourn, R. B. Apudomas of the gut. American Journal of Surgery 1977; 133: 13–22

Welbourn, R. B., Wood, S. M., Polak, J. M., Bloom, S. R. Pancreatic endocrine tumours. In: Bloom, S. R., Polak, J. M., eds. Gut hormones, 2nd ed., pp. 547–554. Edinburgh: Churchill Livingstone, 1981

Welbourn, R. B., Galland, R. B. Endocrine tumours of the gut. In: Taylor, S., Chisholm, G. D., O'Higgins, N. J., Shields, R., eds. Surgery. London: Heinemann Medical (in press)

Zollinger, R. M., Ellison, E. C., Fabri, P. J., Johnson, J., Sparks, J., Carey, L. C. Primary peptic ulcerations of the jejunum associated with islet cell tumors. Twenty-five-year appraisal. Annals of Surgery 1980; 192: 422–430

Index